Wound Healing:
Alternatives in Management

Contemporary Perspectives in Rehabilitation

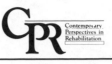

Steven L. Wolf, Ph.D., FAPTA
Editor-in-Chief

PUBLISHED VOLUMES

Thermal Agents in Rehabilitation - Volume 1
Susan L. Michlovitz, M.S., P.T.

Cardiac Rehabilitation: Basic Theory and Application - Volume 2
Frances Brannon, Ph.D., Mary Geyer, M.S., Margaret Foley, R.N.

The Biomechanics of the Foot and Ankle - Volume 3
Robert Donatelli, M.A., P.T.

Pharmacology in Rehabilitation - Volume 4
Charles D. Ciccone, Ph.D., P.T.

Wound Healing: Alternatives in Management - Volume 5
Luther C. Kloth, M.S., P.T., Joseph M. McCulloch, Ph.D., P.T. and Jeffrey A. Feedar, B.S., P.T.

VOLUMES IN PRODUCTION

Thermal Agents in Rehabilitation, 2nd Edition (July 1990) - Volume 6
Susan L. Michlovitz, M.S., P.T.

Electrotherapy in Rehabilitation (November 1990) - Volume 7
Meryl R. Gersh, M.S., P.T.

Wound Healing: Alternatives in Management

Luther C. Kloth, M.S., P.T.
Associate Professor in Physical Therapy
Marquette University
President, Wound Care Resources, Inc.
Vice President,
Preferred Physical Therapy Services of Wisconsin, S.C.
Milwaukee, Wisconsin

Joseph M. McCulloch, Ph.D., P.T.
Associate Professor and Head
Department of Physical Therapy
Director of Rehabilitation Services
Louisiana State University Medical Center
Shreveport, Louisiana

Jeffrey A. Feedar, B.S., P.T.
Vice President and Director, Wound Care Resources, Inc.
President and Director,
Preferred Physical Therapy Services of Wisconsin, S.C.
Milwaukee, Wisconsin

 F.A. DAVIS COMPANY · Philadelphia

Printed in the United States of America

Last digit indicates print number: 10 9 8 7 6 5 4 3

Note: As new scientific information becomes available through basic and clinical research, recommended treatments and drug therapies undergo changes. The author(s) and publisher have done everything possible to make this book accurate, up-to-date, and in accord with accepted standards at the time of publication. However, the reader is advised always to check product information (package inserts) for changes and new information regarding dose and contraindications before administering any drug. Caution is especially urged when using new or infrequently ordered drugs.

Library of Congress Cataloging-in-Publication Data
Wound healing : alternatives in management / [edited by] Luther C. Kloth, Joseph M. McCulloch, Jeffrey A. Feedar.
    p. cm. — (Contemporary perspectives in rehabilitation ; v. 5)
    Includes bibliographical references.
    ISBN 0-8036-5407-3
    1. Wound healing. I. Kloth, Luther. II. McCulloch, Joseph M. III. Feedar, Jeffrey A. IV. Series.
    [DNLM: 1. Wound Healing. W1 C0769NS v. 5 / WO 185 W93815]
RD94.W67 1990
617.1′4—dc20
DNLM/DLC
for Library of Congress   90-3131
                                                      CIP

Dedication

To my wife Doris and children, Eric, Dana, and Diane. Also to Jeffrey Feedar and Joseph McCulloch for their relentless support and expert contributions.
L.C.K.

To my family, friends, and colleagues and to the U.S. Public Health Service for a professional beginning I will always remember.
J.M.M.

To my family: Mom, Dad, Steve, Dave, Rick, and Corky. To my mentor, Luther Kloth, and to my staff.
J.A.F.

Foreword

Not long ago, allied health professionals associated wound healing with debridement, surgery, and pharmacologic management. Typically, only therapists and nurses specially trained in techniques of wound cleansing and debridement had been permitted to care for patients with open or non-healing wounds. Many of these "specialists" were not formally educated about the physiologic, microbiological, and nutritional factors that profoundly influence the healing process. But today, physical therapists and other health professionals play a vital role in the rehabilitation of patients with wounds secondary to trauma, metabolic disorders, or prolonged pressure. Their cutting-edge research has demonstrated the therapeutic value of electrical stimulation, ultrasound, or hyperbaric oxygen to the process of cutaneous and subcutaneous healing.

The co-editors of this volume of *Contemporary Perspectives in Rehabilitation (CPR)* series are among those clinicians/scientists at the forefront of wound healing research and practice. Early on, we appreciated the arduous and systematic manner in which Luther C. Kloth, Joseph M. McCulloch, and Jeffrey A. Feedar sought to upgrade the information base describing the modalities and device-specific techniques being used throughout the world to facilitate wound healing. Because these gentlemen had also gained national reputations as superb teachers who emphasized deductive reasoning in promoting decision making, it seemed obvious that their services be enlisted to write the first book of its kind on the subject of wound healing.

The co-editors have brought to this text an accumulated knowledge base and wisdom aptly complemented by the contributions of other experts in the field. They have done a remarkable job in maintaining a consistent approach to providing referenced information within each chapter and also supplying well-developed case histories in all clinically related chapters. In so doing, *Wound Healing: Alternatives in Management* continues the philosophy of the *CPR* series by seeking to promote understanding and challenging the thinking process of its readers.

This text is well suited to students of physical therapy, nursing, and other disciplines whose teachers recognize the expanding roles and therapeutic options available to health-care professionals responsible for the treatment of wounds. For the older generation of clinicians like me, who were taught debridement and little else in the management of wounds, this text is valuable because it provides a greater scope of treatment alternatives, often using equipment already available in the clinic. Perhaps the most compelling reason for all health-care practitioners to seriously consider this text is because it provides *documented and practical clinical information* that simply is *not published elsewhere*.

Steven L. Wolf, Ph.D., FAPTA
Series Editor

Preface

In the summer of 1986, three physical therapists met with an animated French editor in the exhibit hall of the American Physical Therapy Association (APTA) National Conference in Chicago. We shared our collective concerns over the lack of and need for a comprehensive clinical textbook on chronic wound care for physical therapists. Before the meeting had ended, we found ourselves becoming prospective editors for just such a text. We entered the process much as people do when in buying their first home. The excitement over the possibilities was high. Then the realization of the work set in. We found ourselves "persuading" colleagues to be contributors, setting deadlines, writing, editing, setting new deadlines, and asking ourselves: What did we do? Still the enthusiasm grew. What started out as a sharing with our fellow professionals of what we knew about wound healing and the management of patients with wounds soon became a great learning experience. We learned more and more about all aspects of chronic wounds as the contributing authors shared their knowledge and clinical expertise. Their contributions have been outstanding. We shared their excitement about providing not a technique-oriented but a problem-solving text. It is hoped that this text will bridge the gap between chronic wound etiology and treatment with its extensive coverage of wound evaluation and the clinical decision-making approach to wound care.

As previously stated, the text was originally intended to meet the clinical needs of the physical therapist. It has since taken on a much broader scope and attempts to address many aspects of the management of patients with wounds. Thus, although the primary audience for this text is the physical therapist, the material presented is also intended to be of value to a variety of other health professionals, including physicians, podiatrists, nurses, and especially students in the health professions.

The text is in three parts. Part I, Factors Influencing Wound Healing, includes information from basic and medical sciences that addresses normal and abnormal factors impacting on wound repair. This section provides recent scientific information, the understanding of which is essential for obtaining optimal results from the treatment procedures presented in Part III. Chapter 5, on bacteriology, and Chapter 6, on nutrition, provide clinical decision-making models related to identification of microorganisms and providing optimal nutrition, respectively.

Part II, Evaluation, addresses the needed skills that are critical in applying the decision-making process and in selecting the appropriate treatment of wounds presented to the clinician.

Part III, Principles and Methods of Treatment, is designed to assist the student and clinician in integrating the basic and clinical science concepts presented in Parts I and II with alternative treatment techniques for wound care. Each of the seven chapters in this section provides basic information on the products or instrumentation used to augment wound healing and an extensive review of the literature citing studies that either support or do not support specific treatment approaches. All of the chapters in this section provide clinical decision-making models that will enable the reader to select the technique that is most appropriate for treatment of various types of complicated or uncomplicated wounds.

Chapter 9 discusses factors that interfere with the normal microenvironment and homeostasis of wound tissue. Also addressed in this chapter are various wound debridement techniques and commercial products that may have a deleterious effect on repair of wound tissue. This chapter also provides a thorough discussion of all types of wound dressings and their indications and contraindications. In addition, there is a section on the causes, treatment, and prevention of pressure sores. Special emphasis is placed on the types and appropriate uses of pressure-relieving devices. The chapter closes with two case histories that provide the reader with examples of clinical decisions that must be made when selecting wound dressings and other products or agents for wound care.

Chapter 10 and 11 address the evaluation and treatment of wounds caused by vascular insufficiency and pressure and insensitivity, respectively. In addition to various treatment interventions, these two chapters provide patient case histories with questions and answers pertinent to the evaluation and treatment of patients having these types of wounds.

Chapters 12 through 15 are devoted to specific wound treatment interventions with various physical modalities. Each of these chapters reviews the literature and discusses the theory, rationale, techniques, and protocols for using the specific physical modality in the treatment of chronic wounds. Chapter 12 discusses the use of various types of electrical stimulation to promote wound repair and presents case studies that allow the reader to see how and when electrical currents are most appropriately applied. Chapter 13 is devoted to the role of ultrasound in wound healing. The chapter describes what ultrasound is and how it may be used to facilitate various cellular responses to augment tissue repair. Questions and answers are used in a clinical decision-making model that introduces the reader to the use of this modality. Chapter 14 presents the role of the low-power laser and ultraviolet and infrared radiation in wound healing, and Chapter 15 discusses topical application hyperbaric oxygen to promote tissue healing. Chapter 14 provides experimental protocols that have been used to study the effect of radiant energy on wound tissues, and Chapter 15 provides a case study on the use of and responses to hyperbaric oxygen in the management of a chronic wound.

In the chapters that address treatment interventions, authors have all suggested that additional clinical research is needed to substantiate the efficacy of the specific treatment modality and the protocols described.

Appendices that include lists of some U.S. manufacturers of wound care products and physical modalities are included for Chapters 9, 12, and 15.

Luther C. Kloth, M.S., P.T.

Joseph M. McCulloch, Ph.D., P.T.

Jeffrey A. Feedar, P.T.

Editors

Acknowledgments

The development of this text to its completion has required many months of dedicated hard work by many people. We want to thank the following people for the contributions and assistance they provided as well as for their patience and understanding:

- Each of the 13 contributing authors

- Our reviewers

Christopher Bork, Ph.D., P.T.
Temple University
Philadelphia, Pennsylvania

Susan Michlovitz, M.S., P.T.
Hahnemann University
Philadelphia, Pennsylvania

John Echternach, Ph.D., P.T.
Old Dominion University
Norfolk, Virginia

Elaine Muntzer, P.T.
Hand and Orthopedics Rehabilitation
  Services
Levittown, Pennsylvania

John Eddy, P.T., E.C.S.
University of Pittsburgh
Pittsburgh, Pennsylvania

Charlene Nelson, M.A., P.T.
University of North Carolina, Chapel Hill
Chapel Hill, North Carolina

Althea Jones, M.A., P.T.
Columbia University
New York, New York

Gary Soderberg, Ph.D., L.P.T.
University of Iowa
Iowa City, Iowa

Mary Keehn, P.T.
University of Illinois
Chicago, Illinois

Pamela Unger, B.S., P.T.
Martin, McGough, and Eddy PT Services
Somerset, Pennsylvania

. . . . for their helpful reviews and suggestions for each of the chapters of this text.

- The staff of the Medical Communications Department of the Louisiana State University (LSU) Medical Center, Shreveport, for their support in producing graphics for this text. Special thanks are due to Robert Atkins.

- The patients and fellow staff members in the physical therapy clinics and programs at Marquette University, LSU Medical Center, Wound Care Resources, Inc., and Preferred Physical Therapy Services of Wisconsin, S.C. for their assistance in our research and treatment programs.

- Debbie Blaha, Phyllis Shanks, Joslyn Wade, and May Woodard for their expert word processing and typing of the manuscript.

- The students we have taught at both LSU Medical Center and Marquette University for their questions and concerns regarding wound care.

- Jean-François Vilain of F.A. Davis and Steven L. Wolf of Emory University for their patience, prodding, and encouragement.

L.C.K.
J.M.M.
J.A.F.
Editors

Contributors

James Birke, M.S., P.T.
Chief
Department of Physical Therapy
National Hansen's Disease Center
Carville, Louisiana

Theodore J. Daly, M.D.
Clinical Instructor in Dermatology and Dermatopathology
Metropolitan Hospital Center
New York, New York
and
New York Medical College
Valhalla, New York

John Cummings, Ph.D., P.T.
Professor
Program in Physical Therapy
State University of New York
College of Health Related Professions
Syracuse, New York

Mary Dyson, B.Sc., C. Biol., M.I.Biol., Ph.D.
Reader in Biology of Tissue Repair
Division of Anatomy
Guy's Hospital
University of London
London Bridge, England

Jeffrey A. Feedar, B.S., P.T.
Vice-President and Director
Wound Care Resources Inc.
and
President and Director
Preferred Physical Therapy Services of Wisconsin, S.C.
Milwaukee, Wisconsin

Gail C. Frank, Dr.P.H., M.P.H., L.D.N., R.D.
Nutritional Epidemiologist
Professor of Nutrition
California State University, Long Beach
Long Beach, California

George Hampton, M.P.H., P.T.
Associate Professor and Program Director
Department of Physical Therapy
Louisiana State University Medical Center
New Orleans, Louisiana

Nancy Harkess, Ph.D.
Associate Professor of Medical Technology
Department of Medical Technology
Louisiana State University Medical Center
New Orleans, Louisiana

John Hovde, M.S., P.T.
Director of Work Hardening/Ergonomics Program
Catholic Medical Center of Brooklyn and Queens
Jamaica, New York

Luther C. Kloth, M.S., P.T.
Associate Professor
Program in Physical Therapy
Marquette University
Milwaukee, Wisconsin
President, Wound Care Resources, Inc.
and Vice-President
Preferred Physical Therapy Services of Wisconsin, S.C.
Milwaukee, Wisconsin

Susan B. Kravitz, M.S., P.T.
Private Practice
Englewood Physical Therapy and Pain Management
Englewood, New Jersey

Joseph M. McCulloch, Ph.D., P.T.
Associate Professor and Head
Department of Physical Therapy
and Director of Rehabilitation Services
Louisiana State University Medical Center
Shreveport, Louisiana

Joyce MacKinnon, Ed.D., M.P.T.
Director, Division of Physical Therapy
University of New England
Biddleford, Maine

Katherine H. Miller, R.N.
Patient-Services Coordinator
Staodynamics, Inc.
Longmont, Colorado

Gary D. Mulder, M.S., D.P.M.
Wound Healing Institute
Aurora, Colorado

Helen Price, M.S., P.T.
Associate Professor
Department of Physical Therapy
Louisiana State University Medical Center
Shreveport, Louisiana

TABLE OF CONTENTS

Part I

FACTORS INFLUENCING WOUND HEALING

CHAPTER 1

The Inflammatory Response to Wounding

Luther C. Kloth, M.S., P.T.
Katherine H. Miller, R.N.

Wound healing is a complex process by which all wounds, surgical, indolent, or accidental, heal in the same sequence of events. A combination of vascular responses, cellular and chemotactic activity, and release of chemical mediators within the wounded tissues are inherent, interrelated components of the healing process. There are three overlapping phases in the wound healing process: the inflammatory response, re-epithelialization and contraction, and finally, connective tissue formation. This chapter discusses the first phase, the inflammatory response. The second and third phases are presented in Chapters 2 and 3, respectively.

The initial healing reactions to wounding, the vascular and cellular responses, are manifested as the inflammatory response. Local vasodilation, fluid leakage into the extravascular space, and blocking of lymphatic drainage produce three of the four *cardinal signs of inflammation* including *redness, swelling,* and *heat*. The fourth sign, pain, is produced by distension of tissue spaces from swelling and pressure, and by chemical irritation of nociceptor receptors. In a new wound such as a surgical incision, the acute inflammatory response, which usually lasts 24 to 48 hours and is complete in two weeks,[1] may be misinterpreted by the inexperienced clinician as a bacterial infection process often prevalent in chronic wounds. Following the acute inflammatory response, there is a subacute phase of approximately 2 weeks. Chronic inflammation may last for months or years and may occur from unresolved acute inflammation or gradually from repeated microtrauma or persistent irritation from the presence of a foreign substance in the tissues.

The purpose of this chapter is to acquaint health-care professionals involved in the assessment, evaluation, and treatment of wounds with information that will enable them to describe the characteristics and manifestations of the inflammatory process associated with acute and chronic wounds. This information will enable the practitioner to more effectively evaluate and treat inflammation that occurs in both types of wounds.

ACUTE INFLAMMATORY REACTION

The vascular and cellular activities associated with the acute inflammatory response consist of a complex sequence of highly interrelated events. The primary function of these events is to bring phagocytes to the inflamed area to destroy bacteria and rid the tissue spaces of debris from dead and dying cells so repair processes can begin. The sequence of events that characterize the inflammatory response may vary somewhat, depending on the source of injury (bacterial, chemical, immunologic, ischemic, mechanical, or thermal trauma), the site of injury, the state of local tissue homeostasis, and whether the onset of the injury is acute or chronic. For the purpose of clarification, the interrelated and overlapping events that occur during the acute inflammatory response, including the vascular response, the cellular reactions, and the chemical mediators involved, are discussed separately in this chapter.

The Vascular Reaction

Trauma to soft tissues resulting in physical disruption of blood and lymphatic vessels causes immediate hemorrhage, fluid loss, cell death, and accessibility of the exposed tissues to bacteria and other foreign bodies. All damaged blood vessels (including capillaries, which have no muscular layers) at and contiguous to the site of injury undergo immediate constriction to slow blood loss in the affected area.[2] This initial constriction response by the blood vessels to injury is mediated by norepinephrine and usually lasts from a few seconds to a few minutes. It may be prolonged in small vessels by the powerful vasoconstrictor serotonin contained in the granules of mast cells in connective tissue and in platelets released into the interstitial fluid when injury and bleeding occurs. This secondary prolonged vasoconstriction does not occur unless serotonin release by platelets is triggered by platelet adhesion to naked collagen present in connective tissue, which becomes exposed when the blood vessel endothelial wall is damaged.

A summary of hemostatic mechanisms not dependent on blood coagulation is shown in Figure 1–1. When platelets adhere to collagen, they release their granules, which contain not only serotonin but also adenosine diphosphate (ADP). This chemical causes other passing platelets to adhere to the platelets that first adhered to the exposed connective tissue at the site of injury in the endothelial wall. This aggregation of platelets forms a relatively unstable platelet plug that may temporarily occlude small vessels and slow or stop bleeding.[2] Whether prolonged vasoconstriction occurs or not, areas of microtrauma in the endothelial surface trigger the specific enzyme present in blood known as Hageman factor XII to initiate clotting by converting prothrombin to thrombin, which in turn converts fibrinogen to fibrin.

During the initial vasoconstriction, opposing endothelial surfaces of small vessels of the microcirculation are pressed together. This contact induces a stickiness within the endothelial lining that is capable of occluding these vessels even after active vasoconstriction has started to relax. Almost immediately after injury, leukocytes begin to adhere to the sticky endothelium of venules.[3] Within 1 hour after the onset of inflammation, the entire endothelial margin of venules may be covered with neutrophilic leukocytes. This process is known as neutrophilic margination. Shortly after neutrophilic margination, histamine is released into the area from mast cells, basophils, and platelets, and causes vasodilation and an increase in permeability of the venules.

Histamine action is very short-lived, probably lasting no longer than 30 minutes.[3]

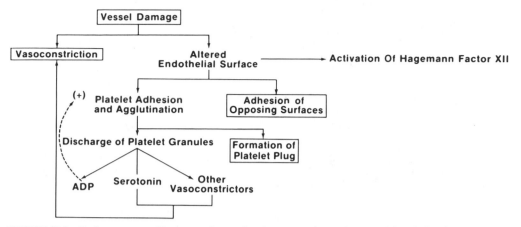

FIGURE 1–1. Summary of hemostatic mechanisms not dependent on blood clotting. Note the role of ADP in platelet adhesion and clumping (Adapted from Vander, Sherman, and Luciano,[2] p. 321).

However, since the increase in vascular permeability lasts long beyond the time of histamine action, other factors may contribute to the longevity of this response. Thus, in the early acute inflammatory period, extravasation of serous fluid containing scant traces of cells and plasma proteins ultimately accumulates as edema in the tissue spaces. This clear transudate edema fluid, which may seep from open wounds, provides fibrinogen, which when acted upon by the enzyme thrombin, forms fibrin. Fibrin plugs then seal damaged lymphatics and confine the inflammatory reaction to a localized area immediately surrounding the injury.[3]

Soon after neutrophils marginate, they begin amoeba-like activity by inserting a narrow amoeboid projection into the space between endothelial cells. By the force of its amoeboid movement, the neutrophil, through the processes of diapedesis and chemotactic attraction for other chemical substances, squeezes through the vessel wall to reach the inflamed extravascular tissues.[2] In the early inflammatory state, neutrophils (which have a survival time in the circulation of only a few hours) and monocytes are the predominant cells at the site of injury.[4] Later in the inflammatory phase, the number of neutrophils declines and macrophages predominate. With increased emigration of leukocytes and lower molecular weight plasma proteins (e.g., albumin) the edema fluid, which was initially clear, serous fluid, becomes a cellular aggregate. When observed as drainage from an open wound this aggregate of cells and debris assumes the appearance and more viscous consistency of the inflammatory edema known as exudate, which is often mistaken for pus. In fact, when large numbers of leukocytes die and are lysed, the exudate actually becomes sterile pus, which may be present in nonbacterial inflammations of open or closed wounds.[3] A diagrammatic representation of the events associated with the formation of edema fluid is presented in Figure 1–2.

In open wounds, the wound exudate that contains the plasma proteins including albumin, globulin, fibrinogen, and gamma globulins, provides a natural environment in which migrating polymorphonuclear leukocytes can ingest bacteria and debris. Within a few days following injury, these cells and the plasma constituents are no longer functional and become incorporated into the desiccated wound crust.[5] In Chapter 9, the importance of maintaining hydration of wound tissues will be explored.

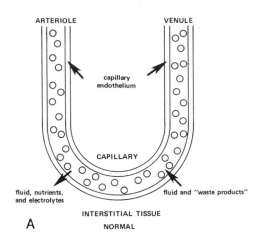

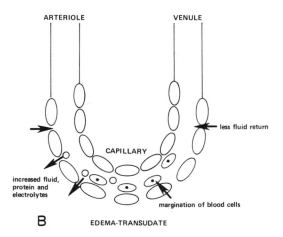

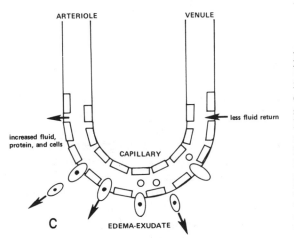

FIGURE 1–2. Edema formation. *A,* Under normal conditions, absorption forces on the venous side of the capillary equal the filtration forces on the arterial side. *B,* When small vessels are damaged, leukocytes marginate, and chemical mediators cause increased capillary permeability and dilatation with edema transudate leaking into the tissue spaces. *C,* As inflammation intensifies, neutrophils and lower molecular weight colloids (albumin) emigrate to the tissue spaces to form edema exudate (From Zarro,[1] p. 7, with permission).

The Cellular Reaction

The circulating blood is composed of specialized cellular elements suspended in liquid known as plasma. The specialized cells are the red blood cells or *erythrocytes*, the white cells or *leukocytes*, and cell fragments called *platelets* derived from megakaryocytes in bone marrow.[2] If the inflammatory reaction is intense, red blood cells may emigrate from capillaries into the tissue spaces along with leukocytes and platelets. Unlike erythrocytes, whose primary functions are exerted within the confines of blood vessels, leukocytes only use the blood vessels as a means of being transported to the extravascular space in response to tissue injury and/or inflammation. Table 1–1 identifies the number and distribution of erythrocytes, leukocytes, and platelets in normal human blood. Interestingly, in one drop of blood, over 99 percent of all the cells are red blood cells.[2]

LEUKOCYTES

Leukocytes are classified according to their structure into *polymorphonuclear leukocytes (granulocytes)* and *mononuclear cells* (Table 1–1). Granulocytes have lobulated nuclei, contain numerous cytoplasmic granules, and are subdivided into three types according to their affinity for various dyes. Granules showing no preference for any dye are called *neutrophils*. Those having an affinity for the red dye eosin are called *eosinophils*. Granules with affinity for basic dye are called *basophils*.[2]

Recall that during the early inflammatory phase, one of the most predominant cells present in the interstitial fluid is the neutrophil whose primary function is phagocytosis of debris particles. When neutrophils are lysed, their lysomes release proteolytic enzymes (proteases) and collagenolytic enzymes (collagenase), both of which begin the early autolytic debridement process of solubilizing necrotic protein and necrotic collagen, respectively.[3] Although neutrophils are the first cells to appear in numbers in wound tissue, in the absence of infection, they are not necessary for wound healing to proceed normally.[6] The eosinophil may also be involved in phagocytosis to some degree, but the basophil is not a phagocytic cell. Basophils contain histamine, which is released locally following injury, to contribute to the early increased vascular permeability.

TABLE 1–1. Number and Distribution of Circulating Blood
Cells per Milliliter of Blood

Total erythrocytes = 5,000,000,000 cells per milliliter of blood
Total leukocytes = 7,000,000 cells per milliliter of blood
Total platelets = 250,000,000 cells per milliliter of blood

Percent of total leukocytes:
    Polymorphonuclear granulocytes:
        Neutrophils 50–70
        Eosinophils 1–4
        Basophils 0.1
    Mononuclear cells:
        Monocytes 2–8
        Lymphocytes 20–40

Adapted from Vander, Sherman, and Luciano, p. 262.

The other type of leukocyte, mononuclear cells, includes *monocytes* and *lymphocytes* (Table 1–1). Monocytes are larger than any of the granulocytes and have a single nucleus and few granules. When monocytes emigrate from the capillary into the tissue spaces, they are transformed into *macrophages*.[1] This cell is considered the most important regulatory cell in the inflammatory reaction as far as tissue healing is concerned.[3]

Unlike neutrophils, which may not need to be present for healing to occur in aseptic wounds, the presence of the macrophage is essential to wound healing.[7,8] Macrophages play a major role in phagocytosis by producing enzymes such as collagenase[9] and proteoglycan degrading enzymes,[10] which also facilitate autolytic wound debridement.[11] A time frame of hemodynamic and phagocytic events is presented in Figure 1–3. Macrophage phagocytic activity is most efficient when oxygen is readily available to wound tissues.[12] However, macrophages tolerate severe hypoxia very well, which may explain why they are usually present in the state of chronic inflammation. In addition, macrophages also release chemotactic factors (for example, fibronectin), which attract fibroblasts to the wound[13] and play a role in localizing the inflammatory process and in adhesion of fibroblasts to fibrin during the later stages of fibroplasia.[3] In this regard, macrophages may enhance collagen deposition[5] because their depletion markedly decreases deposition of collagen in the wound.[8] In the absence of macrophages, fibroblasts migrate to the site of injury in considerably reduced numbers, and those that are found are observed to be somewhat immature.[3] The angiogenic potential of macrophages has also been demonstrated by inducing neovascularization into the avascular cornea of a rat model with macrophage-derived growth factor.[14] Knighton and coworkers[15] have shown that angioblasts follow a gradient of angiogenic factor produced by hypoxic macrophages and that macrophages do not produce angiogenic factor when either fully oxygenated or anoxic. In fact, Banda and colleagues[16] have shown that if the normal gradient of oxygen tension is artificially altered or if macrophages are removed from the tissue spaces, angiogenesis and wound debridement may be temporarily or permanently inhibited. There is strong evidence that the angiogenic potential of macrophages appears to be closely related to the production of macrophage-derived growth factor by these cells.[7]

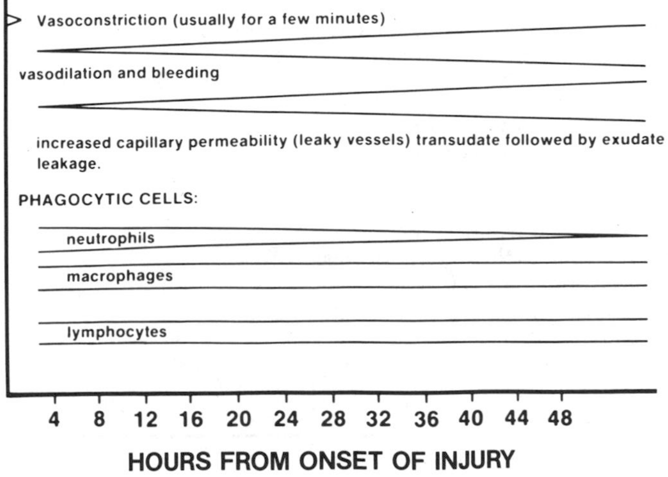

HEMODYNAMIC ACTIVITY:

Vasoconstriction (usually for a few minutes)

vasodilation and bleeding

increased capillary permeability (leaky vessels) transudate followed by exudate leakage.

PHAGOCYTIC CELLS:

neutrophils

macrophages

lymphocytes

4   8   12   16   20   24   28   32   36   40   44   48

HOURS FROM ONSET OF INJURY

FIGURE 1–3. Hemodynamic and phagocytic activity during the early inflammatory phase (Adapted from Evans, P: The healing process at cellular level: A review. Physiotherapy 66:256, 1980).

PLATELETS

Another of the blood constituents involved in the wound repair process consists of cell fragments known as *platelets*. In the early stages of a wound following injury, platelets, which are probably the first cells at the site of injury, form a hemostatic plug to stop bleeding. Platelets and macrophages are considered the regulatory cells in the repair process, probably because both release growth factors. The regulatory protein known as *platelet-derived growth factor (PDGF)* has been shown to be chemotactic and mitogenic for fibroblasts and smooth muscle cells in vitro.[17] There is also evidence that PDGF is chemotactic for macrophages,[18] monocytes, and neutrophils[19] and that thrombin-activated platelets have angiogenic activity.[20] Through these functions, platelets apparently not only play an important role in hemostasis, but also contribute significantly to the control of fibrin deposition, fibroplasia, and angiogenesis.

Chemical Mediators of Inflammation

A number of chemical substances are involved in the initiation and control of the inflammatory reaction. Some are protagonists and others antagonists of inflammation. The actions of some of these substances may be synergistic, but the precise role of most of these substances has not been clearly elucidated.

HISTAMINE

As mentioned earlier, a major source of histamine is the mast cell. The granules of these cells, which are released at the time of injury, contain a number of active materials including serotonin, heparin, and histamine. Recall that the initial short-lived increase in permeability of venules occurs as a result of histamine release. When mast cells are depleted of histamine or histamine receptors are blocked, the early increase in vascular permeability is prevented.[3] The role of the anticoagulant heparin is to temporarily prevent coagulation of the excess tissue fluid and blood components during the early phase of the inflammatory response.

SEROTONIN

Serotonin, or 5-hydroxytryptamine, is a potent vasoconstrictor that has a negligible effect on vascular permeability in humans.[3] However, serotonin appears to be involved in other activities related to the late phase of fibroblastic proliferation and the cross-linking of collagen molecules.[3] Cross-linking of collagen molecules not only affects the tensile strength of newly formed desirable scar tissue, but also accounts for the toughness and lack of resilience of unwanted fibrous adhesions. In addition, serotonin has also been found to stimulate DNA synthesis in granuloma cells. A granuloma is a hard fibrous capsule formed by the laying down of collagen around a foreign substance present in the tissues that cannot be solubilized by autolysis. Most granulomas occur in chronic inflammatory states.

KININS

The kinins are biologically active and nearly indistinguishable peptides that are found in areas of tissue destruction. The most familiar kinin, *bradykinin*, is a potent inflammatory substance that is released in injured tissue from plasma proteins (globu-

lins) by the plasma enzyme, kallikrein.[3,21] The action of the kinins on the microvascula-
ture is similar to that of histamine, causing a marked increase in the permeability of the
microcirculation. Because they are rapidly destroyed by tissue proteases, it appears likely
that kinins are involved in the inflammatory process, primarily during the early phase of
the vascular response.[3]

PROSTAGLANDINS

Prostaglandins are produced by nearly all cells of the body when the cell membrane
is injured. When the cell membrane is altered, its phospholipid content is broken down
by the enzyme phospholipase A_2, which results in the formation of arachidonic acid.
The oxidation of arachidonic acid by the enzyme lipoxygenase forms a series of potent
compounds called *leukotrienes*. Leukotrienes of three different types combine to form a
substance known as *slow-reacting substance of anaphylaxis* (SRS-A), which alters capillary permeability during the inflammatory reaction.[22,23]

Similarly, arachidonic acid is converted by enzymes called cyclooxygenases to
unstable, intermediate compounds known as *cyclic PG endoperoxides* that form prostaglandins (PGs).[24] Other chemically related compounds called *thromboxanes* are also
formed. PGs are extremely potent biologic substances that exert marked effects in very
low doses in a variety of physiologic functions. They are synthesized in most tissues in
response to various stimuli and exert their effects only in localized areas.[23,25] As the
levels of other primary mediators of inflammation decrease, PG levels increase.[3] Specific
classes of PGs appear to control or perpetuate the local inflammatory response. *Prostaglandin E_1* (PGE$_1$) may increase vascular permeability by antagonizing vasoconstriction,
and the chemotactic activity of prostaglandin E_2 (PGE$_2$) may attract leukocytes to the
locally inflamed area.[3] Some PGs are proinflammatory (e.g., PGE$_2$) and synergize the
effects of other inflammatory substances, such as bradykinin. Proinflammatory PGs are
thought to be responsible for sensitizing pain receptors, causing a state of hyperalgesia
associated with the inflammatory reaction.[26] There is also evidence that suggests that
other classes of PGs act as inhibitors of the inflammatory response.[23-27]

Prostaglandins may also regulate repair processes during the early phases of healing by contributing to the synthesis of mucopolysaccharides. Thus, while PGs may be
responsible for the late stages of inflammation, they may also be involved in initiating
the early phases of wound repair.

The primary mode of action of steroids such as prednisone and the nonsteroidal
anti-inflammatory agents like aspirin is the inhibition of PG synthesis by deactivation of
cyclooxygenase.[26] Suppressing the inflammatory response and its associated pain may
be appropriate treatment for chronic inflammation but certainly is not the first choice for
treatment of the normal acute inflammatory response. A summary of prostaglandin
production is given in Figure 1-4.

CHRONIC INFLAMMATION

Most of the symptoms associated with the acute inflammatory response usually
subside within 2 weeks following onset. During the subsequent 2-week period, known
as the *subacute phase*, symptoms continue to wane until they disappear at approximately
1 month from onset. Inflammation persisting for months or years is called *chronic
inflammation*. Chronic inflammation associated with wounds often occurs when a
wound is habitually sealed by necrotic tissue, is contaminated with pathogens, or

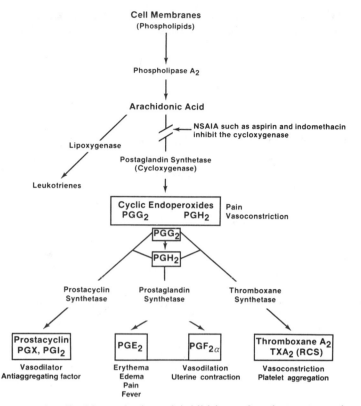

FIGURE 1–4. Prostaglandin biosynthesis and inhibition of cyclooxygenase by aspirin and NSAID (Adapted from Nikander, R, McMahoon, FG, and Ridolfo, AJ: Nonsteroidal anti-inflammatory agents. Annual Review of Pharmacology and Toxicology 19:469, © 1979 by Annual Reviews Inc.).

contains foreign material that cannot be phagocytized or solubilized by granulocytes during the acute inflammatory phase.[28] As granulocytes disappear through lysis and migration during the resolution of the acute inflammatory phase, mononuclear cells, specifically lymphocytes, monocytes, and macrophages, which are more resistant to lysis, increase in numbers and persist at the site of inflammation. Recall that mononuclear cells, especially macrophages, are scavenger cells, particularly of materials in the inflamed area that are not readily solubilized by lysosomal enzymes released by granulocytes. In fact, the persistence of mononuclear cells in chronically inflamed wounds may indicate either the presence of some foreign material or development of delayed hypersensitivity owing to infection. Foreign material may be present in a wound as insoluble fibers from suture, dressings, cotton from cotton swabs, and hydrophilic beads.

The chronic inflammatory response is not characterized by the cardinal signs of inflammation. Rather, the body responds to the presence of persistent foreign material and/or infection by local proliferation of mononuclear cells. In particular, macrophages that have ingested foreign particulate material will remain in inflamed tissue if they are unable to solubilize the material.[3] Through chemotaxis, macrophages attract fibroblasts and, as the chronic inflammatory state continues, large numbers of fibroblasts invade and produce increased quantities of collagen that surrounds the foreign material in a dense fibrous capsule. This hard mass of fibrous tissue is called a *granuloma*, the formation of which is a slow process and is considered a last defense by the body against a foreign material that can not be phagocytized or solubilized.

SUMMARY

The inflammatory response is the first step in wound healing. It consists of a complex process of interrelated events involving vascular reactions, cellular elements, and a number of chemical mediators. The inflammatory response prepares the wounded tissues for the remaining steps in the healing process, namely, repair and reorganization. The acute inflammatory response usually lasts about 2 weeks, followed by the subacute stage that lasts another 2 weeks. Inflammation that lasts for months or even years is termed chronic inflammation. Inflamed wounds may or may not be infected, and infected wounds may or may not be inflamed. The clinician who cares for wounds must be able to recognize the characteristics of inflammation and become familiar with the types of cells and the roles they play during the inflammatory process. The importance of understanding the roles that various cells play in directing and controlling the inflammatory process becomes more evident in later chapters, which describe how various treatment interventions and their timeliness may be used advantageously to enhance or inhibit cellular repair and chemotactic processes.

REFERENCES

1. Zarro, V: Mechanisms of inflammation and repair. In Michlovitz, S (ed): Thermal Agents in Rehabilitation. FA Davis, Philadelphia, 1986, p 12.
2. Vander, AJ, Sherman, JH, and Luciano, DS: Human physiology: The mechanisms of body function, ed 3. McGraw-Hill, New York, 1980, pp 319–324.
3. Peacock, EE: Wound Repair, ed 3. WB Saunders, Philadelphia, 1984, p 13.
4. Kanzler, MH, et al: Basic mechanisms in the healing cutaneous wound. J Dermatol Surg Oncol 12(11):1156, 1986.
5. Pollack, SV: The wound healing process. Clin Dermatol 2(3):8, 1984.
6. Simpson, DM, and Ross, R: The neutrophilic leukocyte in wound repair. A study with antineutrophilic serum. J Clin Invest 51:2009, 1972.
7. Olsen, CE: Macrophage factors affecting wound healing. In Hunt, TK, et al (eds): Soft and Hard Tissue Repair. Biological and Clinical Aspects. Praeger, New York, 1984, pp 343, 352.
8. Leibovich, SJ, and Ross, R: The role of the macrophage in wound repair. A study with hydrocortisone and antimacrophage serum. Am J Pathol 78:71, 1975.
9. Wahl, LM, et al: Collagenase production by endotoxin-activated macrophages. Proc Natl Acad Sci 71:3598, 1974.
10. Laub, R, et al: Degradation of collagen and proteoglycan by macrophages and fibroblasts. Biochem Biophys Acta 721:425, 1982.
11. Diegelmann, RF, Cohen, KI, and Kaplan, AM: The role of macrophages in wound repair: A review. Plast Reconstr Surg 68:107, 1981.
12. Silver, IA: Oxygen and tissue repair. In Ryan, TJ (ed): An Environment for Healing: the Role of Occlusion. Royal Society of Medicine, International Congress and Symposium Series, No. 88, 1984, p 18.
13. Tsukamoto, Y, Hesel, WE, and Wahl, SM: Macrophage production of fibronectin, a chemoattractant for fibroblasts. J Immunol 127:637, 1981.
14. Polverini, PJ, et al: Activated macrophages induce vascular proliferation. Nature 269:804, 1977.
15. Knighton, D, Silver, IA, and Hunt, TK: Regulation of wound-healing angiogenesis—effect on oxygen gradients and inspired oxygen concentration. Surgery 90:262, 1981.
16. Banda, MH, Hunt, TK, and Silver, IA: Fibrosis. Clin Symp 37:12, 1985.
17. Grotendorst, GR, et al: Attachment of smooth muscle cells to collagen and their migration toward platelet-derived growth factor. Proc Natl Acad Sci 78:3669, 1981.
18. Michaeli, D, Hunt, TK, and Knighton, RD: The role of platelets in wound healing: demonstration of angiogenic activity. In Hunt, TK, et al (eds): Soft and Hard Tissue Repair. Biological and Clinical Aspects. Praeger, New York, 1984, p 392.
19. Deuel, TF, et al: Chemotaxis of monocytes and neutrophils to platelet-derived growth factor. J Clin Invest 69:1046, 1982.

20. Knighton, DR, et al: Role of platelets and fibrin in the healing sequence. Ann Surg 196:379, 1982.
21. Katona, G, and Blengia, JR: Inflammation and anti-inflammatory therapy. Spectrum Publications, New York, 1975, pp 3, 88–92.
22. Buissert, PD: Allergy. Sci Am 247(2):86, 1982.
23. Smith, EL, et al: Principles of Biochemistry: Mammalian Biochemistry, ed 7. McGraw-Hill, New York, 1983, pp 371–386, 393–415.
24. Pike, JE: Prostaglandins. Sci Am 71(225):84, 1971.
25. Anthony, CP, and Thibodeau, GA: Textbook of Anatomy and Physiology, ed 11. WB Saunders, Philadelphia, 1983, pp 66–70, 237–238, 286, 321, 352–354.
26. Wilkerson, GB: Inflammation in connective tissue: Etiology and management. Athletic Training, Winter 1985, p 298.
27. Stryer, L: Biochemistry, ed 2. WH Freeman, San Francisco, 1975, pp 851–854.
28. Bryant, WM: Wound healing. Clin Symp 29:9, 1977.

CHAPTER 2

The Repair Phase of Wound Healing—Re-epithelialization and Contraction

Theodore J. Daly, M.D.

The focus of this chapter is the second, or repair, phase of wound healing with respect to the events that occur during the (1) granulation, (2) re-epithelialization, (3) neovascularization, and (4) contraction phases of the wound healing process.

The initial vascular and lymphatic responses to injury discussed in Chapter 1 create the necessary framework to enable the wound healing process to erect a new external barrier against further insult.[1-18] Cellular activity reaches a frenzied pace and an integration of inherent biochemical, synthetic, and regenerative processes results in repair of the traumatized tissue. The energy expended in yielding these reparative results must be used in the most efficient manner possible. This energy-efficient requirement is fulfilled by recreating a permeability barrier (*re-epithelialization*) and reducing the wound surface area (*contraction*) to accelerate the wound healing process. A new blood supply (*neovascularization*) and replacement and reinforcement of the injured tissue (*fibroplasia*) are also fundamental processes involved in the repair phase of wound healing. The final stage of wound healing, matrix formation and remodeling, is discussed in Chapter 3. The three overlapping phases of wound healing are shown in Figure 2–1.

GRANULATION TISSUE FORMATION

When the wound is essentially clear of foreign substances, when infectious agents have been eliminated, and when an infiltrate of macrophages and fibroblasts is present, wound healing can proceed. At this time, polymorphonuclear cells are absent or are present in small numbers. A gel-like matrix of collagen, hyaluronic acid, and fibronectin contains a newly formed vascular network to nourish the macrophages and fibroblasts that have migrated to the tissue defect (Table 2–1). Lymphatics have also formed in this matrix, preventing wound edema and reducing the possibility of resultant infection.

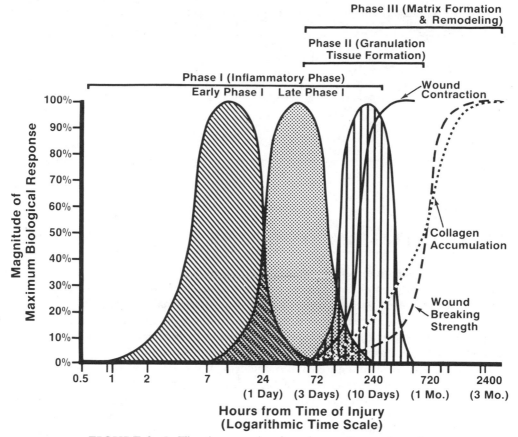

FIGURE 2–1. The three overlapping phases of wound repair.

The individual elements forming this granulation tissue appear to form in the wound space simultaneously. The macrophage clearly has an important role in the wound repair process, but the chemical and cellular substances initiating and promoting granulation tissue formation have not yet been specifically identified and are subjects of intense research.[19-21] Various biologically active substances and the geometric structure of the wound are suspected to play a prominent role in wound repair (Table 2–2).

TABLE 2–1. Matrix and Cellular Constituents Involved in the
Late Inflammatory Phase (Late Phase I) and the Early Granulation
Phase (Early Phase II) of Wound Healing

Wound Matrix Constituents	Cellular Constituents
• Enzymes	• Endothelial cells
• Glycosaminoglycans	• Macrophages
• Elastin	• Fibroblasts
• Proteoglycans	• Lymphocytes
• Type III/I collagen	• Platelets
• Fibrin	• Epidermal cells
• Fibronectin	
• Hyaluronic acid	

TABLE 2–2. Known Factors Responsible for Initiating and Promoting the Repair Phase (Phase II — Granulation Tissue Formation) of Wound Healing

- Chemotactic factors
- Structural macromolecules
- Degradative enzymes
- Tissue geometry (e.g., free edge effect)
- Fibrin
- Collagen
- Fibronectin
- Transforming growth factor–beta (TGF-β)
- Thrombospondin

RE-EPITHELIALIZATION OF THE WOUND SURFACE

The re-establishment of an epidermis in superficial wounds[15] is initiated within hours after the injury occurs.[21] The environmental stress on the cutaneous defect will be reduced or eliminated with the reformation of an epidermal barrier.

The first change noted is a morphologic alteration of the epidermal and adnexal (hair follicle and sweat gland) basal cells at the wound periphery. These epidermal basal cells initially flatten, lose their intercellular attachments (desmosomes, the "links" that maintain the structural integrity of the epidermis), retract their intracellular tonofilaments (the structural girders of the cell), and form actin filaments (a component of muscle) at the edge of the cytoplasm of the cell.[22] These changes occur rapidly and provide epidermal cells with the ability to migrate toward the area of cell deficit due to (1) the loss of rigid cellular structures, and (2) the development of pseudopodia (actin filaments) on the basolateral (side of wound cell deficit, or *free edge*) aspect of the epidermal basal cell.

Re-epithelialization of the wound surface may occur in several ways.[23] The classical mechanism of epithelial cell migration over the wound surface is the leap frog model.[24,25] The epidermal cell migrates no more than two or three cell lengths from its initial position and "slides" or "rolls" over epidermal cells previously implanted in the wound surface. The migrating cell then becomes fixed at this site, and other epidermal cells successively migrate over these cells. An epidermal layer four to six cells thick would progressively advance and close the epithelial defect.

A single layer of epidermal cells can resurface a wound if frictional trauma to the site is prevented during the first week of healing. This method of re-epithelialization suggests that an epidermal cell may migrate across a wound surface with a "train" of epidermal cells behind it, each cell maintaining its original position in the chain, until migration is halted by contact with other epidermal cells or by a complete re-epithelialization of the wound surface. A "leap frog" mechanism that produces an epidermal cell monolayer is a possible but less likely explanation.

The stimuli for re-epithelialization have not been clearly delineated. The "free edge effect," or the loss of cellular contact inhibition at the area of cell deficit at the wound edge, involves chalones, a group of tissue-specific substances that are synthesized by all normal tissues and inhibit biologic events.[26] Wounded tissue would not produce chalones, adjacent normal tissue would not be under its inhibitory effect, and cell division would occur. When the wound was healed, the tissue would again produce chalones and the wound healing process would cease. On the contrary, cellular proliferation is not necessary for cell migration.[27] Epidermal growth factor (EGF) is a polypeptide that stimulated epidermal proliferation.[28-30] Enhanced phosphorylation of endogenous cellular proteins is thought to be the mechanism whereby EGF stimulates epidermal cell proliferation.[30,31] Epibolin and platelet-derived growth factor (PDGF) are also thought to play a role in stimulating re-epithelialization.[32,33]

Next in sequence is the formation of the basement membrane. Bullous pemphigold antigen is always present on the basement plasma membrane of epidermal cells and is the first detected component of the basement membrane.[32-34] Laminin[33,34] and type IV collagen[33,35] are the next components of the basement membrane detected and are synthesized after the epidermal cells have ceased migrating. The basement membrane is first laid down at the wound periphery and then progresses to the center of the wound.

The epidermal basal cells traverse the wound surface guided by various substances in the matrix. Fibronectin,[33,36-39] fibrin,[33,37,40] and type IV collagen[41] provide a framework for migration. When an eschar, or scab, is present on the wound surface, it impedes rapid re-epithelialization. Therefore, crust formation should be minimized by keeping the wound surface hydrated. This fact is discussed in Chapter 9 under microenvironmental dressings.

The epidermal cells finally assume their original cuboidal or rectangular shape when re-epithelialization is complete and the basement membrane is in the final stages of synthesis.[42,43] A rapid re-formation of hemidesmosomes creates a strong bond between the epidermal cells and the newly formed basement membrane to complete the process of re-epithelialization (Fig. 2-2).

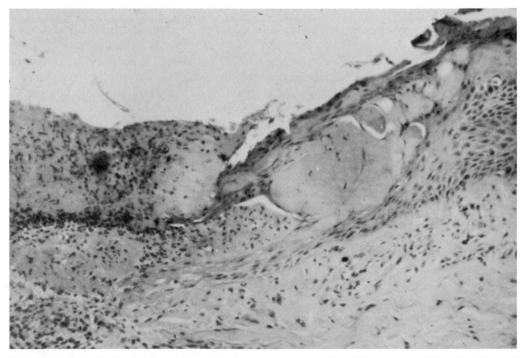

FIGURE 2-2. Re-formation of hemidesmosomes creating bond between epidermal cells and basement membrane (From Rook, A, Wilkinson, DS, and Ebling, FJG: Textbook of Dermatology. Blackwell Scientific Publications, Oxford, England, 1986, p 595, with permission).

FIBROPLASIA

The dermal fibroblasts initially undergo a phenotypic change whereby the cellular organelles retract and the "myofibroblast," a spindle-shaped cell, proliferates and migrates into the wound space.[44-46] Actin filaments align along the cell periphery to allow movement and contractile strength.[45,46] The myofibroblast provides structural macromolecules and synthesizes fibronectin, collagen, glycosaminoglycans (GAGs), various enzymes, thrombospondin, and other molecules in this altered shape.[45,47] The cellular trigger(s) that induce the fibroblast to change shape and synthesize matrix are not well understood. Fibroblast growth factors (FGFs)[48-62] and chemoattractants[63-68] are likely inducing factors.[60,62,69-74] Fibroblast proliferation and migration into the wound space are modulated by the interaction of numerous known and unknown factors.[60,62,69-74] PDGF,[75] EGF,[76-78] FGF, and serum factors play numerous and complex roles in promoting fibroplasia.[62,69,70,72,74]

The myofibroblast initially synthesizes a gel-like extracellular matrix as it moves into the wound.[79] The glycoprotein fibronectin[80,81] is a major component of the gel-like cellular secretion and itself provides for enhanced myofibroblast activity.[47,79,82,83] Thrombin[50-52] and probably EGF[57,84] stimulate fibronectin synthesis and secretion[85] and also promote fibroblast proliferation. Fibronectin allows fibroblasts to bind to the extracellular matrix, providing an adherent base for cell migration,[83] allowing fibroblasts to attach to collagen,[86-88,89] fibrin, and hyaluronic acid.[8] The vectors of fibroblast migration into the wound are chemotactically[13,66,67] and physically[90,91] directed by fibronectin's molecular and gross fibrillar structure, respectively.[36,73,92] Fibronectin therefore has a critical and important role to play in the speed and direction of the dermal repair process in wound healing.

Hyaluronic acid[93] is also found in the extracellular matrix or "ground substance" of the wound. This polysaccharide or GAG classified molecular[93,94] is nonsulfated,[95] is found in the highest amounts in the first 4 to 5 days of healing, and stimulates fibroblast proliferation[95-100] and migration. Hyaluronic acid can absorb large amounts of water, producing tissue edema.[101] This "swelling"[11] of the wound matrix provides additional space to permit increased migration of fibroblasts into the wound.[101-104] Hyaluronidase[105] enzymatically degrades the hyaluronic acid in the early wound, allowing the sulfated GAGs to chemically stimulate the process of fibroplasia.

The sulfated GAGs chondroitin-4-sulfate and dermatan sulfate on days 5 to 7 eventually replace hyaluronic acid as the major GAG.[106,107] These sulfated GAGs promote collagen synthesis and maturation.[95]

Sulfated GAGs have a protein core and are called proteoglycans.[93,94] They provide a more stable and resilient matrix that inhibits cell migration and proliferation.[94] Proteoglycans regulate collagen fibrillogenesis[108-110] and accelerate polymerization of collagen monomers.[108] Heparan sulfate proteoglycan controls cell division,[111] inhibits the growth of smooth muscle cells,[112] and regulates cell function and proliferation.[113]

Myofibroblasts therefore secrete an extracellular matrix that initially consists of fibronectin and hyaluronic acid, inducing cell migration and proliferation, and subsequently synthesize proteoglycans that stimulate collagen formation and increase tissue resilience and tensile strength.

Collagen production begins about 5 days after myofibroblast migration into the wound space.[114] At least three classes of this glycoprotein[115] occur in the connective tissue. Type I collagen (adult), type II collagen (cartilage), and type III collagen (embryonic) are fibrillar collagens. Type IV collagen comprises a part of the basement membrane. Type V collagen is located pericellularly. These collagen types are further discussed in Chapter 3.

The synthesis of collagens is known to be Type III initially, and then Type I, which is similar to mature connective tissue.[79,116-121] Type IV collagen is not fibrillar in nature and composes a portion of the basement membrane. Type V collagen forms a network structure to reinforce cellular arrangement and is deposited around the cells.[122]

The helical fibrillar structure of collagen provides a stiff framework for further healing. The wound breaking strength increases when collagen synthesis begins at day 5,[114,123] and by day 21, the wound strength has increased to only 20 percent of its previous strength.[114] A repaired wound at best attains only 70 percent of the strength of unwounded skin.[114,124]

Wound tensile strength is a result of collagen deposition[125,126] and the remodeling of smaller collagen bundles, with larger bundles forming.[110] Increased collagen synthesis occurs in the first 6 months. Collagen synthesis returns to its normal state within 6 to 12 months after the injury occurs.[127] Collagen acts as a fibroblast chemoattractant[64] and has an effect on fibroblast,[128] epithelial,[129] and endothelial cell[130] functions.

Elastin is a connective tissue protein that also contributes to the remodeling phase of wound healing. Its precise function is unknown.[23]

NEOVASCULARIZATION

There are at least three ways angiogenesis occurs in wounds: (1) the generation of a de novo vascular network in the wound space; (2) the anastomosis to pre-existing vessels—that is, naturally occurring grafts; and (3) the coupling or recoupling of vessels throughout the wound space.[23] Neovascularization involves a phenotypic alteration of the endothelial cell, its directed migration, and various mitogenic stimuli. A pre-existing extracellular matrix and "free edge effect" or the absence of neighboring endothelial cells are essential for new vessel formation to occur.[131,132]

Cytoplasmic pseudopodia extend from endothelial cells on the second wound day.[133] Collagenase is secreted and migration into the perivascular space occurs.[133] A macrophage-derived growth factor[15] and growth factors from the epidermis[134] and wound tissue[135] act together with other growth factors[136-138] to induce angiogenic migration and mitotic activity. Thrombospondin also seems to play a role in neovascularization.[139] Lactic acid,[140] biogenic amines,[141] and low oxygen tension[142] also stimulate neovascularization.

The extracellular matrix provides growth controlling factors[143-147] that affect endothelial cell proliferation and migration. Platelet-derived factors,[148-149] adult tissue extracts,[150] heparin,[151] and fibronectin provide stimuli for directed angiogenesis.

Vascular endothelium secretes prostacyclin, growth factors, proteases and other enzymes, as well as structural macromolecules. Lymphatic vessels are also regenerated in the wound space and are essential to allow for wound drainage and to prevent an edematous, easily infected wound.[152] Neural tissue may also be regenerated along with lymphatic vessels and the new vascular plexus.

WOUND CONTRACTION

Contraction versus Contracture (Scar Formation)

Contraction is the process that closes wounds after loss of tissue. *Contracture* is the end result of wound contraction that may be the result of contraction itself, fibrosis, adhesions, or muscle or other tissue damage.[23]

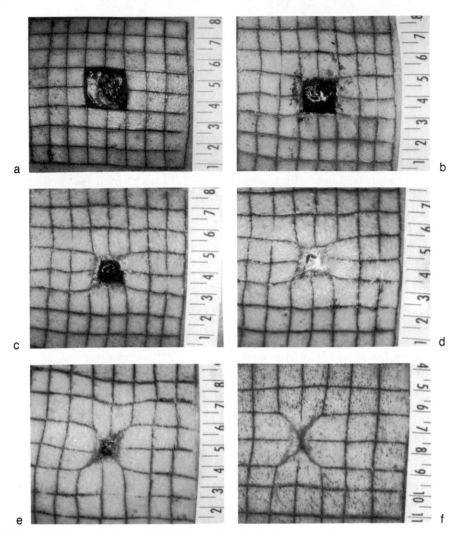

FIGURE 2–3. Photographs of full-thickness excisional wound made on an 8 x 8 cm tattooed grid on domestic pig skin. This sequence depicts healing by both granulation and contraction. (a) Day 0 day of wounding. (b) Day 8 after wounding. (c) Day 12 after wounding. (d) Day 20 after wounding. (e) Day 30 after wounding. (f) Day 45 after wounding. Note the alterations in the shape of each of the grids immediately surrounding the wound. (From Fitzpatrick: Dermatology in General Medicine. McGraw Hill, New York, 1987, p. 330, with permission).

The wound space area is decreased during contraction. This dermal process causes closure of the wound, with or without prior epithelialization.[153] In fact, much of the epithelium is ultimately lost in the fully contracted wound.[154] Contraction involves movement of pre-existing tissue centripetally and not formation of new tissue. Contraction does not always go to completion, except occasionally in small wounds (Fig. 2–3).

Contractures usually present functional problems in the healed wound. They allow healing of the wound to proceed to completion, but often prevent normal movement or physiologic activity of the injured area.

THE MECHANISM OF WOUND CONTRACTION
Contraction begins soon after wounding and peaks at 2 weeks. The myofibroblast is the predominant mediator of this contractile process[155] because of its ability to extend

and retract.[156] Cellular actin contains microfilaments,[45,46] and myofibroblasts contain one of the highest concentrations of actinomyosin of any cell.[157] This muscle-like contraction of myofibroblasts is mediated by prostaglandin F_1, 5-hydroxytryptamine, angiotensin, vasopressin, bradykinins, epinephrine,[158,159] and norepinephrine.

The interaction of the extracellular matrix and cellular components of granulation tissue result in a contractile unit called a *fibronexus*.[160] Extracellular matrix fibrils composed of fibronectin,[160] Types I and III collagen, cytoplasmic actin,[160] and vinculin[161] are the major constituents of this cohesive complex. Cytoplasmic actin binds to extracellular fibronectin and in this way seems to effect contraction.[162] The rate of contraction is proportional to the cell number and inversely proportional to the lattice collagen concentration.[163] Cytoplasmic pseudopodia extend and attach to collagen fibers and retract, drawing the collagen fibers to the cell, thereby producing wound contraction.

The end result of contraction is a stable wound with a constant turnover of collagen with remodeling of the matrix (Fig. 2–3). This topic is covered further in Chapter 3. The synthesis and deposition of collagen initially is more random and the continuity of stresses and strains on the tissue causes an alignment of collagen fibers to occur, which strengthens the wound. Wounds that are under stress heal more securely at an earlier date. Allowing patients to move about freely after the initial stages of wound repair are completed seems reasonable. Wound contraction then continues into the third phase of wound healing, matrix formation and remodeling (see Chapter 3).

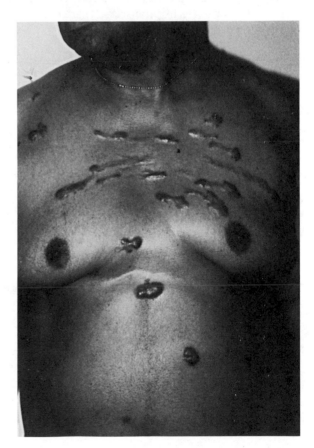

FIGURE 2–4. Patient with multiple keloid scars.

KELOIDS AND HYPERTROPHIC SCARS

Abnormal responses to wound healing can sometimes result in a hyperreactive production of collagen. Keloids and hypertrophic scars are a manifestation of this process. *Keloids* are defined as an overgrowth or extension of the connective tissue of a wound, involving the injured as well as the uninjured normal peripheral wound skin. Figure 2–4 illustrates keloids. *Hypertrophic scars* are thought to be a reactive fibroplasia involving only the injured area of the wound. Hypertrophic scars are popularly thought to resolve within a year or two, while keloids persist indefinitely or for extremely long periods.[156] Recent studies[164] have disputed these concepts and it appears that keloids and hypertrophic scars may occur in varied morphologic or temporal patterns that are often overlapped. The presence of acellular thick bundles of collagen when a biopsy of a scar is performed is the accepted criteria for an undisputed diagnosis of keloid formation.[156] Their absence, along with the presence of numerous whorled cellular formations of connective tissue in the dermis, supports the diagnosis of a hypertrophic scar. Keloids and hypertrophic scars rarely occur in prepubescent or elderly individuals. They tend to occur in areas of skin tension, such as on the chest or shoulder.

Collagen production is increased in both keloids and hypertrophic scars.[156] They occur in all races and show no sex predominance. Familial inheritance is sometimes observed. The presence of earlobe keloids does *not* predict their occurrence on other body sites. Keloid formation and hypertrophic scarring are further addressed in Chapter 3.

Treatment modalities are limited and often produce poor results. Steroid injections, cryotherapy, laser surgery, radiation, pressure dressings, and topical tretinoin cream (especially for hypertrophic scars[164]) are currently used. Excision results in regrowth the majority of the time.

RE-EPITHELIALIZATION AND CONTRACTION UNDER CHRONIC CONDITIONS

Normally, the acute inflammation phase of wound healing is essentially complete after 10 to 14 days. Inflammation may continue due to many factors. Subacute inflammation occurs within a month or two of the injury and chronic inflammation occurs thereafter. The main criteria for acute inflammation is the presence of neutrophils. The presence of monocytes, lymphocytes, histocytes, and macrophages indicates chronic inflammation. Subacute inflammation shows a mixture of all these cells.

If the wound is delayed in its inflammatory phase, signs of inflammation such as tenderness, erythema, edema, and warmth can be seen. When these signs persist after more than 2 to 3 weeks, some factor is probably preventing resolution of the inflammatory phase. A review of the pertinent factors involved in the clinical treatment of wounds is recommended. Most likely, a foreign body or infection is the culprit.

Re-epithelialization of a primarily closed wound (one closed by sutures or with close approximation of the edges) is usually easily accomplished. A chronically inflamed or infected wound may be covered by a viable epithelium. When the normal wound surface is fully covered, multiple changes occur. The neovascular tissue undergoes partial resorption, the granulation tissue reduces in size and the fibroblasts cease to proliferate in the wound and regress. Keloids and hypertrophic scars, the most notable exceptions to these changes, have already been discussed. This new epithelial cover is only several cells thick but continues to develop a normal epithelial complement of cells until it is as thick as uninjured epithelium. Its nutrition is derived from the wound surface below and possibly from oxygen in the ambient air; thus, hypertrophic oxygen may facilitate epithelial growth. Repeated trauma to the wound surface through dressing changes (wet to dry) or flexed skin (skin at a joint or under excessive tension) interferes with establishing an adequate wound epithelium.

Often a raised epithelial edge can be seen in wounds that have chronically been unable to completely re-epithelialize. A "hypertrophic edge" occurs with little advancement over the wound. The wound is unable to close properly due to adverse conditions, some of which will be discussed in the next section.

FACTORS AFFECTING WOUND EPITHELIALIZATION AND CONTRACTION

Local factors adversely affecting wound healing include poor surgical technique[165] such as occurs with application of excessive tension to devitalized tissue; vascular disorders such as arteriosclerosis or venous stasis; tissue ischemia; bacterial,[166] mycobacterial, fungal, or yeast infections; medications such as local anesthetics,[167,168] topical steroids,[169] or antibiotics;[169-173] extravasation of antineoplastic drugs[174,175] or hemostatic agents such as aluminum chloride or ferric subsulfate;[176-178] factitial or other sources of chronic trauma; foreign body reactions; or an adverse wound microenvironment (such as dry versus semiocclusive dressings or photoaged skin).[179,180] Decubitus ulcers, tumor (Marjolin's ulcer), mal perforans ulcers (neuropathic ulcers), and chronic radiation injury[181] all adversely affect wound healing[179] (Table 2–3).

Systemic factors that may be detrimental to wound healing[182] include malnutrition,

TABLE 2–3. Effect of Local Factors on the Promotion or
Impairment of Wound Healing

Local Factors	Promotion of Wound Healing	Impairment of Wound Healing
Surgical technique	Close approximation of wound edges	Excessive tension Devitalized tissue
Blood supply	Patent	Atherosclerosis Venous stasis Tissue ischemia
Infection	None	Bacteria Mycobacteria Fungi or yeast
Medications	Some topical antibiotics (e.g. mupirocin — Bactroban)	Topical steroids Many systemic and topical antibiotics Antineoplastic drugs Hemostatic agents (aluminum chloride or Monsel's solution)
Trauma	None	Chronic trauma Foreign body Factitial trauma
Microenvironment	Occlusive dressings	Dry dressings Photoaged skin Radiation injury
Ulcer type	—	Decubitus ulcers Tumor (Marjolin's ulcer) Neuropathic ulcers (mal perforans ulcers)

TABLE 2–4. Effect of Systemic Factors on the Promotion or
Impairment of Wound Healing

Systemic Factors	Promotion of Wound Healing	Impairment of Wound Healing
Nutrition	No deficiencies	Deficiency of protein, calories, vitamins (especially A and C), trace metals (especially zinc and copper)
Age	Young	Advanced
Illness	None	Chronic illness (hepatic, renal, hematopoietic, cardiovascular, autoimmune, carcinoma) Endocrine disease (e.g., diabetes mellitus, Cushing's disease) Systemic vascular disorders (periarteritis nodosa, vasculitis, granulomatosis, atherosclerosis) Connective tissue disease (e.g., Ehlers-Danlos syndrome)
Systemic medications		Corticosteroids, aspirin, heparin, coumadin, penicillamine, nicotine, phenylbutazone, and other nonsteroidal anti-inflammatory drugs; antineoplastic agents

protein deprivation,[183] and vitamin A and C deficiency.[179] Systemic medications such as corticosteroids,[169] aspirin, heparin, Coumadin, penicillamine, nicotine, phenylbutazone, other nonsteriodal anti-inflammatory drugs,[174,175,184–186] and antineoplastic agents interfere with the wound healing process at various stages and often arrest its progress, resulting in a poorly healing or nonhealing wound (Table 2–4). Topical substances applied to wounds have also been shown to inhibit tissue repair.[187–189] Chronic debilitating illness (hepatic, renal, hematopoietic, cardiovascular, dysfunctional autoimmune, oncologic),[179] endocrine disorders (i.e., diabetes mellitus, Cushing's syndrome), systemic vascular disorders (periarteritis nodosa, leukocytoclastic vasculitis, granulomatoses, antherosclerosis, and so on), as well as connective tissue disease (e.g., Ehlers-Danlos syndrome) often have severely adverse effects on wound healing. Finally, advancing age is a factor that contributes to poor wound healing in largely unknown ways.[190,191]

SUMMARY

Understanding the fundamentals of wound healing is essential to anticipate and prevent adverse results in this process. This chapter discussed the second, or repair, phase of the wound healing process, including granulation, re-epithelialization, fibroplasia, neovascularization, contraction, and scar formation. This review of the basic biology of wound healing should provide a foundation upon which new insights and technologic advances in wound healing can be based to optimize and accelerate the regeneration of injured tissue in the wound repair process.

REFERENCES

1. Cotran, RS and Majno, G: A light and electron microscopic analysis of vascular injury. Ann NY Acad Sci 116:750, 1964.
2. McLean, AEM, et al: Cellular permeability and the reaction to injury. Ann NY Acad Sci 116:986, 1964.
3. Joris, I, et al: Endothelial contraction in vivo: A study of the rat mesentery. Virchows Arch (Cell Pathol) 12:73, 1972.
4. Karnovsky, MT: The ultrastructural basis of capillary permeability studied with peroxidase as a tracer. J Cell Biol 35:213, 1967.

5. Weeks, JR: Prostaglandins. Annu Rev Pharmacol Toxicol 12:317, 1972.

6. Pike, JE: Prostaglandins. Sci Am 225:84, 1971.

7. Hurley, JV: Substances promoting leukocyte emigration. Ann NY Acad Sci 116:918, 1964.

8. Clark, RAF: Cutaneous tissue repair: Basic biologic considerations. J Am Acad Dermatol 13:701–725, 1985.

9. Marchesi, VT: The site of leukocyte emigration during inflammation. Q J Exp Physiol 46:115, 1961.

10. Hunt, TK: Wound healing and wound infection: Theory and surgical practice. Appleton-Century-Crofts, New York, 1980.

11. Leibovich, SJ, and Ross, R: The role of macrophages in wound repair. Am J Pathol 78:71, 1975.

12. Newman, SL, Henson, JE, and Henson, PM: Phagocytosis of senescent neutrophils by human monocyte derived macrophages and rabbit inflammatory macrophages. J Exp Med 156:430–442, 1982.

13. Tsukamoto, Y, Helsel, WE, and Wahl, SM: Macrophage production of fibronectin, a chemoattractant for fibroblasts. J Immunol 127:673–678, 1981.

14. Leibovich, SJ: Production of macrophage-dependent fibroblast-stimulating activity (M-FSA) by murine macrophages. Exp Cell Res 113:47–56, 1978.

15. Martin, BM, et al and Stimulation of nonlymphoid mesenchymal cell proliferation by a macrophage-derived growth factor. J Immunol 126:1510–1515, 1981.

16. Lachman, LB: Human interleukin I: Purification and properties. Fed Proc 42:2639–2645, 1983.

17. Humes, JL, et al: Macrophages synthesize and release prostaglandins in response to inflammatory stimuli. Nature 269:149–151, 1977.

18. Rouzer, CA, et al: Secretion of leukotriene C and other arachidonic acid metabolites by mouse pulmonary macrophages. J Exp Med 155:720–733, 1982.

19. Wahl, LM, et al: Prostaglandin regulation of macrophage collagenase production. Proc Natl Acad Sci USA 74:4955–4958, 1977.

20. Werb, A and Gordon, S: Secretion of a specific collagenase by stimulated macrophages. J Exp Med 142:346–360, 1975.

21. Werb, A and Gordon, S: Elastase secretion by stimulated macrophages. J Exp Med 142:361–377, 1975.

22. Morland, B and Kaplan, G: Macrophage activation in vivo and in vitro. Exp Cell Res 108:279–288, 1977.

23. Alvarez, OM, et al: Wound healing. In Fitzpatrick, T (ed): Dermatology in General Medicine, ed 3. McGraw-Hill, New York, 1987, pp 321–336.

24. Krawczyk, WS: A pattern of epidermal cell migration during wound healing. J Cell Biol 49:247, 1971.

25. Winter, GD: Epidermal regeneration studied in the domestic pig. In Maibach, HI, Rovee, DT (eds): Epidermal Wound Healing. Year Book Medical Publishers, Chicago, 1972.

26. Hunt, TK, et al: Anaerobic metabolism and wound healing: A hypothesis for the initiation and cessation of collagen synthesis in wounds. Am J Surg 135:328, 1978.

27. Krawczyk, WS: A pattern of epidermal cell migration during wound healing. J Cell Biol 49:247–263, 1971.

28. Cohen, S: Isolation of a mouse submaxillary gland protein accelerating incisor eruption and eyelid opening in the newborn animal. J Biol Chem 237:1555–1562, 1962.

29. Cohen, S: The stimulation of epidermal proliferation by a specific protein (EGF). Dev Biol 12:394–407, 1965.

30. Brown, GL, et al: Enhancement of epidermal regeneration by biosynthetic epidermal growth factor. J Exp Med 163(5):1319–1324, 1986.

31. Carpenter, G, King, L, Jr, and Cohen, S: Rapid enhancement of protein phosphorylation in A-431 cell membrane preparation by epidermal growth factor. J Biol Chem 254:4884–4891, 1979.

32. Stanley, JR, et al: Detection of basement membrane zone antigens during epidermal wound healing in pigs. J Invest Dermatol 77:240–243, 1981.

33. Clark, RAF, et al: Fibronectin and fibrin provide a provisional matrix for epidermal cell migration during wound reepithelialization. J Invest Dermatol 70:264–269, 1982.

34. Stanley, JR, et al: Detection of basement membrane antigens during epidermal wound healing in pigs. J Invest Dermatol 77:240, 1981.

35. Hinter, H, et al: Expression of basement membrane zone antigens at the dermo-epibolic function in organ culture of human skin. J Invest Dermatol 74:200–205, 1980.

36. Repesh, LA, Fitzgerald, TJ, and Furcht, LT: Fibronectin involvement in granulation tissue and wound healing in rabbits. J Histochem Cytochem 30:351–358, 1982.

37. Donaldson, DJ and Mahan, JT: Fibrinogen and fibronectin as substrates for epidermal cell migration during wound closure. J Cell Sci 62:117–127, 1983.

38. Kariniemi, A-L, et al: Cytoskeleton and pericellular matrix organization of pure adult human keratinocytes cultured from suction-blister roof epidermis. J Cell Sci 58:49–61, 1982.

39. Kubo, M, et al: Human keratinocytes synthesize, secrete, and deposit fibronectin in the pericellular matrix. J Invest Dermatol 82:580–586, 1984.

40. Odland, G and Ross, R: Human wound repair. I. Epidermal regeneration. J Cell Biol 39:135–151, 1968.

41. Stenn, KS, Madri, JA, and Roll, FJ: Migrating epidermis produces AB_2 collagen and requires continued collagen synthesis for movement. Nature 277:229–232, 1979.

42. Winstanley, EW: Changes in epithelial thickness during the healing of excised full thickness skin wounds. J Pathol 114:155, 1974.

43. Gipson, IK, et al: Hemidesmosome formation in vitro. J Cell Biol 97:849–857, 1983.

44. Gabbiani, G, Chapponnier, C, and Huttner, I: Cytoplasmic filaments and gap junctions in epithelial cells and myofibroblasts during wound healing. J Cell Biol 76:561–568, 1978.
45. Mayno, G: The story of the myofibroblasts. Am Surg Pathol 3:535–542, 1979.
46. Gabbiani, G: The role of contractile proteins in wound healing and fibrocontractive disease. Methods Achiev Exp Pathol 9:187–206, 1979.
47. Grinnell, F, Billingham, RE, and Burgess, L: Distribution of fibronectin during wound healing in vivo. J Invest Dermatol 76:181–189, 1981.
48. Gospodarowicz, D: Purification of fibroblast growth factor from bovine pituitary. J Biol Chem 250:2515–2520, 1975.
49. Zetter, BR, Chen, LB, and Buchanan, JM: Effects of protease treatment on growth, morphology, adhesion, and cell surface proteins of secondary chick embryo fibroblasts. Cell 7:407–412, 1976.
50. Pohjanpelto, P: Stimulation of DNA synthesis in human fibroblasts by thrombin. J Cell Physiol 95:189–194, 1978.
51. Glenn, KC and Cunningham, DD: Thrombin-stimulated cell division involves proteolysis of its cell surface receptor. Nature 278:711–714, 1979.
52. Hall, WM and Ganguly, P: Differential effects of thrombin on growth of human fibroblasts. J Cell Biol 85:70–82, 1980.
53. Liebovich, SJ and Ross, R: A macrophage dependent factor that stimulates the proliferation of fibroblasts in vitro. Am J Pathol 84:501–513, 1976.
54. Heldin, CH, Westermark, B, and Wasteson, A: Platelet-derived growth factor: Purification and partial characterization. Proc Natl Acad Sci USA 76:3722–3726, 1979.
55. Vogel, A, Ross, R, and Raines, E: Role of serum components in density-dependent inhibition of growth of cells in culture: Platelet-derived growth factor is the major-serum determinant of saturation density. J Cell Biol 85:377–385, 1980.
56. Antoniades, HN and Williams, LT: Human platelet-derived growth factor: Structure and function. Fed Proc 42:2630–2634, 1983.
57. Carpenter, G and Cohen, S: ^{125}I-labeled human epidermal growth factor (HEGF): Binding, internalization, and degradation in human fibroblasts. J Cell Biol 71:159–171, 1976.
58. Rinderknecht, E and Humbel, RE: Polypeptides with nonsuppressible insulin-like and cell-growth promoting activities in human serum: Isolation, chemical characterization, and some biological properties of forms I and II. Proc Natl Acad Sci USA 73:2365–2369, 1976.
59. Adams, SO, et al: and Development patterns of insulin-like growth factor-I and -II synthesis and regulation in rat fibroblasts. Nature 302:150–153, 1983.
60. Oppenheimer, CL, et al: Insulin action rapidly modulates the apparent affinity of the insulin-like growth factor II receptor. J Biol Chem 258:4824–4830, 1983.
61. Assoian, RK, et al: Transforming growth factor-B in human platelets: Identification of a major storage site, purification, and characterization. J Biol Chem 258:7155–7160, 1983.
62. Assoian, RK, et al: Transforming growth factor-B controls receptor levels for epidermal growth factor in NRK fibroblasts. Cell 36:35–41, 1984.
63. Postlethwaite, AE, Snyderman, R, and Kang, AH: Chemotactic attraction of human fibroblasts to a lymphocyte-derived factor. J Exp Med 144:1188–1203, 1976.
64. Postlethwaite, AE, Seyer, JM, and Kang, AH: Chemotactic attraction of human fibroblasts to type I, II, and III collagens and collagen-derived peptides. Proc Natl Acad Sci USA 75:871–875, 1978.
65. Postlethwaite, AE, Snyderman, R, and Kang, AH: Generation of a fibroblast chemotactic factor in serum by activation of complement. J Clin Invest 64:1379–1385, 1979.
66. Gauss-Muller, V, et al: Role of attachment factors and attractants in fibroblast chemotaxis. J Lab Clin Med 96:1071–1080, 1980.
67. Postlethwaite, AE, et al: Induction of fibroblast chemotaxis by fibronectin: Localization of the chemotactic region to a 140,000 molecular weight non-gelatin binding fragment. J Exp Med 153:494–499, 1981.
68. Seppa, HEJ, et al: The platelet-derived growth factor is a chemoattractant for fibroblasts. J Cell Biol 92:584–588, 1982.
69. Wrann, M, Fox, C, and Ross, R: Modulation of epidermal growth factor receptors on 3T3 cells by platelet-derived growth factor. Science 210:1363–1365, 1980.
70. Bowen-Pope, D, Discorleto, P, and Ross, R: Interactions between receptors for platelet-derived growth factor and epidermal growth factor. J Cell Physiol 96:679–683, 1983.
71. Stiles, C, et al: Dual control of cell growth by somatomedins and platelet-derived growth factor. Proc Natl Acad Sci USA 76:1279–1283, 1979.
72. Rozengurt, E, et al: Inhibition of epidermal growth factor binding to mouse cultured cells by fibroblast-derived growth factor. J Biol Chem 257:3680–3686, 1982.
73. Clemmons, DR, Van Wyk, JJ, and Pledger, WJ: Sequential addition of platelet factor and plasma to Balb/c 3T3 fibroblast cultures stimulates somatomedin-C binding early in cell cycle. Proc Natl Acad Sci USA 77:6644–6648, 1980.
74. Grotendorst, GR: Alteration of the chemotactic response of NIH/3T3 cells to PDGF by growth factors, transformation, and tumor promoters. Cell 36:279–285, 1984.
75. Ross, R, et al: Platelet-derived growth factor: Its potential roles in wound healing, atherosclerosis, neoplasia, and growth and development. Ciba Found Symp 116:98–112, 1985.

76. Buckley A, et al: Epidermal growth factor increases granulation tissue formation dose dependently. J Surg Res 43(4):322–328, 1987.
77. Franklin TJ, et al: Acceleration of wound healing by recombinant human urogastrone (epidermal growth factor). J Lab Clin Med 108(2):103–108, 1986.
78. Roberts AB, et al: Transforming growth factor-beta: Potential common mechanisms mediating its effects on embryogenesis, inflammation-repair, and carcinogenesis. Int J Rad Appl Instrum [B] 14(4):435–439, 1987.
79. Kurkinen, M, et al: Sequential appearance of fibronectin and collagen in experimental granulation tissue. Lab Invest 43:47–51, 1980.
80. Pospisilova, J, et al: Fibronectin—its significance in wound epithelialization. Acta Chir Plast 28(2):96–102, 1986.
81. Martin, DE, et al: Tissue debris at the injury site is rated by plasma fibronectin and subsequently removed by tissue macrophages. Arch Dermatol 124:226–229, 1988.
82. Cheng, CY, et al: Fibronectin enhances healing of excised wounds in rats. Arch Dermatol 124:221–225, 1988.
83. Yamada, K and Olden, K: Fibronectin-adhesive glycoproteins of cell surface and blood. Nature 275:179–184, 1978.
84. Chen, LB, et al: Control of a cell surface major glycoprotein by epidermal growth factor. Science 197:776–778, 1977.
85. Mosher, DF and Vaheri, A: Thrombin stimulates the production and release of a major surface-associated glycoprotein (fibronectin) in cultures of human fibroblasts. Exp Cell Res 112:323–334, 1978.
86. Doillon, CJ, et al: Collagen deposition during wound repair. Scan Electron Micros (Pt 2):897–903, 1985.
87. Klebe, RJ: Isolation of a collagen-dependent cell attachment factor. Nature 250:248–251, 1974.
88. Pearlstein, E: Plasma membrane glycoprotein which mediates adhesion of fibroblasts to collagen. Nature 262:497–500, 1976.
89. Grinnell, F, Feld, M, and Minter, D: Fibroblast adhesion of fibrinogen and fibrin substrate: Requirement for cold-insoluble globulin (plasma fibronectin). Cell 19:517–525, 1980.
90. Ali, U and Hynes, RO: Effects of LETS glycoprotein on cell motility. Cell 14:439–446, 1978.
91. Hsieh, P and Chen, LB: Behavior of cells seeded in isolated fibronectin matrices. J Cell Biol 96:1208–1217, 1983.
92. Clark, RAF, et al: Blood vessel fibronectin increases in conjunction with endothelial cell proliferation and capillary ingrowth during wound healing. J Invest Dermatol 79:269–276, 1982.
93. Silbert, JE: Structure and metabolism of proteoglycans and glycosaminoglycans. J Invest Dermatol 79(Suppl):31–37, 1982.
94. Hascall, VC and Hascall, GK: Proteoglycans. In Hay, EB (ed): Cell biology of extracellular matrix. Plenum Press, New York, 1981, pp 39–63.
95. Balazs, A and Holmgren, HJ: The basic dye-uptake and the presence of growth inhibiting substance in the healing tissue of skin wounds. Exp Cell Res 1:206–216, 1950.
96. Tomida, M, Koyama, H, and Ono, T: Hyaluronic acid synthetase in cultured mammalian cells producing hyaluronic acid: Oscillatory change during the growth phase and suppression by 5-bromodeoxyuridine. Biochem Biophys Acta 338:352–363, 1974.
97. Hopwood, JJ and Dorfman, A: Glycosaminoglycan synthesis by cultured human skin fibroblasts after transformation with simian virus 40. J Biol Chem 252:4777–4785, 1977.
98. Toole, BP and Gross, J: The extracellular matrix of the regenerating newt limb: Synthesis and removal of hyaluronate prior to differentiation. Dev Biol 25:57–77, 1971.
99. Toole, BP and Trelstad, RL: Hyaluronate production and removal during corneal development in the chick. Dev Biol 26:28–35, 1971.
100. Toole, BP: Hyaluronate turnover during chondrogenesis in the developing chick limb and axial skeleton. Dev Biol 29:321–329, 1972.
101. Toole, BP: Glycosaminoglycans in morphogenesis. In Hay, EB (ed): Cell biology of extracellular matrix. Plenum Press, New York, 1981, pp 259–294.
102. Culp, LA, Murray, BA, and Rollins, BJ: Fibronectin and proteoglycans as determinants of cell-substratum adhesion. J Supramol Struct 11:401–427, 1979.
103. Lark, MW, Laterra, J, and Culp, LA: Close and focal contact adhesions of fibroblasts to fibronectin-containing matrix. Fed Proc 44:394–403, 1985.
104. Rollins, BJ and Culp, LA: Glycosaminoglycans in the substrate adhesion sites of normal and virus-transformed murine cells. Biochemistry 18:141–148, 1979.
105. Bertolami, CN and Donoff, RB: Identification characterization and partial purification of mammalian skin wound hyaluronidase. J Invest Dermatol 79:417–421, 1982.
106. Dorner, RW: Glycosaminoglycans of regenerating tendon. Arthritis Rheum 10:275–276, 1967.
107. Anseth, A: Glycosaminoglycans in corneal regeneration. Exp Eye Res 1:122–127, 1961.
108. Wood, GC: The formation of fibrils from collagen solutions: Effect of chondroitin sulfate and other naturally occurring polyanions on the rate of formation. Biochem J 75:605–612, 1960.
109. Armitage, PM and Chapman, JA: New fibrous long spacing form of collagen. Nature (NB) 229:151–152, 1971.
110. Kischer, CW and Shetlar, MR: Collagen and mucopolysaccharides in the hypertrophic scar. Connect Tissue Res 2:205–213, 1974.

111. Kraemer, PM and Tobey, RA: Cell-cycle dependent desquamation of heparan sulfate from the cell surface. J Cell Biol 55:713–717, 1972.
112. Castellot, JJ, et al: Vascular endothelial cells produce a heparin-like inhibitor of smooth muscle growth. J Cell Biol 90:372–379, 1981.
113. Letourneau, PC, Ray, PN, and Bernfeld, MR: The regulation of cell behavior by cell adhesion. In Goldberger, R (ed): Biological Regulation and Development. Vol 2. Plenum Press, New York, 1980, pp 339–376.
114. Levenson, SM, et al: The healing of rat skin wounds. Ann Surg 161:293–308, 1965.
115. Prockop, DJ and Guzman, NA: Collagen diseases and the biosynthesis of collagen. Hosp Pract 12:62–74, 1977.
116. Holund, B, et al: Fibronectin in experimental granulation tissue. Acta Pathol Microbiol Immunol Scand 90:159–165, 1982.
117. Viljanto, J, Penttinen, R, and Raekallio, J: Fibronectin in early phases of wound healing in children. Acta Chir Scand 147:7–13, 1981.
118. Furthmayr, H and von der Mrak, K: The use of antibodies to connective tissue proteins in studies on their location in tissue. In Furthmayr, H (ed): Immunochemistry of the Extracellular Matrix. Vol II. CRC Press, Boca Raton, FL, 1982, pp 89–117.
119. Epstein, EH, Jr: [a₁(III)]₃ human skin collagen: Release by pepsin digestion and preponderance in fetal life. J Biol Chem 249:3225–3231, 1974.
120. Clore, JN, Cohen, LK, and Diegelmann, RF: Quantitation of collagen types I and III during wound healing in rat skin. Proc Soc Exp Biol Med 161:337–340, 1979.
121. Gay, S, et al: Collagen types in early phases of wound healing in children. Acta Chir Scand 144:205–211, 1978.
122. Gay, S, et al: Collagen molecules comprised of 1 (V)-chains (B chains): An apparent localization in the exocytoskeleton. Cell Res 1:53–58, 1981.
123. Doillon, CJ, et al: Collagen fiber formation in repair tissue: Development of strength and toughness. Coll Relat Res 5(6):481–492, 1985.
124. Scott, PG, et al: Experimental wound healing: Increased breaking strength and collagen synthetic activity in abdominal fascial wound healing with secondary closure of the skin. Br J Surg 72(10):777–779, 1985.
125. Gabbiani, G, et al: Collagen and myofibroblasts of granulation tissue: A chemical, ultrastructural, and immunologic study. Virchows Arch (Cell Pathol) 21:133–145, 1976.
126. Madden, JW and Peacock, EE, Jr: Studies on the biology of collagen during wound healing. I. Rate of collagen synthesis and deposition in cutaneous wounds of the rat. Surgery 64:288–294, 1968.
127. Barnes, MJ, et al: Studies on collagen synthesis in the mature dermal scar in the guinea pig. Biochem Soc Symp 3:917–920, 1975.
128. Bell, E, et al: The reconstitution of living skin. J Invest Dermatol 81(Suppl):2–10, 1983.
129. Sugrue, SP and Hay, ED: Response of basal epithelial cell surface and cytoskeleton to solubilized extracellular matrix molecules. J Cell Biol 91:45–54, 1981.
130. Madri, JA, et al: Capillary endothelial cell cultures: Phenotypic modulation by matrix components. J Cell Biol 97:153–165, 1983.
131. Arnold, F, et al: Wound healing: The effect of macrophage and tumour derived angiogenesis factors on skin graft vascularization. Br J Exp Pathol 68(4):569–574, 1987.
132. Schwartz, SM, Gajdusek, CM, and Owens, GK: Vessel wall growth control. In Nossel, HL and Vogel, HJ (eds): Pathobiology of the Endothelial Cell. Academic Press, New York, 1982, pp 63–78.
133. Kalebic, T, et al: Basement membrane collagen: Degradation by migrating endothelial cells. Science 221:281–283, 1983.
134. Wolf, JE and Harrison, RG: Demonstration and characterization of an epidermal angiogenic factor. J Invest Dermatol 61:130–141, 1973.
135. Banda, MJ, et al: Isolation of a nonmitogenic angiogenesis factor from wound fluid. Proc Natl Acad Sci USA 79:7773–7777, 1982.
136. Sidky, YA and Auerbach, R: Lymphocyte-induced angiogenesis: A quantitative and sensitive assay of the graft-vs-host reaction. J Exp Med 141:1084–1111, 1975.
137. Brown, RA, Weiss, JB, and Tomlinson, IW: Angiogenic factor from synovial fluid resembling that from tumors. Lancet 1:682–685, 1980.
138. D'Amore, PA, et al: Angiogenic activity from bovine retina: Partial purification and characterization. Proc Natl Acad Sci USA 78:3068–3072, 1981.
139. Raugi, GJ, Olerid, JE, and Gown, AM: Thrombospondin in early human wound tissue. J Invest Dermatol 89:551–554, 1987.
140. Imre, G: Studies on the mechanism of retinal neovascularization: Role of lactic acid. Br J Ophthalmol 48:75–82, 1964.
141. Zauberman, H, et al: Stimulation of neovascularization of the cornea by biogenic amines. Exp Eye Res 8:77–83, 1969.
142. Remensnyder, JP and Majno, G: Oxygen gradients in healing wounds. Am J Pathol 52:301–319, 1968.
143. Haudenschild, CC, et al: Human vascular endothelial cells in culture: Lack of response to serum growth factors. Exp Cell Res 98:175–183, 1976.
144. Gospodarowicz, D, Moran, JS, and Braun, DL: Control of proliferation of bovine vascular endothelial cells. J Cell Physiol 91:377–386, 1977.

145. Wall, RT, et al: Factors influencing endothelial cell proliferation in vitro. J Cell Physiol 96:203–214, 1978.
146. Clemmons, DR, Isley, WL, and Brown, MT: Dialyzable factor in human serum of platelet origin stimulates endothelial cell replication and growth. Proc Natl Acad Sci USA 80:1641–1645, 1983.
147. King, GL and Buchwald, S: Characterization and partial purification of an endothelial cell growth factor from human platelets. J Clin Invest 73:392–396, 1984.
148. Wall, RT, Harker, LA, and Striker, GE: Human endothelial cell migration: Stimulated by a released platelet factor. Lab Invest 39:523–529, 1978.
149. Bernstein, LR, Antoniades, H, and Zetter, BR: Migration of cultured vascular cells in response to plasma and platelet-derived factors. J Cell Sci 56:71–82, 1982.
150. Glazer, BM, et al: Adult tissues contain chemoattractants for vascular endothelial cells. Nature 288:483–484, 1980.
151. Bowersox, JC, and Sorgente, N: Chemotaxis of aortic endothelial cells in response to fibronectin. Cancer Res 42:2547–2551, 1982.
152. Schoefl, GI: The migration of lymphocytes across the vascular endothelium in lymphoid tissue: A reexamination. J Exp Med 136:568, 1972.
153. Leipziger, L, et al: Dermal wound repair: Role of collagen matrix implants and sympathetic polymer dressings. J Am Acad Dermatol 12:409–419, 1985.
154. Peacock, EE and Van Winkle, W: Contraction. Peacock, EE and Van Winkle, W (eds): Wound Repair, ed 2. WB Saunders, Philadelphia, 1976, p 54.
155. Majno, G, et al: Contraction of granulation tissue in vitro: Similarity to smooth muscle. Science 173:548, 1971.
156. Murray, JC, Pollack, SV, and Pinnell, SR: Keloids: A review. J Am Acad Dermatol 4:461–470, 1981.
157. Majno, G, et al: Contraction of granulation tissue in vitro: Similarity to smooth muscle. Science 173:548–550, 1971.
158. Ryan, RB, et al: Myofibroblasts in human granulation tissue. Hum Pathol 5:55–67, 1974.
159. Gabbiani, G, et al: Granulation tissue as a contractile organ: A study of structure and function. J Exp Med 135:719–734, 1972.
160. Singer, II: The fibronexus: A transmembrane association of fibronectin-containing fibers and bundles of 5 nm filaments in hamster and human fibroblasts. Cell 16:675–685, 1979.
161. Singer, II and Paradiso, PR: A transmembrane relationship between fibronectin and vinculin (130 kd protein): Serum modulation in normal and transformed hamster fibroblasts. Cell 24:481–492, 1981.
162. Singer, II, et al: In vivo co-distribution of fibronectin and actin fibers in granulation tissue: Immunofluorescence and electron microscope studies of the fibronexus at the myofibroblast surface. J Cell Biol 98:2091–2106, 1984.
163. Bell, E, Ivarsson, B, and Merrill, C: Production of a tissue-like structure by contraction of collagen lattices by human fibroblasts of different proliferative potential in vitro. Proc Natl Acad Sci USA 76:1274–1278, 1979.
164. Daly, TJ, Golitz, LE, and Weston, WL: A double-blind placebo-controlled efficacy study of tretinoin cream 0.05% in the treatment of keloids and hypertrophic scars. J Invest Dermatol 86:470, 1986.
165. Maitra, AK, et al: Use of sterile gloves in the management of sutured hand wounds in the A&E department. Injury 17(3):193–195, 1986.
166. Leyden, JJ: Effect of bacteria on healing of superficial wounds. Clin Dermatol 2(3):81–85, 1984.
167. Chvapil, M, et al: Local anesthetics and wound healing. J Surg Res 27:367, 1979.
168. Morris, T and Tracey: J: Lignocaine: Its effects on wound healing. Br J Surg 64:902, 1977.
169. Corball, M, et al: The interaction of vitamin A and corticosteroids on wound healing. Ir J Med Sci 154(8):306–310, 1985.
170. Brennan, SS, et al: The effect of antiseptics on the healing wound: A study using the rabbit ear chamber. Br J Surg 72(10):780–782, 1985.
171. Geronemus, RG, et al: Wound healing: The effects of topical antimicrobial agents. Arch Dermatol 115:1311, 1979.
172. Eaglstein, WH and Mertz, PM: "Inert" vehicles do affect wound healing. J Invest Dermatol 74:90, 1980.
173. Marks, JG, et al: Inhibition of wound healing by topical steroids. J Dermatol Surg Oncol 9:819, 1983.
174. de Roy van Zuidewijn, DB, et al: Healing of experimental colonic anastomoses: Effect of antineoplastic agents. Eur J Surg Oncol 13(1):27–33, 1987.
175. Capone, A, Jr, et al: In vivo effects of 5-FU on ocular surface epithelium following corneal wounding. Invest Ophthalmol Vis Sci 28(10):1661–1667, 1987.
176. Epstein, E: Effects of tissue-destructive technics on wound healing [letter]. J Am Acad Dermatol 14(6):1098–1099, 1986.
177. Armstrong, RB, et al: Punch biopsy wounds treated with Monsel's solution or a collagen matrix. Arch Dermatol 122(5):546–549, 1986.
178. Harris, DR and Youkey, JR: Evaluating the effects of hemostatic agents on the healing of superficial wounds. In Maibach, HI, and Robee, DT (eds): Epidermal Wound Healing. Year Book Medical Publishers, Chicago, 1972, p 343.
179. Irvin, TT: Wound Healing: Principles and Practice. Chapman and Hall, London, 1981, p 34.
180. Strickland, PT: Abnormal wound healing in UV-irradiated skin of Sencar mice. J Invest Dermatol 86(1):37–41, 1986.

181. Isaacs, JH, Jr, et al: Postoperative radiation of open head and neck wounds, Part I. Laryngoscope 97(3):267–270, 1987.
182. Pollack, SV: Systemic drugs and nutritional aspects of wound healing. Clin Dermatol 2(3):68–80, 1984.
183. Modolin, M, et al: Effects of protein depletion and repletion on experimental open wound contraction. Ann Plast Surg 15(2):123–126, 1985.
184. Almekinders, LC, et al: Healing of experimental muscle strains and the effects of nonsteroidal antiinflammatory medication. Am J Sports Med 14(4):303–308, 1986.
185. Smith, RW, et al: Effects of vinblastine, etoposide, cisplatin, and bleomycin on rodent wound healing. Surg Gynecol Obstet 161(4):323–326, 1985.
186. Lawrence, WT, et al: The reversal of an Adriamycin induced healing impairment with chemoattractants and growth factors. Ann Surg 203(2):142–147, 1986.
187. Hallmans, G, et al: The effect of topical zinc absorption from wounds on growth and the wound healing process in zinc-deficient rats. Scand J Plast Reconstr Surg 19(2):119–125, 1985.
188. Schwartzkopff, T, et al: Topical indomethacin: Inhibition of corneal wound healing in guinea pigs after severe alkali burn. Cornea 4(1):19–24, 1985–1986.
189. Lawrence, WT, et al: Doxorubicin-induced impairment of wound healing in rats. JNCI 76(1):119–126, 1986.
190. Adzick, NS, et al: Comparison of fetal, newborn, and adult wound healing by histologic, enzyme-histochemical, and hydroxyproline determinations. J Pediatr Surg 20(4):315–319, 1985.
191. Chvapil, M and Koopmann, CF: Age and other factors regulating wound healing. Otolaryngol Clin North Am 15:259, 1982.

CHAPTER 3

Connective Tissue in Wound Healing

Helen Price, M.S., P.T.

Connective tissue is the group of elements that provide strength, elasticity, substance, and density to the body. A variable composition of cells and extracellular matrix determines the specific characteristics of connective tissue at any given location of the body, but only the dense irregular connective tissue found in the dermis is discussed here. This chapter highlights connective tissue structure, biosynthesis of collagen and elastin, wound repair, and factors affecting wound healing.

Connective tissue cells and matrix constitute a significant proportion of the dermal skin layer. The connective tissue cells play a role in extracellular local body defense mechanisms and fiber production. The connective tissue matrix is composed of fibers, which determine the biomechanical properties of the dermis, and ground substance, which determines the compliance and integrity of the dermis. Table 3–1 reviews the principal connective tissue cells, with a description of the general characteristics and function for each element.[1,2]

CONNECTIVE TISSUE CELLS

Connective tissue cells are continually active in the turnover of tissue within the dermis. Wounding creates additional cellular demands for phagocytosis, contraction, generation, and remodeling of new extracellular matrix. Cellular responses during the inflammatory process, epithelialization, and contraction have been considered in Chapters 1 and 2.

A most important connective tissue cell for wound healing is the fibroblast, which produces extracellular elements. While the fibroblasts are primarily responsible for fiber production, the interaction of all of the connective tissue cells determines the rate of wound healing and the eventual result of the wound.[1,2]

TABLE 3–1. Principal Connective Tissue Cells

Cell	Characteristics	Function
Fibroblasts	Fusiform or spindle shape; flat with irregular outline	Produce extracellular material— particularly collagen, elastin, and proteoglycans
Myofibroblasts	Specialized fibroblasts with contractile actomyosin	Cause wound contraction
Macrophages	Stationary cells have irregular outline; motile cells have rounded outline	Phagocytose bacteria and damaged tissue
Lymphocytes	Small cells with rounded, heterochromatic, indented nuclei	Produce antibodies
Mast cells	Round or oval cells found in loose connective tissue	Release histamine
Fat cells, pigment cells, reticular cells	Spherical, oval, or polygonal cells	Have specialized function not related to the skin

CONNECTIVE TISSUE MATRIX

Connective tissue matrix can be subdivided into fibrous components and ground substance. Collagen, elastin, and reticulin are the fibrous elements. The nonfibrous elements of ground substance can be glycosaminoglycan (GAG), glycoprotein, or proteoglycan.[3] The function, structure, and biosynthesis of the connective tissue matrix is presented here.

Collagen

Collagen is the principal structural body protein providing strength and stiffness to dermal tissue, constituting approximately 70 percent of the dry weight of skin.[3] Collagen fibers, with diameters from 2 to 15 μm, form finely woven networks in the papillary layer of the dermis or thick bundles paralleling the skin surface. These bundles are relatively inextensible and nonelastic, and thus give dermis a high tensile strength.[3,4]

Five major types of collagen are currently identified and vary only in amino acid constructs. Type I collagen is found in adult dermis, fascia, and bone; type II collagen in adult cartilage; type III collagen in embryonic connective tissue, aorta, deep dermis, and wounds; and types IV and V collagen in basement membrane.[1-3,5]

Only types I and II collagen are found in dermis and are involved in wound healing. The relative proportions of types I and III collagen appear to vary with chronologic age, such that type III collagen is gradually replaced by type I collagen with aging. The diameters of collagen fibers appear to systematically vary throughout dermal depth. Type I collagen fibrils range from 100 to 500 nm and type III collagen fibrils from 40 to 60 nm in diameter,[6] and the proportion of larger size fibrils ultimately determines the skin tissue tensile strength.[7] Type III collagen is found at deepest levels.[8] Tajima and Nagai[9] suggest that skin predominantly bearing heavy loads consists of smaller diameter fibrils, which have good creep resistance when compared with those of skin that

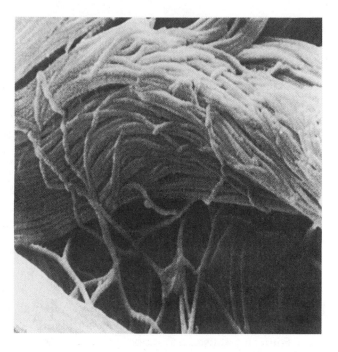

FIGURE 3–1. Normal skin collagen magnified about 10,000X. Note the definition of the collagen fibrils and the large fibers (From Hunt and Dunphy,[10] p. 24, with permission).

withstands shearing loads. Tissue creep, the ability to withstand a load over time, and tissue resilience, the ability to return to original shape, are dependent upon the number and distribution of small diameter fibers.[7] Thus, connective tissue is not as homogeneous as once proposed. In general, 80 percent of dermal collagen is type I and 15 percent is type III.[4]

Biochemically, collagen can be described in a generic fashion as being composed of three polypeptide alpha chains arranged in a triple helix, several of which are cross-linked together to form collagen fibrils.[5] While both type I and type III collagen have the same procollagen precursor, differentiation occurs such that type I collagen is formed by two identical alpha-1 chains and a third alpha-2 chain, and type III collagen consists of three identical alpha-1 chains.[6,10] The collagen fibrils then twine together to form collagen fibers. Dermal collagen fibers, while inherently inelastic and inextensible, form a loose interlacing and deformable network, able to align in directions that accommodate applied stress,[1,4] and therefore allow skin to stretch (Fig. 3–1).

Elastin

Elastin is a highly hydrophobic structural protein providing extensibility in the dermis and comprising only 2 percent of the protein in dermis.[11] Elastin, lipids, and glycoproteins bind to form microfibrils that serve as the scaffolding for future fiber orientation. Microfibrils are infiltrated and surrounded by elastin, which then fuses to form solid elastic fibers 1 to 3 μm in diameter. The characteristically wavy elastin fibers are entwined among those of collagen, and their orientation varies from a horizontal arrangement at the lower dermis to a vertical arrangement at the epidermal margin. Elastic is thus able to inherently and functionally be elastic, providing good recoil, and extensible, providing tissue length by unwinding the fiber wave.[11,12]

Reticulin

The least prevalent fiber found in connective tissue substrate is reticulin. Reticulin fibers are finer collagen-like fibrils and are 0.2 to 1 μm in diameter. These fibers form a supporting framework for many organs and glands. Reticulin may also form an early framework upon which collagen fibers are laid down. They have been found in very small numbers in normal skin and in significant numbers in early phases of the healing wound.[2,3]

Ground Substance

Ground substance, an amorphous viscous gel occupying the spaces between the connective tissue fibers, functionally provides density to tissue and reduces friction between connective tissue fibers during tissue stress or strain. The substrates of ground substance are glycoproteins and mucopolysaccharides, particularly glycosaminoglycans (GAG). Most likely, saccharide chains in the chondroitin sulphate–protein complex cross-link to collagen fibers, and the cross-linkage allows for departmental or small tissue area shifts in pressure, much like an hydraulic dampening, therefore contributing to integrity and force transduction in skin.[4,8]

Flint and colleagues[7] report proportional differences in GAG content in human skin. GAG content progressively decreases from fetal development to maturity in non–weight-bearing skin areas, whereas weight-bearing skin areas, such as the sole of the foot, show minimal change. GAG content, particularly chondroitin sulfate levels, is proportionally increased in Dupuytren's contracture nodules and in hypertropic scarring, both being pathologic states of altered skin composition.

Blood Supply

Connective tissue has a limited blood supply, although the vessels course through this tissue to supply other structures. Lymph vessels are more numerous and vary in distribution throughout the body. They serve as the initial drainage sites for lymph into major vessels and nodes.[1]

BIOSYNTHESIS OF CONNECTIVE TISSUE

In normal skin, connective tissue turnover is a continual process. All components of connective tissue are phagocytized and replaced with new cells perpetually. The fibroblast is responsible for production of replacement collagen throughout life. With wounding, the process of biosynthesis is potentiated. In the inflammatory phase, macrophages digest denatured collagen, thus removing noncollagenous proteins, and excrete useful amino acids and simple sugars for future synthesis.[13] During the fibroblastic phase, about day 10 after wounding, fibroblasts, which have increased in population, begin synthesizing at a higher rate (Fig. 3–2).

Within the fibroblast nucleus, transcription from DNA to messenger RNA occurs. The specific alpha chain configuration having been identified, transfer RNA adds specific amino acids to the polypeptide chain during transportation from the nucleus to the Golgi apparatus. Magnesium and zinc are trace minerals needed for translation. Two

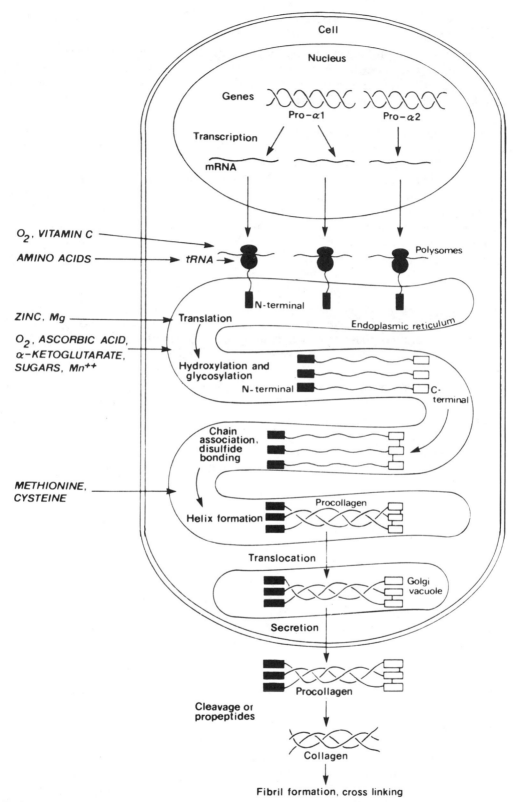

FIGURE 3–2. Diagrammatic representation of steps in collagen synthesis from translation to secretion. Important nutrients at certain steps are noted on the left (From Hunt and Dunphy,[10] p. 36, with permission).

of the amino acids, proline and lysine, when added to the polypeptide chain, require hydroxylation. This process requires use of available oxygen, ferrous iron, and ascorbic acid (vitamin C). Hydroxylation occurs on the ribosome. Without ascorbate, underhydroxylated collagen is produced that fails to aggregate into collagen fibers. Without oxygen, hydroxylation does not occur and collagen production ceases.[14,15]

Following hydroxylation, the polypeptide chains aggregate into a triple helix and are joined by galactose. This molecule, now called procollagen, is released from the fibroblast. Once procollagen is extracellular, three events must occur. First, the terminal propeptides, which have prevented early fibrilogenesis, are removed by peptidases. The resulting molecule is termed *tropocollagen*. Second, the tropocollagen molecules line up in a quarter staggered array reflected as a helix and are initially united by hydrogen bonding. Finally, stable covalent cross-links both intramolecularly and intermolecularly are formed, creating collagen fibrils. The intermolecular cross-links are believed to be responsible for tensile strength.[16] Fibrils combine to form collagen fibers where they align according to lines of stress.[14,17]

The first collagen to be produced in normal wound repair is highly disorganized and more gel-like in construction, yielding poor wound strength. This collagen is structurally akin to type III collagen. With wound closure, a gradual turnover occurs during the maturation phase of wound healing, lasting 6 months to a year, with type III collagen being broken down and turgorous type I collagen being synthesized.[5] The stimulus for conversion of type III collagen to type I collagen may be the biomechanical stress and strain placed across a closed wound. These forces also seem to direct realignment of all connective tissue fibers. The collagen fibers under tension appear to be resistant to action of collagenase while the random fibers not under tension are susceptible to lysis. During collagen turnover, new tropocollagen molecules deposit along lines of the remaining tension-oriented fibers[16] (Figs. 3–3 and 3–4). The resultant healed tissue approximates only 80 percent of normal skin's tensile strength.

FACTORS AFFECTING CONNECTIVE TISSUE REPAIR

Connective tissue repair is affected by available blood supply; available proteins, minerals, amino acids, and enzymes; circulating hormones; and infection.[18] Lack of needed oxygen or connective tissue fiber substrate impedes wound healing time and the strength of the resultant tissue. The hypoxia that usually occurs without neovascularization reduces energy production. Amino-acid bonding in the collagen chain will be retarded without available adenosine triphosphate (ATP).

Vitamins and Minerals

Whether collagen biosynthesis is retarded or potentiated depends upon available minerals, proteins, and vitamins. Lack of available ascorbic acid (vitamin C) can impede the hydroxylation needed during collagen synthesis. Additionally, reopening of very old wounds has been documented in the scorbutic patient.[15] Zinc depletion reduces the rate of epithelialization and retards cellular proliferation.[19] Vitamin A potentiates epithelial repair and collagen synthesis by enhancing inflammatory reactions, particularly macrophage availability.[20] The role of vitamin E remains questionable, with research findings alluding to both positive and negative effects on wound healing.

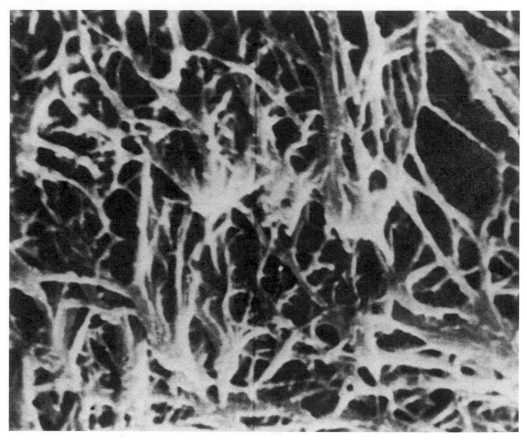

FIGURE 3–3. Wound collagen at 10 days by scanning electron microscopy. Note the lack of definition of collagen fibrils and the smaller fibers (From Hunt and Dunphy,[10] p. 37, with permission).

Steroids

The influence of estrogens and androgens remains unclear. These hormones are known to have a minimal anabolic effect and might be expected to assist the healing process.[21] The neovascularization occurring in early stages of healing appears to be positively affected by progesterone, although this event has not been proven to be a significant change. Neovascularization appears to be adversely affected by estrogen. A combination of estrogen and progesterone, such as that found in antifertility agents, has been shown to delay the healing process.[10]

Brincat and coworkers[22] have shown that while estrogen replacement in postmenopausal women can reverse the typically reduced collagen levels, estrogen administered during wound healing has little conclusive effect.

There is a direct relationship between available macrophages and fibroblast production. In fact, if the initial inflammatory process is blocked by the use of anti-inflammatory steroids during the first 3 days after wounding, healing time and the resultant skin turgor are both retarded.[13] Research has shown that wound healing suppressed by anti-inflammatory steroids can be ameliorated with administration of vitamin A, locally or systematically.[20] Last, the mitotic activity of fibroblasts itself is also suppressed by steroids.

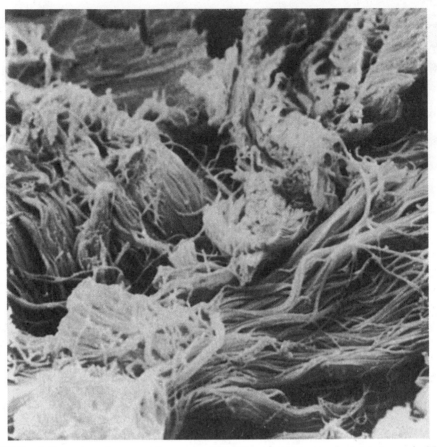

FIGURE 3–4. Scanning electron microscopy of collagen near a rat colon anastomosis. Note the relatively disorderly new collagen fibrils interlacing with the more densely packed and orderly older fibers (From Hunt and Dunphy,[10] p. 38, with permission).

Pathogens

Infections obviously retard healing due to degradation of new tissue and interference with collagen synthesis. This occurrence lengthens normal healing time or may actually cause the wound to extend beyond original boundaries.[10]

Diabetes Mellitus

Many diabetic patients have some particular vulnerability for healing problems. Experimentally induced diabetes has caused changes in the mechanical properties of skin—namely, a resulting increase in tissue stiffness and strength. Insulin replacement restored normal collagen–ground substance proportions and a subsequent normalization of skin mechanical properties.[23]

Increased tissue stiffness is thought to be a function of increased hydration concurrent with diabetes. Biochemically, an osmotic swelling around collagenous fibers could occur and thus prevent normal extensibility. This polyol-hydration of the collagen in the endoneurium cuff surrounding nerve fibers can be the mechanism leading to diabetic neuropathies.[24] Clinical investigations inhibiting excess hydration, most frequently with the administration of Sorbinil, have been inconclusive.

The small vessel disease accompanying diabetes, manifested by endothelial proliferation in small arterioles and by basement membrane capillary thickening, compromises oxygen availability needed for hydroxylation. This prevents normal collagen synthesis.[25]

When suppressed, insulin levels, essential for fibroblastic activity, limit collagen deposition. This diminished collagen synthesis leads to poor tissue tensile strength and consequently a less than desirable healed wound. Experimentally, insulin replacement appears most vital in the fibroblastic phase of healing.[25]

The precise cause of impaired wound healing remains unclear. Researchers concur that optimal diabetic control is the most important factor in determining collagen integrity and wound results.[26]

Concomitant neuropathies and hypoesthesias, typically experienced by diabetic patients, allow for healing sites to be retraumatized. Further, diabetic patients are especially vulnerable to wound infection. All of these factors compound the healing process for the diabetic patient who is frequently the individual presenting with ulcers and decubiti.

ULCERS

Chronic ulcers have not been extensively studied regarding typical and compounding healing characteristics. Wound healing has long been thought to be somehow impaired in denervated tissue.[27] Localdo, Lowman, and Gibson[28] report that while contraction and epithelialization are not affected by denervation, altered vascular growth and deranged phagocytosis may be compromised, thus diminishing collagen synthesis.

While the edges of a typical venous ulcer show normal activity through secondary intention healing, deep and central portions frequently show delayed or resistant healing. Adair[29] suggests that poor cellular adhesion and connective tissue abnormalities may contribute to retarded epithelialization.

COLLAGEN IMBALANCES

Throughout the healing process, there is constant collagen lysis and synthesis. In the early weeks of healing, synthesis occurs more rapidly than lysis at a rate of up to 41 times that in normal skin. This repair is followed by a reverse activity level, such that lysis occurs more rapidly than synthesis. An imbalance can occur where collagen lysis cannot accommodate collagen synthesis, resulting in overdeposition of collagen. This cosmetically noticeable scar is called *hypertrophic scarring* or *keloid*. Hypertrophic scarring is defined as the scar resulting when collagen deposition remains within the area of the original wound, whereas keloid is excessive collagen deposition extending beyond the initial wound edge into originally healthy tissue. This biosynthetic imbalance has no known predictive etiology but can be modified through chemical and mechanical mediation.[10,30]

During the maturation stage of scar formation, when immature scar is converted to mature scar, intracollagen molecular linkage changes from weak hydrogen bonding to strong covalent bonding (Fig. 3–5).[31] Hydrogen bonding occurs through the attraction

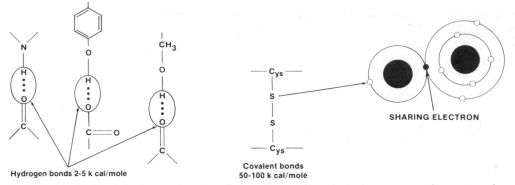

FIGURE 3–5. Weak hydrogen bonding links collagen fibers in immature scar. Strong covalent bonds link collagen fibers in mature scar (Adapted from Cummings, Crutchfield, and Barnes,[32] p. 30).

of positively and negatively charged atoms creating a relatively weak electrostatic bond. This bond is believed to allow collagen in immature scar to be stretched out with gentle, steady stress applied to the scar. In covalent bonding, atoms share electrons, creating a much stronger bond between the molecular structure of collagen and between the collagen fibrils and the ground substance.[32] Thus, mature scar is more dense and tough and less resilient than immature scar, not only because mature scar has more collagen fibers than immature scar but also because the molecular bonding does not yield readily to applied stress. Practically speaking, collagen fibers can be made to reorganize while scar is maturing such that the fibers are absorbed, replaced, and altered in their alignment. When stress is applied to collagen fibers, they produce small voltages or potentials.[33] Substances that produce voltages in response to mechanical stress are called *piezoelectric substances*. These small stress-generated voltages, called *streaming potentials*, may be responsible for the production, maintenance, alignment, and absorption of collagen fibers. In the past 10 years, the piezoelectric mechanism associated with collagen response to stress has been put to use in the treatment of immature burn scar that has the potential to develop into hypertrophic scar. The treatment simply involves applying constant pressure or stretching to the new scar while it is maturing (Fig. 3–6).

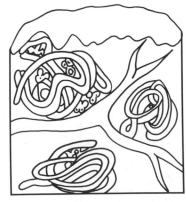

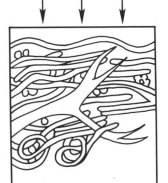

COLLAGEN WHORLS IN UNCONTROLLED HYPERTROPHIC SCAR

COLLAGEN FIBERS RUNNING IN ORDERLY FORMATION DURING PRESSURE APPLICATION

FIGURE 3–6. Reorganization of hypertrophic scar by application of constant pressure to the scar (Adapted from Burn-Scar Management A-V materials. Jobst Institute, Toledo, OH, 1979).

In this regard, pressure gradient garments may be worn by burn patients who are vulnerable to developing hypertrophic scarring to minimize scar volume and thus allow for improved function.

SUMMARY

Dermal skin is primarily composed of connective tissue, particularly collagen. Following injury, a complex yet systematic healing process is activated, with collagen being the major fiber deposited. This wound healing is initially dependent upon oxygen, nutrients, and minerals, and the importance of these elements has been realized for many years. Any condition or pathology affecting the availability of these elements can prevent or retard healing.

Recently, the influence of external environmental factors has been considered. The resultant healed skin is significantly affected by biomechanical stresses placed across the tissue during healing. Force, stress, strain, and motion each direct collagen fiber and proteoglycan alignment. Forrester and associates[34] concluded that Wolff's law is as applicable to connective tissue deposition as it is to osseous alignment. This belief suggests that allowing early gentle movement of tissue during healing would reduce the fragility so typically seen during immobilized healing.

Various therapeutic interventions can potentiate the healing process, and a thorough understanding of wound healing should direct the clinician to the appropriate needs.

REFERENCES

1. Williams, PL and Warwick, R (eds): Gray's Anatomy, ed 36. WB Saunders, Philadelphia, 1980.
2. Lever, W and Schaumberg-Lever, G: Histopathology of Skin, ed 6. JB Lippincott, Philadelphia, 1983.
3. Stewart, WD, Danto, JL, and Maddin, S: Dermatology. CV Mosby, St Louis, 1974.
4. Booth, BA, Polak, KL, and Uitto, J: Collagen biosynthesis by human skin fibroblasts. Biochim Biophys Acta 607:145–160, 1980.
5. Burgeson, RE: The collagens of the skin. Curr Probl Dermatol 17:61–75, 1987
6. Fleischmajer, R: Collagen fibrillogenesis: A mechanism of structural biology. J Invest Dermatol 5:553–554, 1986.
7. Flint, MH, et al: Collagen fibril diameters and glycosaminoglycan content of skins: Indices of tissue maturity and function. Connect Tissue Res 13:69–81, 1984.
8. Parry, DAD and Craig, AS: Growth and development of collagen fibrils in connective tissue. In Ruggeri, A and Motta, PM (eds): Ultrastructure of the Connective Tissue Matrix. Martinus Nijhoff Publishers, Boston, 1984.
9. Tajima, S and Nagai, Y: Distribution of macromolecular components in calf dermal connective tissue. Connect Tissue Res 7:65–71, 1980.
10. Hunt, TK and Dunphy, JE (eds): The Fundamentals of Wound Management. Appleton-Century-Crofts, New York, 1979.
11. Braveman, IM and Fonferko, E: Studies in cutaneous aging: I. The elastic fiber network. J Invest Dermatol 78:434–443, 1982.
12. Mier PD and Cotton, DWK: Biology of the Skin. Blackwell Scientific, London, 1976.
13. Lambert, WC, et al: Cellular and molecular mechanisms in wound healing: Selected concepts. Clin Dermatol 2(3):17–23, 1984.
14. Carrico, TJ, Mehrhof, AI, and Cohen, IK: Biology of wound healing. Surg Clin North Am 64(4):721–733, 1984.
15. Kanzler, MH, Gorsulowsky, DC, and Swanson, NA: Basic mechanisms in the healing cutaneous wound. J Dermatol Surg Oncol 12(11):1156–1164, 1986.
16. Cuono, CB: Physiology of wound healing. In Dagher, FJ (ed): Cutaneous Wounds. Futura Publishing, New York, 1985.
17. Fraser, RDB, and MacRae, TP: Molecular packing in type I collagen fibrils. J Mol Biol 193:115–125, 1987.
18. Pollack, SV: Wound healing: A review. J Dermatol Surg Oncol 5(5):389–393, 1979.
19. Bobel, LM: Nutritional implications in the patient with pressure sores. Nurs Clin North Am 22(2):379–390, 1987.

20. Hunt, TK: Vitamin A and wound healing. J Am Acad Dermatol 15(4):817–821, 1986.
21. Peacock, EE: Wound Repair, ed 3. WB Saunders, Philadelphia, 1984.
22. Brincat, M, et al: Skin collagen changes in postmenopausal women receiving different regimens of estrogen therapy. Obstet Gynecol 70(1):123–127, 1987.
23. Andreassen, TT, Seyer-Hansen, K, and Oxlund, H: Biomechanical changes in connective tissues induced by experimental diabetes. Acta Endocrinol 98:432–436, 1981.
24. Eaton, RP: The collagen hydration hypothesis: A new paradigm for the secondary complications of diabetes mellitus. J Chron Dis 39(10):763–766, 1986.
25. Goodson, WH and Hunt, TK: Studies of wound healing in experimental diabetes mellitus. J Surg Res 22:221–227, 1977.
26. Yue, DK, et al: Effects of experimental diabetes, uremia, and malnutrition on wound healing. Diabetes 36:295–299, 1987.
27. Constantian, MB (ed): Pressure Ulcers: Principles and Techniques of Management. Little, Brown, Boston, 1980.
28. Localdo, SA, Lowman, E, and Gibson, J: Wound healing in the paraplegic patient. Surgery 44:625, 1958.
29. Adair, HM: Repair in acute and chronic ulcers. Ann R Coll Surg Engl 60:393–398, 1978.
30. Cohen, JK, Diegelman, RF, and Keiser, HR: Collagen metabolism in keloid and hypertrophic scar. In Longacre, JJ (ed): The Ultrastructure of Collagen: Its Relation to the Healing of Wounds and the Management of Hypertrophic Scar. Charles C Thomas, Springfield, IL, 1976.
31. Peacock, EE and Van Winkel, W: Wound Repair, ed 2. WB Saunders, Philadelphia, 1976.
32. Cummings, GS, Crutchfield, CA, and Barnes, MR: Orthopaedic Physical Therapy. Vol I: Soft Tissue Changes in Contractures. Stokesville Publishing, Atlanta, GA, 1983.
33. Longacre, JJ: Scar tissue: its use and abuse in light of recent biophysical and biochemical studies. In Longacre, JJ (ed): The Ultrastructure of Collagen. Charles C Thomas, Springfield, IL, 1976.
34. Forrester, JC, et al: Wolff's law in relation to the healing skin wound. J Trauma 10:770–771, 1970.

CHAPTER 4

Factors Complicating Wound Repair

Gary D. Mulder, M.S., D.P.M.

DELAYED AND CHRONIC CLOSURE

This chapter provides the reader with information to help determine why wound repair might be impaired. The more recognized factors complicating repair, particularly infection, malnutrition, and factors indigenous to the wound and/or associated with various pathologies, are adequately covered in other chapters of this text. In this chapter, emphasis is on factors that are often overlooked or underemphasized. The examiner should be aware of the problems and concerns listed in this chapter when analyzing the patient, and of the specific pathology in the clinical setting. Once the general medical status has been established by a thorough and complete history and physical, the examiner can then determine whether interfering or disrupting factors have been neglected. One must remember that the following information is most applicable to chronic wounds or to those undergoing delayed closure.

The definitions of delayed and chronic wounds are often misinterpreted by the clinician or examiner involved in wound care. *Delayed closure* of a dermal ulcer simply implies that a wound is taking longer than expected to heal. The rate of closure is determined by multiple interrelated factors including wound size (area, volume), location, etiology, and quality. Patient medical status, medications, nutrition, and applied modalities will also affect rate of closure. These factors must be examined when attempting to determine why a wound is closing at a slower rate than expected. The examiner must decide whether the delay is caused by (1) an intrinsic factor related to patient's general physical/mental condition, (2) environmental factors (external modality or treatment) including medically administered drugs and therapies, or (3) iatrogenic factors, such as the way the wound is being physically managed.

Delayed closure involving conservative treatment should not be confused with delayed surgical closure in which a wound is allowed to heal by secondary intention. In such circumstances, especially when infection and drainage are involved, a surgical wound is not sutured and is allowed to granulate and re-epithelialize on its own.

The term *chronic wound* is best defined as a wound that has not responded to

43

conservative or surgical treatment. This occurrence does not necessarily mean the wound will not heal. Conservatively treated wounds that become chronic are often responsive to surgical care, although surgical wounds may themselves become chronic. When treatment of any nature fails, one must again review all previous care to ascertain that no factor complicating closure has been overlooked.

In summary, one must determine if a wound is chronic or is closing in a delayed manner. Both types of lesions are affected by factors considered disruptive to wound repair. Once the cause is discovered and eradicated, the wound is more likely to close.

Aging and Wound Repair

Like other tissues and organs, skin undergoes numerous changes with advancing age (Table 4–1). Increased susceptibility to injury and delay in repair once damage has been incurred contribute to impaired wound healing.

Although increased vulnerability to injury is of importance to wound prevention, wound closure once injury has been sustained is of equal concern. Factors affecting repair in the aged are shown in Table 4–2.

Cellular activity, specifically that of the fibroblast, is critical for collagen production. Collagen is a major structural protein responsible for most of the integument's strength. Greater organization and cross-linking of collagen has been found in young men than in older men.[1] Decreased wound tensile strength could be expected to result in greater vulnerability to trauma. Therefore, delayed closure can be expected when a healing wound is subjected to distortion from mishandling during care. Healed tissue is also more fragile. One must be cautious in handling the wound and periwound tissue. Tapes and adhesive dressings may damage the skin surrounding the original lesion, thereby producing new ulcerations.

A study by Sandblum and coworkers[2] on wound breaking strength in relation to aging suggested that less force was required to disrupt the wound in individuals older than age 70 compared with those younger than age 70. This study correlates well with the data of Mendoza and associates,[3] who reported the rate of wound dehiscence to be two to three times higher in patients older than 60 years of age.

Changes in cellular activity are further reflected in biochemical and structural changes in dermal collagen and elastin. Alterations in production of the latter two products results in less soluble and more sclerotic connective tissue.[4]

The vascular supply to ulcers and other wounds delivers cells important to wound repair. Regression and disorganization of cutaneous small vessels have been associated with aging.[5] Decreased or disrupted vascular supply will have an adverse effect on wounds and result in chronic delayed closure.

Diminished blood flow causes decreased clearance of metabolites, bacterial, and

---

TABLE 4–1. Changes that Occur in the Skin with Advanced Aging

- Diminished perception of pain
- Increased vulnerability to injury
- Decreased epidermal proliferation
- Attenuated inflammatory response
- Decrease in dermal clearance
- Decreased barrier properties
- Decreased vascularity

TABLE 4–2. Recognized Effects that Aging Has
on Wound Healing

- Delayed wound contraction
- Decreased wound breaking strength
- Decreased epithelialization
- Attenuated metabolic response
- Diminished biosynthetic activity of components
- Delayed cellular migration and proliferation
- Decreased rate of wound capillary growth
- Delayed collagen remodeling
- Increased rate of wound dehiscence

foreign materials, all of which impede closure. This insult is potentiated by a decreased inflammatory response.[4] A noxious substance introduced to an open wound is less likely to be rapidly cleared. Thus, the elderly appear to be more vulnerable to environmental insults. Once damage is done, the elderly may develop chronic wounds because of decreased cellular turnover and ability to heal.

Animal model studies support more rapid and effective healing in adolescents than in the elderly.[6–8] However, despite age-associated differences in wound healing, surgical experience shows that the elderly and the young may heal equally well.

Surgeries are frequently performed on the elderly without adverse repair or closure. A low rate of wound complications defies what one would expect from research and experimental data.

What, if any, precautions, then, should the clinician or care giver consider when treating chronic wounds in the elderly? Tissue friability is perhaps the most important. As mentioned earlier, damaging intact skin in an overzealous effort to close a wound should be avoided. Forceful scrubs, manual debridement, and frequent dressing changes on clean wounds may inflict more damage than was originally present. Adhesive tapes and materials may remove healthy tissue and cause contact dermatitis. Caustic agents may further irritate skin and cause inflammation. If possible, povidone iodine, acetic acid, Daken's solution, sodium hydrochloride, and hydrogen peroxide at high concentrations should be avoided, and sterile water or saline solution should be used. Wet-to-dry dressings should be limited to necrotic wounds needing debridement. In summary, the following questions must be addressed when treating wounds on geriatric patients:

1. When treating a wound in a geriatric patient, what other skin considerations must one address? (Status of periwound tissue; friable tissue may easily be disrupted and damaged by aggressive adhesives and tapes.)
2. Would frequent scrubs (cleansing) be indicated on a 70-year-old bedridden patient with decreased vascularity? (No; frequent scrubs may further damage friable tissue. Poor circulation to the damaged area may increase ulcer size.)
3. An 80-year-old patient presents with a 30 × 30 cm ischemic ulcer without necrotic tissue. The wound base is clean with a healthy-appearing red base. What is the best cleansing solution for such a lesion? (Sterile water or saline solution.)
4. A 75-year-old patient presents with multiple right-hip pressure ulcers. All lesions are covered with loose necrotic and fibrotic tissue. Although there are no indications of infection, a small amount of yellow serous fluid is seen draining from the wound. Sinus tracts are absent. What is the appropriate dressing to use on such lesions, if manual debridement is not indicated? (b.i.d. or t.i.d. wet-to-dry dressings with a 1 : 1000 dilution of povidone iodine.)

TABLE 4–3. Drugs Affecting Wound Repair

- Nonsteroidal anti-inflammatory drugs (NSAIDs)
- Steroids
- Immunosuppressive agents
- Antineoplastic drugs
- Anticoagulants
- Antiprostaglandins

5. Why should wounds with dry necrotic bases be debrided with caution in geriatric patients with poor vascular perfusion? (There is a high risk of increasing ulcer size.)

MEDICATIONS

Patients with chronic and open wounds frequently have a host of unrelated medical problems for which they may be taking medications (Table 4–3). Often clinicians apply various treatments to the wound without considering the medications taken by the patient. What medications are being prescribed? Do they have any negative effects that may complicate wound closure?

Nonsteroidal Anti-Inflammatory Drugs

Nonsteroidal anti-inflammatory drugs (NSAIDs) are prescribed for a variety of problems ranging from arthritis to chronic pain. Each drug may differ in its effect on the repair process.

Colchicine, an NSAID often used in the treatment of gout, has been reported to reduce the tensile strength of connective tissue.[9] Effects of short-term, low-dose therapy have not been clinically established.[10] There is suspicion that colchicine may have numerous effects including reduced blood supply to the wound resulting from vasoconstriction and a modification of the early inflammatory phase of wound healing. Topically applied NSAIDs (indomethacin,[12] ibuprofen, and meclofenamate sodium) were found not to influence re-epithelialization or dermal collagen biosynthetic capacity when studied on superficial wounds of domestic pigs.[11] However, topical indomethacin has been shown to delay corneal re-epithelialization.[12]

The NSAIDs most often seen clinically are taken orally, not applied topically. The major goal in prescribing them is to reduce the inflammatory response, thereby reducing pain. Inflammation, important in the initial stages of wound repair and in acute wounds, may not be important in chronic wounds. Therefore, NSAIDs may be less significant when administering care to chronic wounds.

Steroids

Before attempting any treatment regimen, a clinician should always determine if the patient is receiving any form of steroid treatment. Documented effects of corticosteroids administered before or soon after injury include inhibition of collagen synthesis and retardation of wound healing.[13,14] Wound tensile strength and healing of open wounds are also affected by steroid treatment.[15] Steroids may impair wound repair by inhibiting important factors in the repair process including fibroblast function[16-18] and resultant collagen synthesis. The deleterious influence of steroids on related cellular components would affect antibacterial and phagocytic components of wound repair and closure. The overall effect is one of delayed chronic or altered wound repair, which often frustrates and confuses the clinician who has failed to note the high dose of corticosteroids taken by a patient. One should not judge the effectiveness of a newly marketed wound-care product based on its results when given to a patient undergoing steroid treatment.

Topical steroids are frequently used to treat damaged skin. A prime example is the practice of applying steroids to skin of patients with venous stasis dermatitis. When applying the corticosteroid, caution should be taken to avoid applying the topical agent to the ulcer surface. Topical anti-inflammatory corticosteroids have varying effects on epidermal resurfacing and dermal collagen synthesis.[19] One effect may be to retard wound closure and thus alter the wound quality.

Immunosuppressive Drugs

In one study, cyclosporin, an immunosuppressive drug often used in transplant patients, did not affect hydroxyproline content (collagen-level indicator) and macrophages as much as did methylprednisolone.[20] Another research group, however, has presented data suggesting that cyclosporin does impair wound healing.[24] Azathioprine and prednisone therapy have both been associated with a significant reduction in breaking strength of cutaneous wounds and are believed to create unwanted problems in the healing process.[22]

The most important factor to be derived from these studies is that a patient receiving immunosuppressive drugs may not respond to conventional wound therapy. Extra care must be taken not to compromise the wound environment by causing externally inflicted trauma or by application of caustic agents during treatment.

Other drugs having an implied effect on wound repair include anticoagulants, antineoplastics, and antiprostaglandins.[23,24] A thorough investigation of the patient's medication intake is always justified before choosing a wound treatment modality to determine whether wound repair will be affected by one or more of the patient's drugs.

WOUND CLOSURE ATTRIBUTED TO CYTOTOXICITY

A 36-year-old paraplegic man with a 5.0 × 3.0 cm partial thickness sacral pressure ulcer is being treated with an immunosuppressive drug for acquired immune deficiency syndrome (AIDS). The wound has not responded to conventional therapy including whirlpool, wet-to-dry dressings with a 50/50 combination of povidone iodine and water, wet-to-moist dressings with saline, polyurethane dressings, and pressure relief pads. (The failure of this wound to respond may be attributed primarily to environmental causes, although iatrogenic factors cannot be excluded.) The cytotoxic effect of povidone iodine will further delay closure (iatrogenic effect).

Occlusive hydrocolloid dressings would be appropriate for treatment of this patient's wound. Dressings of this type can be left on for extended periods of time and will further promote healing by decreasing the number of times a wound is disturbed.

ACQUIRED IMMUNE DEFICIENCY SYNDROME

The increasing number of acquired immune deficiency syndrome (AIDS) patients in both outpatient and inpatient settings has resulted in a greater number of patients with this primary diagnosis who are treated by wound-care personnel. Patients with AIDS are not necessarily more predisposed to developing ulcers than other patient populations. However, once a dermal lesion has developed, patients with AIDS are more likely to develop wounds that deteriorate rapidly and become chronic. The poor response of the wound to treatment can be attributed to the immunocompromised state of the individual. Recall that immunosuppression affects fibroblast function, collagen synthesis, and phagocytic action in the wound. A depressed ability to fight off bacterial infection results in an optimal environment for bacterial proliferation and sepsis. Special care must be taken to keep these wounds sterile while avoiding further tissue trauma. Host organisms are normally only contaminants in the nonimmunosuppressed patient and may not have any noticeable effect on wound closure. On the other hand, AIDS patients are very vulnerable to hospital-transmitted organisms that may cause rapid wound colonization and subsequent systemic spread.

The precise mechanism in which AIDS affects wound repair is unknown. Human immunodeficiency virus (HIV) proliferates in the lymphocytes. T-cell depletion is believed to impair wound breaking strength and wound collagen deposition.[25] T cells also have important roles in cellular immunity.[26] A T-cell defect creates a very profound effect on the wound repair process by suppressing the body's ability to fight off infection.

Abnormalities in AIDS patients include evidence of atypical dermal vessels that not only may be potential sites of Kaposi's sarcoma[27] but also possibly may contribute to ulcer development and impaired healing. A depressed defense mechanism coupled with impaired healing will affect almost all aspects of the repair process,[28] including fibroblast collagen production, macrophage activity, and ultimate wound closure. Until more is known about the AIDS virus, the best treatment for the patient's wound is to optimize the wound environment for healing with the most appropriate dressing and to decrease the pain associated with the lesion.[29] This approach might involve selection of an occlusive dressing that would prevent further outside contamination and not disrupt the wound.[30] An occlusive dressing that could be left on for many days might prove most effective. When considering an occlusive dressing, the clinician must keep in mind the following considerations:

1. An occlusive dressing would prevent external contamination while not necessarily promoting an increase in bacterial burden. An initial culture of the wound might indicate a varied and high bacterial burden (no evidence currently exists that proves that occlusion of a "noninfected" wound promotes infection). Caution must be taken with AIDS patients to avoid introducing new bacteria into a wound during dressing changes.
2. The differences in oxygen permeability of a hydrocolloid (impermeable) versus polyurethane (oxygen permeable) membrane should not be important. Either type dressing will function well. Dressing selection should depend on ease of use, cost, and effectiveness.
3. Personal experience should outweigh manufacturer choice, although manufacturer's indications and contraindications should be carefully noted.

Clinicians and health-care professionals treating AIDS patients should remain updated on current AIDS literature addressing the disease, its treatment, and patient

TABLE 4–4. Recommendations/Precautions for Care of Wounds in HIV-Positive Patients

- Always use gloves
- Avoid wound contact
- Avoid forceful flushing
- Use sterile dressings and instruments
- Minimize sharp debridement
- Choose dressing that contains fluids
- Dispose of all contaminated materials according to AIDS guidelines
- Avoid wound disruption
- Minimize dressing changes on noninfected wounds

care. Some recommendations and precautions for care of the AIDS wound are listed in Table 4–4.

TREATMENT INTERVENTIONS

Antimicrobial Toxicity

One of the greatest detriments to wound healing is the assumption that common treatment interventions are beneficial to the patient. Among these treatments, povidone iodine, hydrogen peroxide, and acetic acid are widely used in hospitals, care centers, and homes across the country. Their negative impact is demonstrated by the following case presentation:

A paraplegic man had a chief complaint of a left-buttock pressure ulcer that would not heal. The patient had been free of other medical problems and had no other medical complications.
Examination revealed an otherwise healthy 34-year-old wheelchair-bound patient with a 2.5 × 1.5 cm clean, red ulcer extending down to, but not through, the dermis. The lesion was free of drainage, purulence, necrosis, and clinical signs of infection. A complete review of previous treatment history revealed that the patient had been treating the wound for the past 8 months with half-strength povidone iodine solution applied twice daily via soaked gauze. His new treatment program included discontinuing the povidone iodine solution and covering the wound with a polyurethane occlusive dressing. This dressing was changed every 5 days, and the wound was cleansed with sterile saline between dressings. At the initial evaluation, the wound was chronic in nature. Closure was apparently delayed by the cytotoxic effects of povidone iodine on healthy tissue. Povidone iodine applications are inappropriate on this wound, which was not clinically infected and had a clean, healthy, red-tissue base. Once the extrinsic (environmental) factor was removed, the wound healed completely in 15 days.

Considering that almost all chronic ulcers (venous insufficiency, diabetic, and pressure-induced) are contaminated but not necessarily infected, one must weigh the advantages against the disadvantages of using antimicrobial agents. Clinicians should ask themselves (1) if use of an antimicrobial agent is warranted (is the wound truly infected?), (2) what will using the antimicrobial agent accomplish?, and (3) if used, is there an appropriate agent concentration? The antimicrobial concentration may significantly influence the agent's effect on wound healing.

Antibiotics and topical antiseptics have bactericidal and cytotoxic effects.[31,32] Betadine is *not* cytotoxic when reduced to a 0.001 dilution.[31]

In view of the questionable value of antimicrobials on contaminated wounds, use of sterile saline solution in sterile water is more prudent. Until evidence is available to support the safe, effective, and beneficial use of commercially available topical antimicrobial agents on wounds, their use should be limited to infected—not contaminated—wounds.

Radiation

Patients being treated in a wound clinic and simultaneously undergoing radiation therapy may present a challenge to standard treatment. A complete history should include determination of whether radiation therapy is in the patient's treatment regimen.

The effect of radiation is dependent on a number of factors including dose, frequency, and location of the irradiated area in relation to the wound site. A wound distal to a site treated with low-dose irradiation may not be as severely affected as one proximal to a high-dose irradiated site.

Radiotherapy has numerous negative influences on wound repair. Impairment to healing results from a combination of multiple effects, including injury to fibroblasts and endothelial cells, decreased collagen production and content in skin, destruction of cells in mitosis, vascular damage, and decreased ability of tissue to withstand sepsis.[33,34] These effects are summarized in Table 4–5. Since cells in a wound are undergoing repair and cell division, they are the ones more likely to be damaged by radiation.

The consequences of radiation therapy are not easily reversed. Again, one must make all attempts to optimize the wound environment and prevent further damage to already fragile and friable tissue. Choice of a treatment that will disrupt the tissue as little as possible and allow the wound to remain undisturbed will be of greatest benefit.

Chemotherapy

Data on the effect of chemotherapeutic agents on wound repair are not accurate indicators of how specific drugs will affect the repair process. Effects depend on the drugs used and their dosage. Experimental data from animal studies cannot be expected to provide equal results when applied to humans.

The degree to which different agents are detrimental to wound healing is unclear and more studies are warranted. More information on chemotherapeutic drugs is available.[35,36]

Risks from chemotherapy include increased susceptibility to infection, altered fibroblast function, collagen synthesis and metabolism, and interference with myofibroblast function.[36]

Chemotherapeutic agents may affect wound repair in varying degrees. However, one must look beyond the drug to other factors that, when combined with the chemo-

TABLE 4–5. Effects of Radiotherapy

- Injury to fibroblasts
- Injury to endothelial cells
- Decreased collagen production
- Destruction of cells in mitosis
- Vascular damage
- Decreased tolerance of bacterial burden

therapeutic drugs, may be the contributing impediments to repair. These factors include, but are not limited to, malnutrition, other medications such as corticosteroids, and vascular status. Several other considerations are listed elsewhere in this text.

SUMMARY

Wound repair may be complicated by multiple intrinsic and extrinsic factors. Health professionals involved in wound care must have a thorough knowledge of the patient's medical history including nutritional status, medications, and prescribed treatment regimens for unrelated medical problems. Aside from intrinsic considerations, one must be fully aware of extrinsic influences causing complications in wound closure. Caustic and cytotoxic external agents, harmful therapeutic treatment interventions, and disruptive dressings may all be part of a standard treatment regimen that care givers may not recognize as being potentially harmful. The clinician should question the benefit, effect, and consequence of every therapy administered in the general and specific treatment of any patient's wound.

REFERENCES

1. Holm-Pedersen, P and Viidik, A: Tensile properties and morphology of healing wounds in young and old rats. Scand J Plast Reconstr Surg 6:24, 1972.
2. Sandblom, PH, Peterson, P, and Muren, A: Determination of the tensile strength of the healing wound as a clinical test. Acta Chir Scand 105:252, 1953.
3. Mendoza, CB, Postlethwait, RW, and Johnson, WD: Veterans Administration Cooperative Study of Surgery for Duodenal Ulcer. II. Incidence of wound disruption following operation. Arch Surg 101:396, September, 1970.
4. Grove, GL: Physiologic changes in older skin. Clin Dermatol 4:425, 1986.
5. Carter, DM and Balin, AK: Dermatological aspects of aging. Med Clin North Am 67:531, 1983.
6. Goodson, WH and Hunt, TK: Wound healing and aging. J Invest Dermatol 73:88, 1979.
7. Cohen, BJ, Damon, D, and Roth, GS: Wound repair in mice as influenced by age and antimacrophage serum. J Gerontol 42:295, 1987.
8. Eaglestein, WH: Wound healing and aging. Clin Dermatol 4:481, 1986.
9. Boucek, RJ: Factors affecting wound healing. Otolaryngol Clin North Am 17(2):243–264, 1984.
10. Flower, RJ, Moncada, S, and Vane, JR: Analgesic antipyretics and anti-inflammatory agents: Drugs employed in the treatment of gout. In Gilman, AG, Goodman, LS, and Gilman, A (eds): The Pharmacologic Basis of Therapeutics. Macmillan, New York, 1980, p 718.
11. Alvarez, OM, et al: Effect of topically applied steroidal and nonsteroidal anti-inflammatory agents on skin repair and regeneration. Fed Proc 43:2793, 1984.
12. Schartzkopff, T, Kewitz, H, and Pahlitzsch, T: Topical indomethacin: Inhibition of corneal wound healing in guinea pigs after severe alkali burns. Cornea 4:19, 1985–1986.
13. Corball, M, O'Dwyer, P, and Brady, MP: The interaction of vitamin A and corticosteroids on wound healing. Irish Journal of Medical Science 154:306, 1985.
14. Ehrlich, HP and Hunt, TK: The effects of cortisone and vitamin A on wound healing. Ann Surg 167:324, 1968.
15. Ehrlich, HP, Tarver, H, and Hunt, TK: Effect of vitamin A and glucocorticoids upon inflammation and collagen synthesis. Ann Surg 177:222, 1974.
16. Van Story-Lewis, PE, and Tennenbaum, HC: Glucocortic inhibition of fibroblast contaction of collagen gels. Biochem Pharmacol 35:1283, 1986.
17. Priestley, GC: Effects of corticosteroids on the growth and metabolism of fibroblasts cultured from human skin. Br J Dermatol 99:253, 1978.
18. Ponec, M, et al: Effects of glucocorticoids on primary human skin fibroblasts. I. Inhibition of proliferation of culture of primary human skin and fibroblasts. Arch Dermatol Res 259:117, 1977.
19. Eaglestein, WH, et al: Current wound management: A symposium. Clin Dermatol 2:134, 1984.
20. Nemlander, A, et al: Effect of cyclosporine on wound healing. Transplantation 36:1, 1983.
21. Fishel, R, et al: Cyclosporine A impairs wound healing in rats. J Surg Res 34:572, 1983.
22. Eisinger, D and Sheil, AGR: A comparison of the effects of endosporin and standard agents on primary wound healing in the rat. Surg Gynecol Obstet 160:135, 1985.

23. Reed, BR and Clark, RAF: Cutaneous tissue repair: Practical implications of current knowledge. II. J Am Acad Dermatol 13:929, 1985.
24. Pollack, SV: Systemic medications and wound healing. Int J Dermatol 21:489, 1982.
25. Peterson, MJ, et al: Significance of T-lymphocytes in wound healing. Surgery 102:300, 1987.
26. Kottra, CJ: Wound healing in the immunosuppressed host. Association of Operating Room Nurses 35:1142, 1982.
27. DeDebbeleer, G, et al: Clinically uninvolved skin in AIDS: Evidence of atypical dermal vessels similar to early lesions observed on Kaposi's sarcoma. Ultrastructural study in four patients. J Cutan Pathol 14:154, 1987.
28. Daynes, R: What is the relationship between the status of a patient's host defense mechanisms, his metabolic response, and his ability to respond to injury? Trauma 24:S84, 1984.
29. Witt, MD (ed): AIDS and Patient Management: Legal, Ethical and Social Issues. National Health Publishing, Owings Mill, MD, 1986.
30. Institute of Medicine, National Academy of Sciences: Confronting AIDS. National Academy Press, Washington, DC, 1986, p 374.
31. Lineaweaver, W, et al: Topical antimicrobial toxicity. Arch Surg 120:267, 1985.
32. Rodeheaver, G, et al: Bactericidal activity and toxicity of iodine containing solutions in wounds. Arch Surg 117:181, 1982.
33. Shamberger, R: Effect of chemotherapy and radiotherapy on wound healing: Experimental studies. Recent results. Cancer Res 98:17, 1985.
34. Ormiston, MCE: A study of rat intestinal wound healing in the presence of radiation injury. Br J Surg 72:56, 1985.
35. Falcone, RE, and Nappi, SF: Chemotherapy and wound healing. Surg Clin North Am 64:779, 1984.
36. Carter, SK, Batkowski, MT, and Hellman, K: Chemotherapy of Cancer. John Wiley and Sons, New York, 1977, pp 67–69.

CHAPTER 5

Bacteriology

Nancy Harkess, Ph.D.

Of the many factors that affect wound healing, bacterial infection is the most commonly encountered. The effects of bacterial infection of a wound vary greatly. At the least serious end of the clinical spectrum, wound healing is delayed, often leading to a temporary disability at the site of the infection. Consequences of the delayed healing and disability may include a prolonged hospital stay and loss of productive activity for the patient. At the opposite end of the spectrum of effects, wound infection can lead to the death of the patient. The most common cause of death in patients with burn injuries is infection.[1] Infection is also a leading factor in deaths following implantation of prosthetic devices during cardiovascular surgery.[2]

The mechanism by which bacteria interfere with wound healing is not completely understood. However, evidence gained from studies with laboratory animals suggests that the principal effect is at the level of collagen metabolism. Bacteria have been shown to decrease the synthesis[3] and increase the lysis of collagen.[4-6] These effects are related to elaboration of toxins, enzymes, and waste products by bacteria that they secrete or excrete into the environment. Moreover, studies have shown that many bacteria decrease the amount of oxygen available to infected tissues.[7,8] Competition of the cells present at the infected wound site for the available oxygen can lead to decreased metabolism and eventually death of the cells involved in the repair process. The result of these activities is reduced collagen content of the wound, delayed growth and migration of epithelial cells into the area of the wound, cellular necrosis, and microvascular thrombosis.[9]

A goal of health professionals is to prevent bacterial contamination of wounds so that rapid and proper healing occur. Health professionals should also understand how to deal with infections when they occur and be able to prevent contamination of themselves and other patients when caring for persons with infected wounds. An understanding of the field of bacteriology is an important step toward achieving these goals. The remainder of this chapter focuses on a discussion of some basic concepts of bacteriology, including methods of culturing wounds for identification of the infecting organism, laboratory methods used in the identification of bacteria, sources of wound infections, and methods by which bacteria are transmitted and treated.

THE WORLD OF MICROBIOLOGY

Bacteria belong to a large group of organisms known collectively as *microorganisms.* The term *microorganism* includes the viruses, chlamydia, rickettsia, mycoplasmas, fungi, and protozoa, as well as the bacteria. These unicellular organisms vary in size and complexity from the small and structurally simple viruses to the larger and more complex fungi and protozoa. Bacteria are intermediate in size and complexity as are the rickettsia, chlamydia, and mycoplasmas. The criteria of structural arrangement and complexity are used to divide cells into two groups: the *prokaryotes* and *eukaryotes.* The prokaryotes are simpler in structure in that they lack a nuclear membrane and mitochondria. Other differences between eukaryotic and prokaryotic cells are listed in Table 5–1.

These unicellular microorganisms also vary in their ability to exist outside of a host cell. Viruses, chlamydia, and most of the rickettsia lack certain metabolic machinery or possess defective structural components that prevent them from functioning independent of a host cell. Because of their requirement of a host cell for multiplication and metabolic function, this group of microorganisms are referred to as obligate, intracellular parasites. Most bacteria and the mycoplasmas, fungi, and protozoa can multiply and function freely in the environment in a saprophytic existence. However, these microorganisms are capable of an intracellular or parasitic existence when introduced into a susceptible host and may cause damage to that host. These and some other distinguishing features that vary among the different kinds of microorganisms are listed in Table 5–2.[10]

NORMAL FLORA

Many areas of the body are colonized by a variety of microbes that constitute a group of microorganisms referred to as the normal flora (Table 5–3).[11] The skin and mucous membranes of newborns become colonized within a few hours after birth. Colonization of these areas is maintained throughout life with variations in the type and

TABLE 5–1. Characteristics Distinguishing Prokaryotic and Eukaryotic Cells

Characteristic	Eukaryotic	Prokaryotic
Nuclear membrane	Present	Absent
Genetic material	Arranged in linear strands of DNA; more than one present per cell	Arranged as a circular molecule of DNA; one present per cell
Protein associated with genetic material	Present	Absent
Mitochondria	Present	Absent
Size and location of ribosomes	80S;* located on the endoplasmic reticulum	70S;* found free in the cytoplasm
Mode of reproduction	Meiosis and mitosis	Binary fission
Site of respiration	Mitochondria	Cell membrane
Sterols in cell membrane	Usually present	Usually absent
Peptidoglycan in cell wall	Absent	Present

*S = Svedberg units, a measure of size that is determined by the rate of sedimentation during centrifugation.

TABLE 5–2. Comparison of Properties of Microorganisms

Property	Viruses	Chlamydia	Rickettsia	Mycoplasma	Bacteria	Fungi
Prokaryotic or eukaryotic*		P	P	P	P	E
Nucleic acids present	DNA or RNA	DNA and RNA	DNA and RNA	DNA and RNA	DNA and RNA	DNA and RNA
Growth outside the host	−	−	−†	+	+	+
Mode of reproduction	Direction of host cell machinery	Fission	Fission	Fission	Fission	Meiosis and mitosis
Independent protein synthesis	−	+	+	+	+	+
Generate metabolic energy	−	−	+	+	+	+

*P = prokaryotic; E = eukaryotic
†Except *Rochalimea quintana*
Adapted from Davis et al,[10] p 917.

TABLE 5–3. Bacteria that Normally Inhabit the Human Body*

Skin	**Lower Intestine**
Corynebacterium species (diphtheroids)	*Alcaligenes faecalis*
Propionibacterium acnes	Anaerobic staphylococci and streptococci
Staphylococcus aureus	*Bacteroides* species
Staphylococcus epidermidis	*Clostridium* species
Conjunctiva	*Escherichia coli*
Corynebacterium species	*Eubacterium* species
Hemophilus species	*Fusobacterium* species
Nares	*Klebsiella* species
Branhamella catarrhalis	*Lactobacillus* species
Corynebacterium species	*Proteus* species
Hemophilus species	*Pseudomonas aeruginosa*
Staphylococcus aureus	*Staphylococcus aureus*
Staphylococcus epidermidis	*Streptococcus faecalis* (enterococci)
Streptococcus pneumoniae	Viridans streptococci
Viridans streptococci	**External Genitalia**
Mouth	Anaerobic streptococci
Actinomyces species	*Bacteroides* species
Anaerobic staphylococci and streptococci	*Corynebacterium* species
Bacteroides species	*Escherichia coli*
Branhamella catarrhalis	*Fusobacterium* species
Corynebacterium species	*Mycobacterium smegmatis*
Fusobacterium species	*Staphylococcus epidermidis*
Lactobacillus acidophilus	*Streptococcus faecalis* (enterococci)
Neisseria species	*Streptococcus* species
Spirillum species	**Vagina**
Staphylococcus epidermidis	*Acinetobacter calcoaceticus*
Treponema dentium	Anaerobic staphylococci and streptococci
Veillonella species	*Bacteroides* species
Viridans streptococci	*Corynebacterium* species
Pharynx	*Escherichia coli*
Actinomyces israelii	*Hemophilus* species
Anaerobic streptococci	*Lactobacillus* species
Bacteroides species	*Propionibacterium* species
Branhamella catarrhalis	*Streptococcus faecalis* (enterococci)
Corynebacterium species	*Veillonella* species
Fusobacterium species	
Hemophilus species	
Klebsiella species	
Neisseria species	
Proteus species	
Streptococcus pneumoniae	
Treponema dentium	
Veillonella species	
Viridans streptococci	

*Not intended to be a complete listing.
Adapted from Myrvik and Weiser, p. 109.

number of organisms present at different times. The type and number of organisms present at any site are influenced by a number of factors. For example, factors that influence organisms present on the skin include the level of hygiene maintained at the site and the proximity of the site to other anatomic features. Culture of skin near the intestine may yield normal intestinal organisms such as *Escherichia coli*, while skin near the mouth or nose may be positive for *Staphylococcus aureus*, which is normally found in this area.

Interpretation of culture results is made difficult when the source of the specimen is a site that possesses a normal flora. Isolation of an organism in this area does not necessarily indicate that it is playing a role in an infectious process. The microbe may have been present at the site only at the time the culture was obtained and should be considered a contaminant. Another consideration in interpreting culture results involves an evaluation of organisms considered to be normal flora. Members of the normal flora serve a number of useful functions.[12] Their presence prevents the colonization and/or invasion of the body by other microbes. These organisms may also immunize the host against microbes that share related antigens. However, some normal flora organisms may assume the role of pathogens under conditions that cause depression of host defense mechanisms.[13] For example, individuals who have been debilitated by surgery are subject to stitch abscesses caused by *Staphylococcus epidermidis*, which is part of the normal skin flora.[14]

Many laboratories attempt to aid in interpreting culture results by indicating the relative numbers of organisms isolated from the sample. These results may be reported by giving the actual number of colonies of each organism identified or by listing organisms according to quantities in either ascending or descending order. The presence of large numbers of bacteria from a properly taken specimen cultured soon after leaving the body is highly suggestive that the isolate is the causative agent in the infectious process. An additional factor in interpreting culture results is the fact that organisms once termed *nonpathogenic* are now being recognized as etiologic agents of infectious diseases. *Staphylococcus epidermidis*, once discarded as a skin contaminant, has been shown to cause a variety of infections including stitch abscesses, endocarditis, peritonitis, and osteomyelitis.[14-16] Repeated isolation of these organisms from a given site in a debilitated individual is considered indicative of a causative role in the infectious process.

PATHOGENESIS OF WOUND INFECTIONS

The first step in the establishment of an infection involves contact between a microbe and a susceptible host. Factors that determine the fate of the initial contact include the number of organisms present, the pathogenic potential of the microbe(s), and the immune status of the host.[17]

Sources of Organisms in Wounds

Humans live in an environment where they are continually brought into contact with microorganisms. Their own normal flora serves as a major source of a variety of organisms, each having the potential of causing an infection within them. Infections caused by these endogenous organisms are seen primarily in individuals with lowered defenses.[18] Many wound infections are caused by these endogenous organisms, particularly bacteria such as *Staphylococcus aureus* and *Pseudomonas aeruginosa*.[19]

Additional sources of infectious agents include the environment and other humans. Direct contact with microorganisms harbored by animate objects or indirect contact with contaminated inanimate objects may also lead to infections in a susceptible host. Directly transmitted infections include venereal diseases such as syphilis and gonorrhea that are transmitted by direct sexual contact. Diseases of the newborn such as rubella, syphilis, and toxoplasmosis that have been transmitted from mother to child at or before birth are also classified as directly transmitted.

Infectious agents are indirectly acquired by (1) inhalation of contaminated aerosols, (2) ingestion of contaminated food or drink, (3) contact with contaminated inanimate objects (fomites), and (4) bites from insects that carry microorganisms (arthropod vectors).[20] The major potential source of infectious agents causing wound infections is fomites. Microorganisms of the environment, including dust and air, or from the respiratory tract, the intestinal tract, or skin may contaminate clothing, bedding, or hospital instruments and equipment. Those microbes afforded the added protection of body secretions may withstand the effects of drying and sunlight and remain viable for long periods of time.

Control of Environmental Organisms

Reduction of environmental sources of infection involves use of physical or chemical agents to inhibit or destroy microorganisms. The proper use of disinfectant and sterilization procedures constitutes a major factor in controlling hospital-acquired (nosocomial) infections. The choice of a specific agent and protocol is determined largely by the level of microbial killing required, the nature of the instrument or device to be treated, and the cost, availability, and ease of use of the agent.[21] For example, sterilization, the complete destruction of all microbial life, is required for objects that are to be introduced into the body. Such objects include scalpels, cardiac catheters, and artificial heart valves. However, sterilization is not required for objects that come in contact with mucous membranes but do not penetrate into the body. Instruments such as respiratory and hydrotherapy equipment may be used after subjecting the equipment to a procedure that destroys disease-producing organisms (disinfection). Protocols that utilize meticulous cleaning followed by treatment with a high-level disinfectant have been shown to render the equipment free of pathogenic organisms.[21-25]

Specific recommendations with regard to the care of hydrotherapy equipment are found in publications from the Centers for Disease Control.[26] Pools should be drained and cleaned every week or two, and tanks after each patient. Pools, pumps, and associated equipment should be scrubbed with a phenolic germicidal detergent and rinsed thoroughly before refilling. Failure to clean the thermometer, drains, and area around the shaft of the agitator unit has been shown to cause infection in persons using hydrotherapy equipment.[27] Chlorination of water is recommended when organic matter is removed by a filtering system. When continuous filtration is not possible, iodine, rather than chlorine, should be used. The bactericidal activity of chlorine is reduced in water contaminated with organic matter from the skin, feces, urine, and nasal discharges. By contrast, iodine retains full bactericidal activity in the presence of organic matter. In addition, the effectiveness of chlorine is significantly reduced if the pH is below 7.2 or above 7.6. The pH level should be monitored and the proper level maintained by adding sodium carbonate when the pH is below 7.2 and sodium hydrogen sulfate when pH is above 7.6.

An additional comment concerns the relationship between bacteria classified in the genus *Pseudomonas* and disinfectant solutions. Most of the pseudomonads are highly resistant to all forms of antimicrobial agents. Moreover, they are usually present whenever water or moisture accumulates around sinks, drains, hydrotherapy equipment, and respiratory therapy equipment.[28] Outbreaks of infections caused by pseudomonads have been traced to use of disinfecting solutions diluted with tap water or nonsterilized distilled water.[29-32] A recommendation that followed this discovery is to make dilutions with sterile water when disinfectant solutions must be diluted. In addition, dilutions should be prepared in small, sterile containers and the unused portion discarded after a few weeks.

Host Defense Mechanisms

The first line of the host's defenses is rendered by the mechanical barrier provided by the skin and mucous membranes. Microorganisms reach the deeper tissues only through breaks in the skin, sweat and sebaceous glands, or hair follicles. Production of lactic acid by sweat glands, fatty acids by sebaceous glands, and metabolic products by the normal flora contribute to the antimicrobial nature of the skin. Additional antimicrobial features include the mucociliary action of ciliated epithelium, the flushing effects of tears and urine, and the acid pH of the stomach. Furthermore, antimicrobial products such as lysozyme and an immunoglobulin called secretory IgA are present in body secretions and are active in inhibiting microbes.[33]

Organisms that penetrate the first lines of defense encounter a second series of processes designed to destroy and/or remove them. The second line of the host's defense is primarily a cellular response utilizing phagocytic cells of tissue and blood. Such cells include blood polymorphonuclear neutrophilic leukocytes and monocytes and tissue macrophages and histiocytes. The classic signs of inflammation including swelling (tumor), redness (rubor), heat (calor), and pain (dolor) at the site of an infection are manifestations of this cellular response.

Microbes that resist the initial effects of the phagocytic process or that have become adapted to an intracellular existence become subject to the immune system.[17] This final defensive tactic by the host is a specific action being directed against specific components of specific organisms. When an infection occurs, cells of the immune system react to microbial components (antigens) to produce either a humoral or cellular response. The humoral response results in the synthesis of antibody by B lymphocytes. Detectable levels of antibody rarely occur before 5 days after a first exposure to the antigen. Subsequent exposure to the same antigen results in a more rapid response. Antibody can initiate direct killing of microbes, neutralize toxic effects of bacterial products, and enhance phagocytosis. A cell-mediated response involves interaction between an antigen and the T lymphocyte. Activated T cells may have direct cytotoxic effects against a variety of cells or release products called lymphokines that activate other cells to control infections.

Pathogenic Properties of Microbes

Microorganisms possess a variety of mechanisms by which they cause disease.[34] Some bacteria, such as *Streptococcus pneumoniae* and *Hemophilus influenzae*, produce capsules that reduce their ability to be phagocytized. By evading phagocytes, these organisms are able to penetrate the deeper tissues, causing diseases such as pneumonia and meningitis. Other organisms, such as *Staphylococcus aureus* and *Clostridium perfringens*, produce leukocidins that are toxic for white blood cells. Some bacteria, like *Pseudomonas aeruginosa* and *Staphylococcus aureus*, survive within phagocytic cells by interfering with lysosomal function and eventually cause death of the phagocytic cell.[17] Many bacteria release toxic substances that produce a variety of effects. The endotoxin of gram-negative cell walls causes fever, hypotension, decreases in leukocyte and platelet counts, hemorrhage, and disseminated intravascular coagulation. Tetanus and botulism toxins interfere with the function of nerve cells, causing paralysis. *Escherichia coli* and staphylococcal enterotoxin cause intestinal cells to release large amounts of fluid and electrolytes, which may result in dehydration.

Predisposing Factors to Infections

The human host and bacteria coexist in the normal healthy individual by maintaining a balance between the defense mechanisms of the host and pathogenic properties of the microbe. A compromised host is produced when some process interferes with the host's ability to mount a proper defense. Some of the factors known to predispose an individual to infection include congenital immunodeficiency diseases, surgery, burns, malnutrition, cancer, metabolic diseases such as diabetes mellitus, kidney disease, immunosuppressive drugs, and antibiotic therapy.[18] Special precautions must be taken with these immunocompromised individuals to prevent infections by keeping their environment as free of microorganisms as possible.

AIDS and the Health-Care Professional

Care must also be taken to prevent the transmission of microorganisms from an infected individual to the health-care worker. Of special interest in recent years has been the precautions necessary when caring for individuals with acquired immune deficiency syndrome (AIDS). Guidelines for health-care workers are available in publications of the Centers for Disease Control,[35-40] and are summarized here:

1. Precautions should be taken to prevent exposure of skin and mucous membranes of the health-care worker to the patient's blood and other body fluids. These precautions include wearing gloves when touching blood and other body fluids, mucous membranes, or nonintact skin, and when handling items or surfaces soiled with blood or body fluids. The eyes and face should be protected with glasses and a mask when performing procedures likely to generate droplets of blood or other body fluids. Clothing should be protected with gowns or aprons when performing procedures likely to result in splashing of blood or other body fluids.
2. Any skin surfaces contaminated with blood or other body fluids should be washed immediately. Furthermore, hands should be washed immediately after removing gloves.
3. Extraordinary care must be taken to prevent injuries with any sharp instrument or device contaminated with potentially infectious material.
4. Direct patient care and handling of equipment or devices contaminated with potentially infectious material should be avoided by health-care workers with open lesions until the lesions are healed.
5. A disinfectant solution such as sodium hypochlorite (bleach) should be used to clean spills of blood or body fluids immediately after they occur.

Organisms Commonly Encountered in Wound Infections

When the pathogenic mechanisms of microbial organisms overpower or bypass the defense systems of the host, sepsis occurs. *Wound sepsis* is defined by the United States Institute of Surgical Research as bacterial contamination exceeding 10^5 organisms per gram of tissue.[41]

Bacteria from both endogenous and exogenous sources are commonly involved in postoperative wound infections.[42] The most common agent causing these infections is *Staphylococcus aureus*. The source of infections caused by *S. aureus* is often the infected individual's own skin or anterior nares but it may also come from an exogenous source. Facultative gram-negative rods are commonly implicated in wound infections and include bacteria such as *Escherichia coli, Proteus, Enterobacter,* and *Klebsiella*. These are usually endogenous bacteria causing infection when wounds become contaminated with intestinal contents. Another gram-negative rod that may come from the intestine or from the hospital environment is *Pseudomonas*. Infections of burns are commonly caused by either *Pseudomonas aeruginosa* or *Staphylococcus aureus*.[43] The etiologic agent of infections of deep, traumatic wounds or wounds contaminated with feces or soil is often anaerobes in the genus *Clostridium*.

SPECIMEN COLLECTION

When an infection is recognized, identification of the infecting organism can be accomplished by sending a representative sample of the infected material to the bacteriology laboratory for culture. Proper specimen collection and immediate transport of that specimen to the laboratory are essential to recovery of the etiologic agent of an infection. A poorly collected sample or delay in transport may lead to the isolation of a contaminant rather than the true agent and result in the institution of improper therapy. Some guidelines are given below to aid in properly collecting samples for bacteriologic culture. The first set of guidelines are general in scope and apply to the collection of specimens from any site in the body. These general guidelines are followed by specific principles to use when collecting samples from wound infections.[44,45]

The general guidelines are as follows:

1. Specimens must be collected from the actual site of the infection with the minimal amount of contamination by material from adjacent tissues or secretions. When collecting material from wounds, precautions should be taken to avoid contact with adjacent skin. When culturing deep abscesses, material should be aspirated with a needle or cannula (see specific guidelines further on).
2. Specimens must be collected at a time that is optimal for recovery of the etiologic agent. A knowledge of the natural history of the infectious process aids in determining the optimal time for collection of a specimen. For example, natural concentration of organisms occurs in the lungs and kidneys overnight, leading to the presence of higher numbers of organisms in early morning specimens. Collection of early morning urine or sputum specimens are more likely to yield positive results.
3. A sufficient quantity of specimen must be collected to allow recovery of the etiologic agent. Submission of a dry swab or one with only small amounts of purulent material frequently results in a negative culture. The maximal quantity of purulent secretions should be collected whenever material is submitted for culture.
4. Specimens must be collected with appropriate collection devices and placed in appropriate containers. All collection devices and specimen containers must be sterile. Containers should be easy to use with tightly fitting caps or lids to prevent leakage and/or contamination. When a swab is the collection device, it should be composed of dacron or polyester but not cotton. Cotton fibers contain fatty acids, which may inhibit the growth of some strains of bacteria. Moreover, swabs should not be used when submitting specimens for anaerobic culture. The specimen of choice for anaerobic culture is a wound aspirate collected with a needle and syringe, followed by protection of the specimen from exposure to oxygen.

5. Specimens should be transported to the laboratory as quickly as possible. Some bacteria, like anaerobes, die quickly outside of the body. Moreover, all specimens should be protected from drying. When immediate transport to the laboratory is not possible, the specimen may be inoculated into a tube containing a transport medium that maintains most but not all bacteria for up to 48 hours.

6. Specimens should be collected before the administration of antimicrobial agents whenever possible. The laboratory should be notified whenever antibiotics have been administered and told what type of antibiotics have been given. Some organisms that are unlikely to be recovered after antibiotics have been administered include *Streptococcus pyogenes* from a throat specimen, *Neisseria gonorrhoeae* from the genitourinary tract, or *Hemophilus influenzae* and *Neisseria meningitidis* from cerebrospinal fluid.

7. All specimen containers should be properly labeled. Minimal information needed by the microbiologist to ensure proper culturing techniques is the patient's name and identification number, the source of the specimen, the name of the physician in charge, and the date and time the specimen was collected. Special instructions or requests should also be indicated.

Specific guidelines recommended for the collection of wound cultures are as follows:

1. Purulent material should be aspirated from the depths of a wound with a sterile needle and syringe. The margin of cutaneous lesions or decubitus ulcers are usually contaminated with environmental bacteria and should be decontaminated before collecting the sample. A recommended decontamination procedure is to cleanse the surface of the wound with surgical soap, followed by the application of 70 percent ethyl or isopropyl alcohol. If the specimen can be transported to the laboratory within 30 minutes, the needle cap can be replaced immediately and the syringe sent directly to the laboratory. However, the specimen should be transferred to an anaerobic container if delivery is to be delayed beyond 30 minutes.

2. When material cannot be aspirated with a needle and syringe, the specimen may be collected with a swab. The margin of the wound should be decontaminated as just described. The swab should be introduced deep into the wound with one hand while the margins of the wound are gently separated with the thumb and forefinger of the other hand, which is protected by a sterile glove. When removing the swab, care should be taken not to contaminate the swab by touching the margins of the skin. The swab should be placed in an anaerobic container and transported as quickly as possible to the laboratory.

LABORATORY PROCEDURES USED IN THE IDENTIFICATION OF ORGANISMS

When specimens are received in the laboratory, microbiologists use a variety of techniques to isolate and identify the etiologic agent of an infectious process. Isolation procedures involve inoculating the clinical sample onto various plates and tubes containing nutrients (media) that support the growth of bacteria in the specimen.[44] Because specimens from different body sites vary in the types of bacteria that are present, the media onto which the specimen is inoculated will differ. Media selection is made on the basis of that which will isolate the organisms present in the sample. Laboratories have a wide variety of commercial media available that serve these primary plating needs. Each laboratory selects ones that fit best with the equipment available and protocol developed in that laboratory.

Following growth of the bacteria on the primary plating media, the isolates are identified by evaluating their microscopic, cultural, biochemical, and immunologic characteristics. Moreover, many bacterial isolates are further evaluated for their susceptibility to antimicrobial agents to aid in the selection of an appropriate therapeutic agent. In addition, procedures are now becoming more readily available that are not dependent upon the growth of the organism in the laboratory. These newer methods generally result in a more rapid detection and identification of bacteria present in clinical samples.

Microscopic Characteristics

Visualization of most bacteria in the light microscope requires that they be stained. The primary staining procedure used in the bacteriology laboratory is a differential stain developed by Dr. Christian Gram in 1884. The procedure involves the stepwise addition of crystal violet, Gram's iodine, 95 percent ethanol, and safranin to a heat-fixed sample.[46] Bacteria that retain the purple color of the crystal violet following decolorization with 95 percent ethanol are called "gram positive." Those bacteria that are decolorized when ethanol is added are stained red or pink by the safranin and are called "gram negative." Unreliable gram stain results occur when the recommended timing of the decolorization step is not adhered to or when the bacterial cells are old or dead. For example, decolorization for too long of a time may result in gram-positive cells appearing gram negative while under-decolorization may lead to gram-negative cells appearing gram positive. In addition, old or dead gram-positive cells will stain gram negative.

Gram-positive and gram-negative bacteria differ in many important ways. In addition to their staining reaction, gram-positive and gram-negative bacteria differ in their cell wall composition.[47] The major constituent of the cell wall of gram-positive bacteria is a chemical unique to prokaryotes called peptidoglycan. Gram-negative bacteria also contain peptidoglycan in their cell walls but in much smaller quantities. By contrast, the major component of the cell wall of gram-negative bacteria is lipopolysaccharide (LPS), a compound found only in gram-negative bacteria. The lipid portion of this chemical has toxic properties and when released into tissues or blood causes endotoxic shock or endotoxemia. The polysaccharide portion of the molecule serves as an antigenic marker that can be used to identify specific strains of bacteria in the laboratory.

Gram-positive and gram-negative bacteria also differ in their susceptibility to many antimicrobial agents such as antibiotics and disinfectants. Penicillin G, for example, is effective mainly against gram-positive bacteria and has little or no effect against most gram-negative bacteria. Bacterial cell walls are often a major site of attack for antimicrobial agents to be used inside of the human body because of their unique composition and the fact that human cells lack cell walls. Unlike bacteria that have both a cell membrane and a cell wall, human cells have only a cell membrane. Thus, agents directed against cell walls are selective for bacteria.

Some bacteria fail to stain with the Gram procedure and must be visualized using some other method. For example, mycobacteria contain a waxy material in their cell walls, which prevents the penetration of most dyes. The acid-fast stain is a method used in many laboratories to visualize these bacteria.[46] This procedure uses heat or chemicals to cause penetration of dyes through the waxy coat. The classic procedure uses heat to force carbol-fuchsin into the organism. Once stained, these bacteria resist decolorization with acid alcohol and retain the red of the carbol fuchsin. The red organisms are visible against a blue background when methylene blue is used as the counterstain. Because of their ability to resist acid decolorization, the mycobacteria are called acid-fast bacilli (AFB). Bacteria that exhibit this type of staining characteristic include the etiologic agents of tuberculosis (*Mycobacterium tuberculosis*) and leprosy (*M. leprae*).

Other bacteria that fail to Gram stain are members of the genus *Treponema*, which includes *T. pallidum*, the etiologic agent of syphilis. These organisms can be visualized in unstained preparations using a technique called darkfield microscopy.[44] Darkfield microscopy uses a special condenser to illuminate the field so that light is directed at oblique angles. The diffracted light causes light-colored organisms to be visible against a dark background.

Special staining procedures are also available in some laboratories to make visible certain structures.[44] Capsules that serve as antiphagocytic organelles in microbes can be made visible using a "negative" staining technique. In this procedure, the background is stained while the organism remains unstained. This procedure is used primarily to detect and identify a fungus called *Cryptococcus neoformans*. Flagella and spore stains are also available but are not routinely performed in clinical laboratories. These special stains are used only when knowledge of flagellar arrangement or spore location are needed for bacterial identification. For example, species identification of some members of the genus *Pseudomonas* is dependent upon the number and arrangement of flagella at the cell surface.[48]

Cell morphology is another important criterion that is used by microbiologists to identify and classify bacteria. The morphologic features that are readily detectable in stained preparations are shape and arrangement of organisms and the presence or absence of spores. The shape of bacteria is maintained by the relative rigidity of the cell wall. Medically important bacteria fall into one of three basic shapes: spherical to oval (cocci), rod-shaped (bacilli), or spiral-shaped (spirochetes). Combining the characteristics of Gram reaction and morphology allows separation of most disease-causing bacteria into four major groups as follows: gram-positive cocci, gram-positive bacilli, gram-negative cocci, and gram-negative bacilli.

Recognition of the arrangement of bacterial cells is also useful in identifying bacteria. Bacteria may appear as single cells, in chains, or in clusters. The arrangement of cells is determined by the manner in which they reproduce. Bacteria that divide in a single plane may appear singly, in pairs (diplo-), or in chains (strepto-). Bacteria that divide in more than one plane will appear in clusters (staphylo-) as well as singly or in pairs.

Only two genera of medically important bacteria produce endospores. Endospores develop in these bacteria when conditions become unfavorable for growth, such as during starvation or dehydration. Endospores are not stained by commonly used staining procedures because the dyes are unable to penetrate the thick coat that surrounds the spore. Therefore, detection of nonstaining, round or oval structures in the cytoplasm of a bacterial cell identifies that organism as a member of one of the two spore-forming genera, that is, a member of the genus *Bacillus* or *Clostridium*. Diseases associated with these spore-forming bacteria include anthrax (*B. anthracis*), gas gangrene (*Cl. perfringens* and others), and tetanus (*Cl. tetani*). Additional important features of spore-forming bacteria to health-care professionals is that endospores are commonly present in the environment and are highly resistant to disinfecting and sterilization procedures. Any sample containing bacterial endospores must be treated with high temperatures for long periods of time (autoclaving at 121°C for 20 minutes) or with chemical agents classified as sporocides (8 percent formaldehyde in 70 percent alcohol) to achieve sterilization.

Cultural Characteristics

Growth of bacteria in the laboratory is dependent upon providing the proper environmental conditions and nutritional requirements.[44] Providing the proper environment requires a knowledge of the oxygen and temperature requirements of bacteria that may be present in the sample. Bacteria can be classified into one of three major groups, based on their oxygen requirements. The groups are designated as follows:

1. Strict or obligate aerobes — organisms that grow only when oxygen is present (*Mycobacterium* and *Pseudomonas*)
2. Strict or obligate anaerobes — organisms that grow only when oxygen is essentially absent (*Clostridium* and *Bacteroides*)
3. Facultative anaerobes — organisms that grow best when oxygen is present but are capable of growing in the absence of oxygen (*Escherichia* and *Staphylococcus*)

Special procedures must be followed to isolate organisms classified as anaerobes.[49] Oxygen not only prevents these organisms from growing but may be toxic to them. Laboratories use special media that binds oxygen (e.g., thioglycollate) or use special containers that are filled with an atmosphere that lacks oxygen.

Most laboratory incubators are set at a temperature between 35°C and 37°C. This temperature is optimal for most bacteria that produce disease in humans. However, some bacteria that produce disease fail to grow at this temperature. For example, samples containing the organism *Mycobacterium ulcerans* that produces cutaneous lesions must be incubated below 32°C to achieve isolation and identification.

Bacteria also grow only when provided the proper nutrients. Most bacteria will grow when there is a source of carbon, hydrogen, nitrogen, and sulfur plus some trace metals. Bacteriologic media provide these substances in the form of carbohydrates such as glucose, proteins, (peptones), and water. Bacteria referred to as fastidious have additional nutritional requirements and fail to grow if these added nutrients are not provided. For example, *Hemophilus influenzae* will not grow in media that lacks either hemin or nicotinamide adenine dinucleotide (NAD).

The length of time required to receive the results of a bacteriologic culture is determined largely by the growth rate of the organisms present. Rapidly growing organisms such as members of the family *Enterobacteriaceae* may produce visible colonies in 12 to 18 hours (Fig. 5–1). At the opposite extreme, cultures of *Mycobacterium tuberculosis* may not be positive for 4 to 6 weeks. Most laboratories hold negative wound cultures submitted to the general bacteriology laboratory for a minimum of 2 weeks before discarding them. Specimens submitted for acid-fast studies are usually held for 6 weeks.

Biochemical and Immunologic Characteristics

A preliminary classification of bacteria can be achieved using the morphologic and cultural characteristics described earlier (Table 5–4). However, identification of an isolate as belonging to a particular genus and species usually requires further testing.[44] Biochemical testing involves an evaluation of the metabolic or enzymatic potential of the isolate. These tests are performed by subculturing colonies from the primary isolation plate to a series of reaction vessels containing substrates for enzymatic degradation. Indicators incorporated into the media or added after incubation change color when

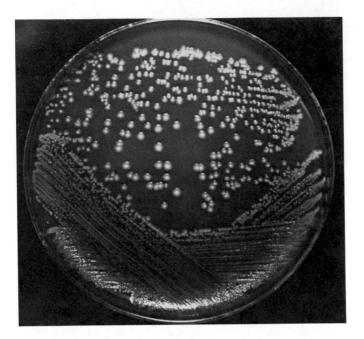

FIGURE 5–1. Colonies of *Escherichia coli* cultured on 5 percent sheep blood agar following incubation at 37°C for 18 hours.

particular products appear. The time required to interpret these results ranges from less than 1 minute to several days.

Complete identification of some bacteria may require detection of surface antigens using commercially prepared antisera. For example, identification of an isolate of *Hemophilus influenzae* as type b requires use of an antiserum containing antibodies to the type b capsular antigen.[50] These types of tests are also useful in epidemiologic surveys to trace the source and spread of a particular infection, such as *Salmonella*.

Non–Growth-Dependent Tests

Several non–growth-dependent methods are now available for the detection of microorganisms in clinical samples.[51] Immunofluorescent (IF) techniques are based on detection of bacterial antigens in tissues using antibodies attached to a fluorescent compound. Examples of IF tests currently used in bacteriology laboratories include the detection of group A streptococci in throat swabs, *Legionella pneumophila* in sputum or lung tissue, and *Bordetella pertussis* in nasopharyngeal aspirates. One of the newest techniques uses nucleic acid probes that are reacted with a treated sample under conditions that allows hybridization of the probe with bacterial nucleic acid.[52] The two tests currently available are probes specific for members of the genus *Legionella* in sputum samples[53] and for *Mycoplasma pneumoniae* in a throat swab.[52] Availability of these types of tests is at present limited, but the kinds of tests and number of organisms detectable by these methods are continually expanding. The major advantage to non–growth-dependent tests is that diagnostic results are often available in less than 2 hours.

Antimicrobial Susceptibility Testing

A number of factors are involved in selecting an appropriate antimicrobial agent to treat an infection. These include (1) the pharmacologic properties of the drug; (2) the nature and site of the infectious process; (3) the conditions present in the host, including

TABLE 5–4.Microscopic and Cultural Classification of Some
Medically Important Bacteria

Gram-Negative Bacilli	**Gram-Positive Bacilli**
Aerobic or Facultative	Non–Spore-Forming (Asporogenous)
Family: *Enterobacteriaceae*	Aerobic or facultative
Arizona	*Corynebacterium*
Edwardsiella	*Erysepelothrix*
Enterobacter	*Listeria*
Escherichia	*Nocardia*
Klebsiella	Anaerobic
Proteus	*Actinomyces*
Providencia	*Arachnia*
Salmonella	*Bifidobacterium*
Serratia	*Eubacterium*
Shigella	Spore-forming (sporogenous)
Yersinia	Aerobic
Family: *Vibrionaceae*	*Bacillus*
Aeromonas	Anaerobic
Plesiomonas	*Clostridium*
Vibrio	**Gram-Positive Cocci**
Others:	Aerobic or facultative
Alcaligenes	*Aerococcus*
Bordetella	*Staphylococcus*
Brucella	*Streptococcus*
Flavobacterium	Anaerobic
Francisella	*Peptococcus*
Hemophilus	*Peptostreptococcus*
Legionella	**Acid-Fast Bacilli**
Pasteurella	*Mycobacterium*
Pseudomonas	**Spiral or Curved Bacteria**
Anaerobic	*Borrelia*
Bacteroides	*Campylobacter*
Fusobacterium	*Leptospira*
Gram-Negative Cocci or Coccobacilli	*Spirillum*
Aerobic or Facultative	*Treponema*
Acinetobacter	
Branhamella	
Moraxella	
Neisseria	
Anaerobic	
Veillonella	

his or her immune status; and (4) the susceptibility of the infecting organism. Bacteriology laboratories are capable of direct measurement of the susceptibility of organisms to a series of antimicrobial agents in use in a particular clinical setting. The two basic methods used to make this determination are called the disk diffusion (Fig. 5–2) and the tube dilution methods. Both techniques require pure cultures of the infecting organism(s) isolated from the clinical material and must be performed in a standardized method to yield reliable results.

Results of the disk diffusion tests are usually reported as sensitive (S), resistant (R), or moderate (M). The results are generally interpreted as follows:[54]

Sensitive—Use of the drug at levels generally achievable in the peripheral circulation should be effective in inhibiting the organism.

Resistant—Use of the drug at levels generally achievable in the peripheral circulation will not be effective in inhibiting the organism.

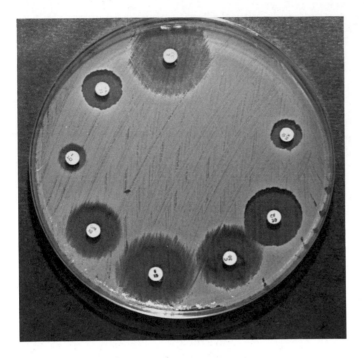

FIGURE 5–2. Disk diffusion antibiotic susceptibility test on *Staphylococcus aureus*. Zones around each filter paper disc represent inhibition of the organism by the antibiotic as it diffuses from the disc.

Moderate—Use of the drug at levels generally achievable in the peripheral circulation cannot be predicted. However, the drug may be effective in areas of the body, such as the urinary tract, where high levels of the drug may be present.

Results of the tube dilution method are often given as a numerical value. These numbers are referred to as the minimal inhibitory concentration (MIC). If the achievable blood level is threefold to fivefold higher than the MIC, the drug should be effective in inhibiting the organism.[55]

Antibiotic resistance due to the presence in bacteria of antibiotic-destroying enzymes can be detected accurately with rapid and simple test procedures. Assays for beta-lactamase are commonly used to detect resistance to penicillin and related drugs in all strains of staphylococci, *Hemophilus influenzae*, *Neisseria gonorrhoeae*, and *Bacteroides species*.[56]

TREATMENT OF WOUND INFECTIONS

A number of different modalities are used in the treatment of wound infections. Infections in the compromised host may involve treatment of the underlying disease, such as control of blood sugar levels in a diabetic. Debridement and/or draining of the wound site is used when necrotic tissue is present and pus has accumulated.

Antimicrobial therapy may not be instituted unless signs of local or systemic spread of the infectious process are evident or the patient is severely immunocompromised. Antimicrobial therapy is normally delayed until results of laboratory testing identify the etiologic agent and its antibiotic susceptibility pattern (antibiogram). Many bacteria carry extrachromosomal genetic elements, called plasmids, that encode for multiple drug resistance. The ability of plasmids to be rapidly transferred from one bacterium to another has resulted in an inability to predict the antibiogram of most bacteria without laboratory testing.

An additional form of therapy in use in some clinical settings is hyperbaric oxygen. Hyperbaric oxygen has been advocated as an adjunct to other types of therapy. This form of treatment involves enclosing the patient in a chamber and increasing the oxygen pressure in that chamber to greater than one atmosphere.[57] Although originally suggested for use in the treatment of anaerobic infections, hyperbaric oxygen therapy is now advocated for infections caused by a variety of aerobic organisms including *Mycobacterium tuberculosis*, *Neisseria meningitidis*, and *Pseudomonas aeruginosa*.[58] Studies using laboratory animals have shown a 92 percent survival rate in experimentally induced infections treated with hyperbaric oxygen, as compared with a 100 percent lethal rate in control animals. A recent study has indicated that the survival rate is due to the increased availability of oxygen for repair by the host tissue rather than an antimicrobial effect against the infecting agents.[59]

CLINICAL DECISION MAKING

Problem. The morning after a sample from a lesion on the lower leg has been sent to the bacteriology laboratory for culture, you call for the preliminary results. The technologist tells you that the direct Gram stain on the previous day had showed numerous gram-positive cocci in clusters. The sample had been plated on a 5 percent sheep blood agar plate and incubated aerobically overnight at 37°C. The aerobic culture was growing a pure culture of approximately 30 white, medium-sized (3 mm in diameter) colonies that were surrounded by a zone of beta-hemolysis. What is the most likely identification of this organism and what is the likely significance of this organism in this sample?

Answer. The most likely identification of this isolate is *Staphylococcus aureus*. The two major groups of gram-positive cocci that grow under aerobic conditions are staphylococci and streptococci. These two groups can often be distinguished by their microscopic appearance because staphylococci tend to occur in clusters while streptococci tend to be in chains. Since the direct Gram stain showed gram-positive cocci in clusters, members of the genus *Staphyloccus* would be more likely. Moreover, the colonial appearance of these two groups of bacteria is usually quite different and the organisms can often be placed in the appropriate genus by looking at the colony. In general, streptococci produce small, pinpoint, colorless colonies while staphylococci produce larger, opaque colonies that are white to yellow. The white, medium-sized colonies favor staphylococci. Moreover, the zone of beta-hemolysis points to identification of the isolate as *Staphylococcus aureus*. Although *S. aureus* is not the only staphylococcal isolate that can be hemolytic, it is the major hemolytic species isolated from human specimens. Confirmation that this organism is *S. aureus* can be achieved in the laboratory by testing for the presence of two enzymes, catalase and coagulase. The presence of catalase confirms the isolate as a member of the staphylococcal group; staphylococci are catalase positive while streptococci are catalase negative. Furthermore, the only member of the genus *Staphylococcus* to produce the enzyme coagulase is *S. aureus*.

The number of colonies that grew from the sample indicates that the isolate is likely to be involved in the disease process. Although *S. aureus* is part of the normal flora of the anterior nares and sometimes other skin sites of approximately 30 percent of the population, the isolation of 30 colonies is indicative of involvement in the disease process. Furthermore, only gram-positive cocci were seen in the direct Gram stain and no other aerobic organisms grew from the same sample. These findings strongly suggest that *S. aureus* is the etiologic agent of the infection.

SUMMARY

A basic concept of which all health professionals must be aware is that microorganisms are everywhere. Potential sources of infection include all areas of the environment, other patients, health-care personnel, and the patient himself or herself. Microbes from an exogenous source can be reduced by sterilizing or disinfecting items that will come in contact with the patient. Items that should be sterilized are those that will bypass the body's first lines of defense and be introduced directly into body tissues. Items that only come in contact with the intact skin and mucous membranes but do not penetrate them may be used after being subjected to a disinfection process. Once an infection has occurred, the etiologic agent can be isolated and identified by submitting material from the infection site to the laboratory. It is essential that the specimen be taken properly and transported immediately to the laboratory to ensure isolation of the infecting agent(s). In addition, the specimen must be labeled as to source so that the microbiologist can select the proper environment and nutrients required by the organisms in the sample.

REFERENCES

1. Evans, AJ: The modern treatment of burns. Br J Hosp Med 13:287, 1975.
2. Gordon-Smith, IC, et al: Management of abdominal aortic aneurysm. Br J Surg 65:834, 1978.
3. Niinikoski, J, Grislis, G, and Hunt, TK: Respiratory gas tensions and collagen in infected wounds. Ann Surg 175:588, 1972.
4. Jackson, DS: Collagen degradation in vivo and in vitro. In Kulonen, E, and Pikkarainen, J (eds): Biology of Fibroblasts. Academic Press, London, 1973, p 411.
5. Irvin, TT: Collagen metabolism in infected colonic anastomoses. Surg Gynecol Obstet 143:220, 1976.
6. Hawley, PR: The aetiology of colonic anastomotic leaks with special reference to the role of collagenase. MS Thesis, University of London, 1969.
7. Smith, IM, et al: Studies on the mechanism of death of mice infected with staphylococci. Infect Dis 107:369, 1960.
8. Bullen, JJ, Cushnie, GH, and Stoner, HB: Oxygen uptake by *Clostridium welchi* type A: Its possible role in experimental infections in passively immunized animals. Br J Exp Pathol 47:488, 1966.
9. Irvin, TT: Wound infection. In Irvin, TT (ed): Wound Healing: Principles and Practice. Chapman and Hall, London, 1981, p 64.
10. Davis, BD, et al: Microbiology, ed 2. Harper and Row, New York, 1973, p 917.
11. Myrvick, QN and Weiser, RS: Fundamentals of Medical Bacteriology and Mycology. Lea and Febiger, Philadelphia, 1988, p 109.
12. Mackowiak, PA: The normal microbial flora. N Engl J Med 307:83, 1982.
13. Miller, CP and Bohnhoff, M: Changes in the mouse's enteric microflora associated with enhanced susceptibility to *Salmonella* infection following streptomycin treatment. J Infect Dis 113:59, 1963.
14. Sewell, CM, et al: Clinical significance of coagulase-negative staphylococci. J Clin Microbiol 16:236, 1982.
15. Karchmer, AW, Archer, GL, and Desmukes, WE: *Staphylococcus epidermidis* causing prosthetic valve endocarditis: Microbiological and clinical observations as guides to therapy. Ann Intern Med 98:477, 1983.
16. Rubin, J, et al: Peritonitis during continous ambulatory dialysis. Ann Intern Med 92:7, 1980.
17. Sherris, JC and Ray, CG: Pathogenesis of infection: Initial defenses, infectivity, virulence, and immune response. In Sherris, JC (ed): Medical Microbiology: An Introduction to Infectious Diseases. Elsevier, New York, 1984, p 59.
18. Mandell, LA, and Feld, R: Infections in the immunocompromised host. In Mandell, LA and Ralph, ED (eds): Essentials of Infectious Diseases. Blackwell Scientific, Boston, 1985, p 337.
19. Phillips, P and Chow, AW: Nosocomial infections. In Mandell, LA and Ralph, ED (eds): Essentials of Infectious Diseases. Blackwell Scientific, Boston, 1985, p 387.
20. Boyd, RF: Host-parasite relationships. In Boyd, RF and Marr, JJ (eds): Medical Microbiology. Little, Brown, Boston, 1980, p 257.

21. Favero, MS: Chemical disinfection of medical and surgical materials. In Block, SS (ed): Disinfection, Sterilization and Preservation, ed 3. Lea and Febiger, Philadelphia, 1983, p 469.
22. Favero, MS: Sterilization, disinfection, and antisepsis in the hospital. In Lennette, EH, et al (eds): Manual of Clinical Microbiology, ed 4. American Society for Microbiology, Washington, DC, 1985, p 129.
23. Block, SS: Federal regulation of disinfectants in the United States. In Block, SS (ed): Disinfection, Sterilization and Preservation, ed 3. Lea and Febiger, Philadelphia, 1983, p 831.
24. Bond, WW, et al: Inactivation of hepatitis B virus by intermediate-to-high level disinfectant chemicals. J Clin Microbiol 18:535, 1983.
25. Walsh, M: Hydrotherapy: The use of water as a therapeutic agent. In Michlovitz, S and Wolfe, S (eds): Contemporary Perspectives in Rehabilitation: Thermal Agents in Rehabilitation. FA Davis, Philadelphia, 1986, p 119.
26. Centers for Disease Control: Suggested Health and Safety Guidelines for Public Spas and Hot Tubs. HHS Pub No 99-960. Centers for Disease Control, Atlanta, 1981, p 1.
27. McMillan, J, et al: Procedure for decontamination of hydrotherapy equipment. Phys Ther 56:57, 1976.
28. Gilardi, GL: Pseudomonas. In Lennette, EH, et al (eds): Manual of Clinical Microbiology, ed 4. American Society for Microbiology, Washington, DC, 1985, p 350.
29. Bassett, DCJ, Stokes, KJ, and Thomas, WRG: Wound infection with Pseudomonas multivorans: A water-borne contaminant of disinfectant solutions. Lancet 1:1188, 1970.
30. Basset, DCJ: The effect of pH on the multiplication of a pseudomonad in chlorhexidine and centrimide. J Clin Pathol 24:708, 1971.
31. Knudsin, RB, Underwood, RH, and Rose, LI: Pseudomonas species ATCC 27330 with 17-dehydrogenase activity: A contaminant in an endocrine laboratory. Appl Microbiol 24:665, 1972.
32. Schaffner, W, Reisig, G, and Verrall, RA: Outbreak of Pseudomonas cepacia infection due to contaminated anaesthetics. Lancet 1:1050, 1973.
33. McNabb, PC, and Tomasi, TB: Host defenses at mucosal surfaces. Annu Rev Microbiol 35:477, 1981.
34. Swanson, J, Sparling, PF, and Puziss, M: Bacterial virulence and pathogenicity. Rev Infect Dis 5:633, 1983.
35. Centers for Disease Control: Acquired immunodeficiency syndrome (AIDS): Precautions for clinical and laboratory staffs. MMWR 31:577, 1982.
36. Centers for Disease Control: Acquired immunodeficiency syndrome (AIDS): Precautions for health-care workers and allied professionals. MMWR 32:450, 1983.
37. Centers for Disease Control: Recommendations for preventing transmission of infection with human T-lymphotropic virus type III/lymphadenopathy-associated virus in the workplace. MMWR 34:681, 1985.
38. Centers for Disease Control: Recommendations for preventing transmission of infection with human T-lymphotropic virus type III/lymphadenopathy-associated virus during invasive procedures. MMWR 35:221, 1986.
39. Centers for Disease Control: Recommendations for preventing transmission of human T-lymphotropic virus type III/lymphadenopathy-associated virus from tears. MMWR 34:533, 1985.
40. Centers for Disease Control: Recommendations for prevention of HIV transmission in health-care settings. MMWR (Suppl) 36:3S, 1987.
41. Robson, M: Management of the contaminated wound: Aids in diagnosis and treatment. In Krizek, T and Hoops, J (eds): Symposium on Basic Sciences in Plastic Surgery. CV Mosby, St Louis, 1976, p 50.
42. Bohnen, JMA and Meakins, JL: Post-operative infection. In Mandell, LA and Ralph, ED (eds): Essentials of Infectious Diseases. Blackwell Scientific, Boston, 1985, p 353.
43. Landis, SJ: Infections in burn patients. In Mandell, LA and Ralph, ED (eds): Essentials of Infectious Diseases. Blackwell Scientific, Boston, 1985, p 371.
44. Koneman, EW, et al: Introduction to Medical Microbiology. In Koneman, EW, et al (eds): Color Atlas and Textbook of Diagnostic Microbiology, ed 2. JB Lippincott, Philadelphia, 1983, p 7.
45. Ronald, AR and Hoban, D: Microbiology for the clinician. In Mandell, LA and Ralph, ED (eds): Essentials of Infectious Diseases. Blackwell Scientific, Boston, 1985, p 3.
46. Henderickson, DA: Reagents and stains. In Lennette, EH, et al (eds): Manual of Clinical Microbiology, ed 4. American Society for Microbiology, Washington, DC, 1985, p 1093.
47. Rogers, HJ: Bacterial Cell Structure. American Society for Microbiology, Washington, DC, 1984, p 20.
48. Appelbaum, PC, et al: Comparison of four methods for identification of gram-negative non-fermenters: Organisms less commonly encountered in clinical specimens. Med Microbiol Immunol 169:163, 1981.
49. Allen, SD: The anaerobic bacteria. In Koneman, EW, et al (eds): Color Atlas and Textbook of Diagnostic Microbiology, ed 2, JB Lippincott, Philadelphia, 1983, p 347.
50. Kilian, M: Haemophilus. In Lennette, EH, et al (eds): Manual of Clinical Microbiology, ed 4. American Society for Microbiology, Washington, DC, 1987, p 387.
51. Tilton, RC (ed): Rapid Methods and Automation in Microbiology. Proceedings of the Third International Symposium on Rapid Methods and Automation in Microbiology, Washington, DC, 1982, p 1.
52. Tenover, FC: Diagnostic dexoxyribonucleic acid probes for infectious diseases. Clin Microbiol Rev 1:82, 1988.
53. Edelstein, PH, et al: Retrospective study of Gen-Prove rapid diagnostic system for detection of Legionella in frozen clinical respiratory tract samples. J Clin Microbiol 25:1022, 1987.
54. Thornsberry, C and Sherris, J: Laboratory tests in chemotherapy: General considerations. In Lennette, EH,

et al (eds): Manual of Clinical Microbiology, ed 4. American Society for Microbiology, Washington, DC, 1985, p 959.

55. Petersdorf, RG, and Plorde, JJ: The usefulness of in vitro sensitivity tests in antibiotic therapy. Annu Rev Med 14:41, 1963.

56. Thornsberry, C, Gavan, TL, and Gerlach, EH: New developments in antimicrobial agent susceptibility testing. In Sherris, JC (ed): Cumitech 6. American Society for Microbiology, Washington, DC, 1977, p 1.

57. Harris, M and Young, D: Hyperbaric medicine: A specialized mode of treatment that is gaining acceptance. Indiana Med 25:258, 1987.

58. Holmes, C and Gargis, L: Effects of hyperbaric oxygen. J Infect Dis 155:1084, 1987.

59. Thom, SR, Lauermann, MW, and Hart, GB: Intermittent hyperbaric oxygen therapy for reduction of mortality in experimental polymicrobic sepsis. J Infect Dis 154:504, 1986.

CHAPTER 6

Nutritional Requirements for Patients with Chronic Wounds

Gail C. Frank, Dr.P.H., M.P.H., L.D.N., R.D.

Undernourished individuals cannot respond physiologically well to any form of rehabilitation. When the patient is experiencing either an acute stage or a continuous high-risk stage of a chronic wound, tailored nutritional care is essential. While all health-care practitioners need to possess a working knowledge of clinical nutrition, the responsibility for determining the nutritional requirements of patients rests primarily with the registered dietitian. The major focus of this chapter is therefore directed toward the registered dietitian and his or her role in the rehabilitation of patients with chronic wounds. Although this material may appear somewhat overwhelming to other health professionals, an attempt is made to address other health professionals' roles in identifying the need for dietary intervention.

THE STRESS OF CELLULAR INJURY

During stress from cellular injury, the body responds with major alterations in energy and protein metabolism directed by hormonal changes. There is an increase in antidiuretic hormone (ADH), adrenocorticotropic hormone (ACTH), catecholamines, and glucagon. In response to these hormonal changes, the body experiences a diminished protein-conserving capacity. As a result, the metabolic rate increases and, although somewhat adverse to need, fat catabolism and ketone utilization are blocked.[1] The response has been depicted as an *ebb and flow* pattern.[2] The immediate response — the *ebb* — is characterized by circulatory insufficiency of protein and energy and is often referred to as *shock*. This response is followed by an increased metabolism or hypermetabolic state coupled with depletion of body protein within 24 to 48 hours after an injury — the *flow*. Nutritional care during stress and wound healing must encompass the unstable or catabolic phase and the anticipated anabolic or recovery phase. In addition, nutrition has a major role in maintaining both homeostasis and the body's resistance to infection while furthering a healthy recovery when chronic wounds exist.

The extent of catabolic response to wounds depends on the severity of the stress.

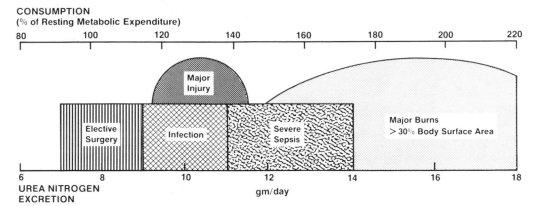

FIGURE 6–1. Rates of hypermetabolism estimated from urinary urea nitrogen excretion (Adapted from Blackburn, et al,[12] p. 11, 1977.).

Figure 6–1 depicts the increasing need for energy to complement the severity of stress and to minimize protein breakdown for energy. Urea nitrogen excretion indicates protein loss.

There is only a slight increase in resting metabolic expenditure with elective surgery, but the demand for energy is 20 to 30 percent above normal needs with infection. Urea nitrogen excretion may be 9 to 11 g per day. Severe sepsis or extensive burns can double or triple the energy demands and double the urea nitrogen excretion of an otherwise normally functioning individual. In the presence of a suboptimal nutritional state, the body's recovery rate is vastly restricted. The ability of the body to defend and to repair itself depends jointly on the extent and frequency of injury and nutritional status. Cellular injury that results from a chronic disease may be recurrent and may require continual vigilance of the body's defenses. Such is the case of the patient with diabetes experiencing recurrent infections often leading to gangrene.

Chronic wounds can overlap several levels of stress depending on the severity of the wound and the stage of healing. For example, a patient presents with a stage I decubitus ulcer with a mild infection. The unbroken skin is pink and feels warm, but blanches on touch. Discoloration lasts several minutes after pressure is released. The energy demands in this patient would be approximately 20 to 30 percent above normal needs.

On the other hand, a patient presents with a stage III decubitus ulcer. The skin is broken and black in areas due to the necrotic tissue. Some of the tissue is yellow and draining. The site of the decubiti makes healing difficult, as the patient lies on the area and brushes it frequently. For this patient the energy demands are doubled to 40 to 60 percent above normal needs.

The age and health habits of the patient are also important. With chronic wounds, patients often experience periods of nutritional deprivation in an effort either to reduce pain (such as occurs with ulceration) or to diminish the side effects of eating (e.g., diarrhea or vomiting). Inadequate nutrition only compounds the problem. During starvation and immobilization, wound healing requires sufficient mobilization of amino acids, nonprotein calories, minerals, and trace elements.[3] If the body stores are low, then nutritious foods or supplements must be provided, with differentiation between an enteral or a parenteral modality, if needed.

This chapter outlines the steps needed to develop a program of tailored nutrition care when managing patients with chronic wounds. The discussion is presented in four stages of program development: planning, assessing, implementing, and monitoring. During the planning stage, clarification of diet order and identification of personnel are essential. Components of a comprehensive nutritional assessment are discussed in two parts: an initial interview conducted during the planning stage, followed by a second, more detailed assessment during the assessing stage if a patient is labeled as high risk. During the implementing stage, the strategies appropriate for the patient's nutritional status are considered. A discussion of parenteral and enteral nutrition includes the benefits and possible complications of each therapy. The final stage, monitoring the success of therapy, improves the continuity of care and provides the vigilance required to restore patients to normal functioning.

In this chapter, nutrition is presented as a substrate for wound healing. Several definitions are pertinent to this concept and discussion. A brief glossary is provided at the end of the chapter for reference and clarity of subject matter.

PLANNING MODEL FOR A TAILORED NUTRITIONAL CARE PROGRAM

Upon hospital admission, certain questions should be asked about the patient. First, "Has there been a recent body weight loss?" If so, "does it amount to 7 to 10 percent or more of current body weight?" Second, "Has there been a recent major procedure such as surgery or chemotherapy, or does a chronic condition exist?" Third, "Has the recent illness been longer than 3 weeks? Has the patient been unable to eat usual foods in average amounts?" If the patient has been hospitalized for 3 days or more, then an additional question is, "Has the patient received intravenous support with dextrose or saline only for 5 or more days?" A positive response to any of these questions should alert medical professionals to a potentially high-risk patient. Further evaluation is necessary to establish the tailored nutrition care program.

Planning

The goal of planning is to establish the framework by which an individual or team can evaluate a patient, implement a therapy, and monitor the patient's progress in a timely fashion. Of equal importance is the assurance of quality care and the continuous updating of procedures as techniques improve. The planning process involves an initial series of steps.

STEP 1: Identify personnel.
STEP 2: Confirm physician's diet order.

Step 1 is basic to the program development and implementation. Specific personnel must be identified to conduct the nutrition care program. If a dietitian coordinates a nutrition care program, the program mimics the skills of that individual. Registered dietitians functioning in a critical-care practice should be highly trained to assume the position. Clarity of the responsibilities of all staff members in carrying out the nutrition care plan is essential. Agriesti-Johnson[4] has specified the roles and responsibilities of nutritional support team members in a questionnaire format.

Nutritional support teams have become an effective approach in many hospital settings and link several professionals: physicians, nurses, pharmacists, and registered dietitians (RD). When a team is functioning, the skill of the dietitian remains pivotal.[5-7]

Within 48 hours after a patient has been admitted to the hospital, the physician has ordered special nutrition care, and steps 2 to 4 should be completed. The dietitian confirms the physician's written diet order, conducts a medical record review, and completes the first patient contact. These initial activities will determine the degree of nutritional support that the patient requires.

Assessing

STEP 3: Conduct medical record review
STEP 4: Schedule initial consultation with patient
STEP 5: Evaluate and/or establish need for additional diagnostic data
STEP 6: Complete assessment

The medical record review should include the following data: body weight on entry and daily weights thereafter; height; serum albumin; complete blood count; serum glucose; blood urea nitrogen (BUN) and creatinine; vital signs; fluid intake and output; and other laboratory data that are disease specific such as amylase for pancreatitis, blood cholesterol and triglycerides for arteriosclerosis, or ammonia for cirrhosis.[8,9] Current medications or treatments such as hemodialysis, chemotherapy, or radiation should be identified. Information regarding bowel habits, gastrointestinal function, presence of edema, obesity, and dental health is important.

Seltzer and colleagues[10] developed an "instant nutritional assessment" to aid decision making with only two parameters: serum albumin and total lymphocyte count. They noted correlations between increased morbidity and mortality and low levels of albumin and lymphocytes. A fourfold increase in complications and a sixfold increase in death was associated with serum albumin concentrations less than 3.5 g per dl. Patients were at a 1.8 times greater risk of developing complications and were 4.0 times more likely to die if total lymphocyte count was less than 1500 per mm^3.[10]

During the initial consultation with the patient, a fairly complete eating behavior history is obtained. Pertinent information includes the patient's physical ability to eat or drink as a result of level of consciousness, pain, dental health, physical impairment, dysphagia, or use of life support equipment.[8] The patient's dietary pattern during the previous 7 days and resulting weight are important variables used to determine the duration of suboptimal nutrition. The dietary history should identify if substance abuse has occurred or if the patient has experienced a roller coaster weight history including bulimia and anorexia.

A 24-hour dietary recall should be included in the diet history. This recall provides a quick measure of total protein and energy intake. From the recall, the dietitian can calculate the percentage of recommended protein and energy actually being consumed. An estimate of usual 24-hour fluid intake from water, carbonated beverage, tea, coffee, milk, and juice is also possible from the recall.

After the initial interview, step 5 involves review of the data. A patient is classified as high risk if the following conditions are noted:[8]

1. Patient has not taken food for more than 7 days
2. During the past 5 days, protein and energy intakes were less than 85 percent of recommended intake for age and sex
3. Current weight is 90 percent or less of desirable body weight

4. Serum albumin concentration is less than 3.5 g per 100 ml
5. Specific diagnosis or treatment warrant further study *or*
6. Complications secondary to the current therapy prolong restricted nutrient intake.

If the status of the patient indicates a high-risk or borderline high-risk situation, then a complete nutritional assessment should be obtained during the next 24-hour period.

The information gathered during step 6 confirms the presence of a suboptimal nutritional condition and is used to determine the appropriate amount, type, and method of nutritional support needed. The patient's blood pressure, temperature, pulse, and respiratory history during hospitalization are reviewed. Serum sodium, potassium, and magnesium levels are monitored, as are more recent blood counts. In addition, the dietitian gathers information regarding the patient's attitudes and practices with food, and the amount of body fat is estimated with simple anthropometric measures. For example, the patient's food intolerances, allergies, and bulimic or anorexic episodes are detailed. Self-prescribed vitamin and mineral supplements and alcohol use by type, frequency, and amount are documented. The patient's ability to provide food, nursing, and medical care is determined. As the nutrition care plan is tailored for the patient, a long-range goal is to establish the capability of the patient to receive appropriate nutritional support at home. Alerting the social services personnel to evaluate the patient for follow-up care early in the patient's hospitalization is recommended to maintain continuity of care.

Anthropometric measures provide a quantitative measure of the composition of the body and can gauge tissue depletion.[11,12] Triceps skinfold and arm circumference measurements are relatively easy to obtain and can be compared with standard percentiles for healthy men and women.[13] The right arm should be used for these measurements.

Procedure for Anthropometric Measures. Arm muscle circumference is the circumference of the inner, upper arm, which is mainly muscle with a small central bone. Since bone is a constant, if muscle mass changes, then a change in muscle circumference indicates protein depletion.[12,14]

To assess arm circumference, the patient stands and bends the right forearm toward the abdomen. The distance between the acromial process of the scapula and the olecranon process of the ulna is recorded. This distance is divided by two to locate the midpoint. The midpoint is marked on the outer curvature of the arm. The circumference is measured at the midpoint to the nearest millimeter using a flexible steel tape.[15,16]

Arm muscle area is a more accurate two-dimensional measurement and is calculated as follows:

$$\text{Arm muscle area (mm}^2) = \frac{\text{Arm circumference (mm}^2)}{4\,\pi}$$

The triceps skinfold is measured with calipers in back of the arm at the midpoint between the acromial and olecranon processes. With the patient's arm hanging in a relaxed position, about 1 cm of skin and fat is picked up above the midpoint. Lange skinfold calipers are placed over the fatfold at the midpoint and released. Without 4 seconds, the reading is taken. The procedure is repeated for two additional readings; then the three measures are averaged.[15] Changes in subcutaneous fat occur slowly and therefore do not reflect acute changes in nutritional status. In chronic malnutrition, however, subcutaneous fat stores become markedly depleted and percent body fat measurements reveal significant changes from published norms.

To further characterize the patient according to the degree of protein catabolism, calculating a catabolic index is useful.[16] This index integrates dietary protein intake represented by nitrogen intake in food (N), urinary urea nitrogen (UUN), and metabolic stress into a single number. The equation is:

$$\text{Catabolic Index} = \text{UUN} - (0.5 \text{ N from intake} + 3)$$

A score of −5 to 0 indicates no stress or mild stress, 0 to +5 is moderate stress, and +5 to 10, severe stress. The catabolic index has been demonstrated as useful in determining whether patients will improve when treated with amino acid solutions enriched with branched-chain amino acids.[17] Moderately to severely catabolic patients with fluid intolerance or organ failure and lower protein intakes demonstrate a reduced net protein catabolism when given branched-chain amino-acid–enriched formulas. On the other hand, a patient with a catabolic index of less than 0 or one who received more than 1 g of protein per kg experiences little benefit from branched-chain amino acids.[17]

The urinary urea nitrogen loss serves as a major indicator of overall stress level. Table 6–1 incorporates seven parameters including urinary nitrogen level to identify stress levels ranging from 0 to 3. With stress and sepsis, alteration in the metabolism of the energy-yielding nutrients occurs. Indicators of the carbohydrate aberrations include insulin resistance and elevated total glucose plus an increase in lactate from the excess carbohydrate.[18] Having a working knowledge of the level of stress of a patient simplifies decisions about the appropriate nutritional support required.

Within the American Dietetic Association, a practice group exists for dietitians in critical-care specialties. Dietitians in this group have outlined problem-specific criteria for the assessment and nutrition management of patients with critical conditions. A booklet entitled, "Suggested Guidelines for Nutrition Management of the Critically Ill Patient" is an excellent resource and reference guide and capsulates extensive information beyond the scope of this chapter. Criteria are outlined for patients with acute respiratory failure, burns, cancer, pressure ulcers, inflammatory bowel disease, multisystem organ failure, sepsis, and surgery.[8]

Role of the Non-nutritionist. Often the medical setting does not have an active evaluation or referral system for nutritional care of patients. In this case, physical therapists or other health professionals who are routinely in contact with patients may suspect that a certain patient needs nutritional evaluation. Their astute observations and inquiries may aid referral of patients with suboptimal nutrition.

What can the non-nutritionist evaluate to see if a patient needs referral to a

TABLE 6–1. Steps for Establishing a Tailored Nutrition Care
Program for High-Risk Patients

Stage	Step	Activity
Planning	1	Identify personnel
	2	Confirm physician's diet order
Assessing	3	Conduct medical record review
	4	Schedule initial consultation with patient
	5	Evaluate and/or establish need for additional diagnostic data
	6	Complete assessment
Implementing	7	Formulate care plan
	8	Implement program
Monitoring	9	Monitor patient progress
	10	Provide discharge and home care instructions

registered dietitian? Answering the following four questions should provide vital information:

1. Are there any visible wounds such as an ulcer or incision or a recurrent infection or lesion? These are direct evidence that a patient's stress level is elevated and that immediate attention is needed.
2. Is the current functional capacity of the gastrointestinal tract limiting nutrient absorption? That is, is the patient experiencing frequent vomiting or diarrhea?
3. What is the result of an "instant nutritional assessment"? Is the lymphocyte count less than 1500 per mm^3 and is the albumin less than 3.5 g per dl?
4. What is the patient's weight history during the past 3 weeks? Is the weight loss more than 10 percent of current body weight?

If any of these questions is answered with a "yes," then the patient should be referred to a registered dietitian immediately.

Implementing

STEP 7: Formulate care plan
STEP 8: Implement program

After completion of steps 3 to 6, the dietitian can proceed to step 7 with the assurance that a comprehensive review of the patient's status has been performed. The stress level as defined in Table 6–1 serves as a reference for tailoring and implementing the nutritional care program, steps 7 and 8.

Table 6–2 identifies the energy and protein needs based on stress level and establishes the important nutrient substrates. The substrates are presented in proportions that decrease the likelihood of complications and increase the chances of recovery.[18]

Caloric requirements are based on the estimated basal energy expenditure (BEE) and injury and activity factors.[19] Adequate energy intake is essential to aid maintenance and/or gain of body weight and lean body mass.[20] The DuBois nomogram and Boothby chart can also be used to determine basal energy requirements.[21] The BEE is sex-specific; is easy to use; and requires only weight in kilograms, height in centimeters, and age in years. This formula correlates well with DuBois' and Boothby's determinations and is used widely as an accurate expression of energy need. The formula is:

BEE male = 66.4730 + [13.7516 × (wt in kg)] +
[5.0033 × (ht in cm) − [6.7550 × (age in yrs)]

BEE female = 655.0955 + [9.5634 × (wt in kg)] +
[1.8496 × (ht in cm) − [4.6756 × (age in yrs)]

Once the total BEE is established, the nutrient composition can be determined. The extent by which BEE must be increased depends on activity and injury. Table 6–2 outlines a progressive increase of BEE with stress level. Long and colleagues[22] established the following formula to include activity and injury variables in calculation of total energy needs:

Total kcal per 24 hr = BEE × activity factor × injury factor

TABLE 6–2. Stratification of Metabolic Stress Needs

Stress Level	Clinical Type	Urinary Nitrogen Loss (g/day)	Plasma Lactate* (m/l)	Plasma Glucose† (mg%)	Insulin Resistance	Oxygen Consumption Index (ml/M2)	Glucagon Insulin Ratio
0	Nonstress starvation	<5	100 ± 50	100 ± 20	−	90 ± 10	2.0 ± 0.5
1	Elective general surgery	5 ± 10	1200 ± 200	150 ± 25	−	130 ± 6	2.5 ± 0.8
2	Polytrauma	10 ± 15	1200 ± 200	150 ± 25	+	140 ± 6	3.0 ± 0.7
3	Sepsis/ hypermetabolic state	>15	2500 ± 500	250 ± 50	+	160 ± 10	8.0 ± 1.5

*with normal lactate : pyruvate ratio
†no diabetes or pancreatitis
From Nutritional Support Services, Vol 4, No 2, Feb 1984, with permission.

Activity factors are 1.2 for "confined to bed" to 1.3 for "out of bed." Injury factors are minor surgery 1 to 1.2, peritonitis 1.2 to 1.5, soft-tissue trauma 1.14 to 1.37, skeletal trauma 1.35, starvation 0.7, and major sepsis 1.4 to 1.8. For each degree of fever above 98.6°F, a factor of 1.07 can be used.[22]

The hypermetabolic patient may require nonprotein calories at 150 to 200 percent of the BEE, but acceptance of substrates is essential. Table 6–3 summarizes the recommended percentage of total calories from glucose, fat, and amino acids by stress level. If a hyperglycemia of 250 mg persists, then carbohydrate calories should be partially replaced with fat calories or adjunct insulin may be required on a sliding scale. Triglyceride levels should be monitored to assess tolerance of fat. Elevated triglycerides may warrant discontinuance of fat until the stress level decreases.

Protein requirements increase as stress level rises. Branched-chain amino acids can improve nitrogen retention, enhance protein synthesis, and reduce proteolysis as mentioned earlier.[23] The branched-chain amino acids are three essential amino acids: leucine, isoleucine, and valine. As stress increases, these amino acids are oxidized for energy and configured for protein synthesis at an increased rate. Apparently, increasing the supply of the branched-chain amino acids serves a twofold purpose. They meet the increased requirement for amino acids while reducing the exogenous supply. The result is an improved clinical profile.[23] A ratio of nonprotein calories to nitrogen is useful in progressing patients to higher levels of protein intake as stress levels increase. For example, a patient at a 0 stress level can still be nutritionally deficient and need 150 kcal per 1 g of nitrogen (see Table 6–2). Nitrogen is determined by dividing total protein intake in grams by 6.25. A patient at stress level 3 may need a reduced nonprotein calorie intake in relation to protein or a ratio of 80 : 1.[18]

Essential fatty acids should provide a minimum of 4 percent of the total caloric intake, otherwise the risk of a fatty acid deficiency increases. This risk is real if nonprotein calories are provided entirely by dextrose. As a safeguard, a minimum of two bottles of 500 ml of 10 percent fat emulsion should be administered weekly if no lipids are included in the nonprotein calories. As much as 40 percent of the total energy intake as fat has been tolerated well by patients at high stress levels.[18]

Electrolyte, vitamin, and trace element needs vary with the presence of other conditions but must be adjusted to achieve or maintain normal levels.[24]

Enteral or Parenteral Therapy? The nature of the nutritional support depends on several factors, including the aggregate evaluation of the patient's condition and his or her ability to ingest foods at the calculated nutrient level. Often the nutritional modality is a combination of solid food, enteral therapy, and/or parenteral therapy. The purpose of each therapy is to provide the necessary nutrient substrate in the form most effectively used by the body.[25] Frequently, therapy will change until the patient achieves an anabolic state. Enteral and parenteral feedings have both demonstrated effectiveness in achieving an anabolic state.[26] The literature is extensive on each topic and only general guidelines are presented herein.

Enteral nutritional therapy is delivering nutrients via the oral route when the patient has a functional gastrointestinal tract. The patient may be unable to eat, however, or it may be anticipated that the patient cannot consume ample solid food to achieve either sufficient calories or the blend of nutrients calculated as essential. Often enteral feeding is a transitional modality, seen as having a major advantage over parenteral therapy due to cost and potential reduction of complications.[27] Further, enteral therapy allows continuous use of the gastrointestinal tract and enhances normal functioning of the intestine, pancreas, and liver.[28,29] A reduced frequency of gastrointestinal bleeding has been noted for patients receiving enteral feeding.[30] In addition,

TABLE 6-3. Summary of Metabolic Stress Needs

| Stress Level | BEE | Total kcal | | | | Nonprotein kcal | | Amino Acids |
		kcal/kg/day	% Amino Acids	% Glucose	% Fat	Ratio to g N	kcal/kg/day	(g/kg/day)
0	1.0 × BEE	28	15	60	25	150:1	25	1.0
1	1.3 × BEE	32	20	50	30	100:1	25	1.5
2	1.5 × BEE	40	25	40	35	100:1	30	2.0
3	2.0 × BEE	50	30	70	35	80:1	35	3.0

Adapted from Table III, Konstantidinis, 1984. From Nutritional Support Services, Vol 4, No 2, Feb 1984, with permission.

delivery of the enteral feeding with a pump has been shown to reduce diarrhea because a steady infusion is possible.[31]

Several metabolic complications may occur with enteral therapy including electrolyte imbalances, potential damage to kidney or liver function if protein intakes are excessive, and elevated lipids if fat intolerance exists.[32,33] Vanlandingham and colleagues[34] followed 100 patients receiving enteral therapy and observed 29 percent developing hyperglycemia and 2 percent hypoglycemia. Both conditions occurred as frequently among diabetics as nondiabetics. Thirty-one percent had hyponatremia compared with 10 percent experiencing hypernatremia. Forty percent experienced hyperkalemia, whereas eight percent had hypokalemia.[34] Metabolic aberrations such as these must be kept to a minimum to stabilize and to progress patients to normal functioning.[18]

Choosing the appropriate commercial product for an enteral feeding requires a comparison of the nutrient content of various products. Manufacturers of enteral formula provide detailed charts of the nutritional content of products. A listing of current manufacturers and their formulas is given in Table 6–4. To create a hospital inventory, a group of products that seem to meet the most frequent demands of patients should be selected. Tailoring for a specific patient involves assessing the product's ability to meet the nutrient needs of the patient, but cost, osmolality, viscosity, lactose content, and other factors should also be considered.[35]

A recent innovation to enteral nutrition is the use of modular feeding or the addition of single nutrients to a base formula. This application allows a tailoring of formula to meet specific alterations in metabolism and should be considered for high-risk patients capable of enteral nutritional support.[36]

If a patient needs a tube feeding, then the feeding route is based on the expected

TABLE 6–4. Manufacturers of Enteral Formula

Manufacturer	Formula
Biosearch	Entrition
Chesebrough-Pond's	Fortison, Magnacal, Microlipid, Propac, Sumacal, Vitaneed
Kendall McGaw	Amin-Aid, Hepatic Aid II, Traum-Aid HBC
Mead Johnson	Casec, Criticare HN, Isocal, Isocal II, Isocal HCN, MCT Oil, Moducal, Portagen, Susta II, Sustacal Liquid, Sustacal HC, Sustagen, Traumacal
Navaco	High Fat Supplement, Liquid Carbohydrate Supplement, ProMix, Pure Carbohydrate Supplement, Isolife
Norwich Eaton	Vivonex High Nitrogen, Vivonex Standard, Vivonex T.E.N
Ross	Enrich, Ensure, Ensure HN, Ensure Plus, Ensure Plus HN, Osmolite, Osmolite HN, Polycose Liquid, Polycose Powder, ProMod, Pulmocare, Ross SLD, TwoCal HN, Vital High Nitrogen, Jevity, Ensure Powder, Glucerna
Sandoz	Citrotein, Compleat Modified, Compleat Regular, Isotein HN, Meritene Liquid, Nutrisource Amino Acids, Nutrisource Amino Acids—HBC, Nutrisource Carbohydrate, Nutrisource Lipid—LCT, Nutrisource Lipid—MCT, Nutrisource Minerals for Amino Acid Formulas, Nutrisource Minerals for Amino Acid Formulas—Electrolyte Restricted, Nutrisource Minerals for Protein Formulas, Nutrisource Minerals for Protein Formulas—Electrolyte Restricted, Nutrisource Protein, Nutrisource Vitamins, Precision High Nitrogen, Precision Isotonic Diet, Precision LR Diet, Resource, Stresstein
Clintec Nutrition	Travasorb, Travasorb Hepatic, Travasorb MCT, Travasorb HN, Travasorb Renal, Travasorb STD

duration of tube feeding, the status of the alimentary tract and any potential for aspiration. For a short-term tube feeding, nasal intubation for gastric or transpyloric feeding is common. If an extended enteral feeding is anticipated and the patient can tolerate surgery, then an ostomy may be considered.[37]

Parenteral nutrition is a method of nutritional support placed directly into the circulatory system, bypassing the gastrointestinal tract.[38] Total parenteral nutrition or intravenous hyperalimentation is a method for direct intravenous or intramuscular administration of all nutrients. Parenteral nutrition is selected as the preferred therapy when a patient cannot ingest adequate nutrients through the gastrointestinal tract. The survival of the patient may depend on selecting this therapy, which is often indicated for chronic vomiting, diarrhea, malabsorption syndromes, prolonged ileus or gastrointestinal obstruction, malignancies, and burns. Fistulas and bowel and renal diseases may warrant parenteral therapy.[27] Use of parenteral therapy is appropriate if the gastrointestinal tract will not be functional or will be limited in function for 7 or more days. If the patient has a functional alimentary tract or if a terminal state exists in which aggressive nutritional treatment is not deemed necessary, then parenteral nutrition may appear useful but should likely not be selected.[38]

Since the parenteral nutrient solutions are usually hypertonic, they can cause phlebitis or thrombosis if infused via peripheral veins. A central venous cannulation is preferred, particularly entry through the superior vena cava. This approach allows the hypertonic solutions to be diluted rapidly into the bloodstream avoiding phlebitis and thrombosis.[38]

There are complications from parenteral nutrition using central venous catheters, including metabolic problems and problems resulting from the catheter itself. The major metabolic problems are hypoglycemia and hyperglycemia, glucosuria, liver enzyme alterations, mineral and electrolyte abnormalities, and nutrient deficiencies.[38] Catheter problems may involve infections resulting from contaminated catheters or solutions; looping or splitting catheters; and difficulties during cannulation such as air embolus, vein laceration, or pneumothorax. If parenteral nutrition therapy is selected, then safe and aseptic catheter insertion, along with preparation of noncontaminated nutrient solutions and routine checks of the delivery process, is essential.[38]

Peripheral hyperalimentation, on the other hand, offers some advantages over the central vein approach. These include the reduction in risks with the catheter placement, ease in caring for the infusion site, and elimination of complications of hyperosmolar glucose infusions.[39] Severely catabolic patients may not be candidates for the peripheral hyperalimentation since usual regimens provide only 50 to 100 g of protein per 24 hours. Generally, the following criteria should be followed for selecting patients for peripheral rather than central venous entry:[39,40]

1. Patient has an acceptable nutritional status
2. The anticipated caloric requirements are not significantly greater than normal or less than 2000 kcal per day
3. Oral intake has been restricted for no more than 7 to 10 days

The nutrient solutions selected for the parenteral feeding must constitute the essential nutrients in the proportions indicated by the stress level and normal requirements. Generally, the most commonly used substrates for carbohydrate, amino acids, and fat are dextrose, crystalline L-amino acids, and intravenous fat emulsions, respectively. Glucose monohydrate is the form of dextrose used and has 3.4 kcal per g rather than 4 kcal per g. Dextrose is available in 5, 10, 20, 25, 50, and 70 percent concentrations. Using the concentration and total volume, the total energy content of a solution can be calculated. For example, 500 ml D50 in water equals 50 g dextrose per 100 ml, or 5 × 50 or 250 g dextrose in 500 ml; 250 g × 3.4 kcal per g = 850 kcal from dextrose.

Amino acids are available as synthetic crystalline L-amino acids and have been shown to allow better nitrogen utilization.[41] Several products are available with various concentrations of protein; for example, Travasol by Clintec Nutrition is available in 3.5, 5.5, 8.5, and 10 percent concentrations.[40] A container of 600 ml of Travasol at 5.5 percent concentration is equivalent to 5.5 g of protein in 100 ml, or 5.5 g × 6 = 33 g protein. This amount equals 33 g × 4 kcal per g, or 132 kcal. Further, 33 g divided by 6.25 g protein per 1 g nitrogen = 5.28 g of nitrogen.

Fat emulsions provide 9 kcal per g and may comprise more than 35 percent of total energy needs but should provide a minimum of 4 percent of the total calories as essential fatty acids. Fat emulsions are more expensive than dextrose and have been shown to provide less protein-sparing effect than glucose in select clinical conditions.[27] Two common intravenous fat emulsions are Intralipid, a soybean product by Clintec Nutrition, and Liposyn, a safflower product by Abbott.

Water, electrolytes, minerals, and vitamins must be added to the parenteral solution to meet the requirements of the patient. Fluid is essential for normal urination, and needs are based primarily on body weight and temperature. For the first 10 kg of body weight, calculate 100 ml per kg. If the patient weighs 11 to 20 kg, then add 50 ml per kg for each kilogram greater than 10 kg. For a patient weighing more than 20 kg, add 20 ml for each kilogram greater than 20 kg.[42,43] In effect, a 58-kg woman would need 100 ml × 10 for the first 10 kg, or 1000 ml. Then she would need 50 ml × 10 for the second 10 kg, or 500 ml. Finally, she would need 20 ml × 38 for the remaining 38 kg, or 760 ml. This amount totals 2260 ml of fluid in a 24-hour period.

If fever is present, then fluid needs should be increased by 360 ml per degree Celsius per 24 hours.[27] Conversely, if the patient has renal insufficiency, significant liver or cardiovascular disease, then fluids may need to be progressively decreased.[42]

The addition of electrolytes and minerals depends on the serum concentrations identified during the assessment stage, losses that are known and the ability of the kidney to function.[27] The ratio of potassium to nitrogen should be 3.5 mEq potassium to 1 g nitrogen to ensure protein synthesis.[44] Because trace mineral deficiencies have been noted for patients receiving total parenteral therapy, the recommendations of the Nutrition Advisory Group of the American Medical Association Department of Foods and Nutrition should be incorporated into the tailored nutritional care plan.[45]

The four most important trace elements are zinc, chromium, copper, and manganese, which are all available in solutions.[39] Zinc is needed for more than 70 different enzymes, promotes wound healing, assists normal skin hydration, and aids the senses of taste and smell. Chromium is one part of the glucose tolerance factor and activates insulin-mediated reactions. Chromium is most important for maintaining normal glucose metabolism and peripheral nerve function. Copper is a cofactor for serum ceruloplasmin, an oxidase needed for transferrin formation. Copper helps form white and red blood cells. Manganese initiates enzymatic reactions involving polysaccharide polymerase, liver arginase, cholinesterase, and pyruvate carboxylase.[46] For patients receiving total parenteral nutrition, the 24-hour recommended dosage of these four trace elements is zinc 2.5 to 4 mg; chromium 10 to 15 μg/per L; copper 0.5 to 1.5 mg per day; and manganese 0.15 to 0.8 g per day.[45,47]

Both fat- and water-soluble vitamins are essential for the patient receiving parenteral therapy.[48] Vitamin C deficiency is known to inhibit wound healing. If a patient's body stores of vitamin C are low, then frank deficiency can occur due to the added stress of illness, requirements of wound healing, and demand for ascorbate to detoxify certain medications or anesthetics.[49] One product, MVI-12, produced by Armour, is composed of the recommended adult dosage of vitamins, except for vitamin K.

As can be recognized from this discussion, skill in calculation of the parenteral solution is essential. Several instructive materials are available and should be completed as inservice by staff members performing this service.[50]

Step 8, or implementation of the nutritional care plan, begins with initiation of an enteral or parenteral therapy after the physician's order has been verified and pertinent assessments and calculations have been completed. Although the medical staff may be knowledgeable in all aspects of each nutritional modality, a standardized form for initiating the therapy is recommended (Fig. 6–2). The form identifies placement, equipment size, administration rate, and other pertinent activities to ensure clarity of instruction and delivery. Established hospital procedures for implementing the nutritional plan should be followed, all pertinent decisions or modifications in the diet composition should be documented, and the calculated diet composition should be enumerated in the patient's chart.

Monitoring

STEP 9: Monitor patient progress
STEP 10: Provide discharge and home care instructions

Monitoring assesses both the effectiveness of therapy and the metabolic response pattern of the patient. The movement from a high stress to a lower stress level can be tracked as well as the onset of sepsis or other complications.[18] The potential for nutrient–drug interaction is possible and a careful, consistent evaluation is needed to minimize any potential complications that could hamper the recovery of the patient.

Andrassy[51] has observed that only 60 to 70 percent of the total calories and protein ordered for patients are actually delivered often due to protocol violations. As few as 40 to 50 percent of recommended nutrients may be given to patients when activities are the responsibility of routine nursing care.[51] In addition, 5 of the 14 "undesirable practices" identified by Butterworth[49] as affecting the nutritional health of patients are germane to understanding that a successful nutritional care program involves all aspects of the medical environment. Common situations influencing nutritional health of patients are:

1. Withholding meals due to diagnostic tests
2. Performing surgical procedures without first making certain that the patient is optimally nourished
3. Failing to provide nutritional support after surgery
4. Failing to appreciate the role of nutrition in the prevention of and recovery from infection, giving unwarranted reliance on antibiotics
5. Delaying nutritional support until the patient is in an advanced state of depletion, which may be irreversible
6. Limiting laboratory tests for nutritional status due to lack of availability of procedures.[49]

Monitoring thereby implies a means of ensuring that the tailored nutritional care program for a patient is, in fact, implemented in all phases of medical care. A summary of the major metabolic and anthropometric variables that should be monitored to complete step 9 is presented in a time line in Table 6–5. Generally, the variables that reflect carbohydrate, fat, and protein metabolism are the most useful.[18] Glucose, insulin,

DATE	TIME	INSTRUCTIONS: PLEASE USE BALLPOINT PEN AND PRESS FIRMLY.

DELETE THOSE ORDERS DENOTED BY AN "X"

Check (√) APPROPRIATE BOX WHERE CHOICE INDICATED

1.   Insert standard feeding tube.

2.   Chest X-ray on initial feeding tube insertion only. Clinical Indications Determine location of feeding tube Start feeding when location verified

3.   Weigh every other day.

4.   I & O.

5.   Every 4 hours (a) Check gastric placement and residual. Utilize 60 ml syringe with leur-lock tip.

         (If more than 150 ml. contact M.D. Replace aspirant.)

         (b) Flush tube with 20 ml H_2O.

         (c) Hang fresh formula.

         (d) Add blue food coloring to feeding.

6.   Flush tube with 20 ml H_2O when feeding stops.

7.   HOB elevated approximately 30° during infusion and for 1/2 hr. after feeding stopped.

8.   Change bag and connecting tubing q 48 hrs.

9.   Continuous drip, infused by enteral pump. Initially_____strength at_____ml/hr.

10.   Formulas: ( ) Elemental

           ( ) 1 Kcal/ml   ( ) Liver Dysfunction

           ( ) 1.5 Kcal/ml   ( ) Renal Dysfunction

           ( ) 2 Kcal/ml   ( ) Pulmonary Dysfunction

11.   Banana Flakes 1 Tbsp. mixed in 30 ml H_2O per feeding tube tid prn diarrhea.

12.   Venous Blood Glucose q_____hrs. x_____days, then q _____ hrs.

13.   Cover venous Blood Glucose determinants with Regular Insulin sub q. per sliding scale:

      ( ) GLUCOSE 200-249 mg% 5 units   ( ) GLUCOSE 200-249 mg%_____ units

                  250-299 mg% 10 units   250-299 mg%_____ units

                  300-349 mg% 15 units   300-349 mg%_____ units

                  350-399 mg% 20 units   350-399 mg%_____ units

                  400 mg% **Call M.D. STAT**   400 mg% **Call M.D. STAT**

14.   LABORATORY STUDIES

        (a) Initially: UA, CBC, Major & Minor Chemistry Profiles, PT, Mg, TIBC.

        (b) Minor Chemistry Profile qd x 3 d.

        (c) CBC, Major & Minor Chemistry Profiles. Mg q Monday.

        (d) 24 hr. urine for Creatinine & Urea Nitrogen q wk. Start at 0600 tomorrow & weekly.

        (e) Anergic Skin Tests.

        (f) Other:_____

15.   PULMONARY FUNCTION: Metabolic Rate and Respiratory Quotient.

16.   Nutritional therapy consultation by Clinical Nutritionist.

17.   Physical Therapy consultation for strengthening and progressive ambulation.

MO	DATE	PAGE 1 OF 1	X	M.D.	DATE	TIME

5   **ENTERAL NUTRITION: INITIATION OF**

FIGURE 6–2. Physician's order form for enteral nutrition (From Schwartz, DB: Enteral Nutrition. In Lang, LE (ed): Nutritional Support in Critical Care. Saint Joseph Medical Center, Burbank, CA, 1982, p. 95, with permission.).

TABLE 6–5. Timeline for Monitoring the Hypermetabolic
Patient on Enteral or Parenteral Nutrition Therapy

Parameter	Initial Measure	Monitoring Schedule				
		Daily	3–4X/wk	2X/wk	Weekly	Monthly
Anthropometrics						
Skinfold	1X					X
Circumference	1X					X
Weight	1X	X				
BUN	Daily			X		
Coagulation	1X				X	
Creatinine	Daily			X		
Electrolytes						
Sodium	Daily		X			
Potassium	Daily		X			
Calcium	3–4X				X	
Magnesium	3–4X				X	
Phosphorus	3–4X				X	
Fluid balance	Daily	X				
Insulin level	Daily	X				
Liver function	1X				X	
Nitrogen balance	1X				X	
Oxygen consumption	1X			X		
Prealbumin	1X				X	
Serum albumin	2X					X
Serum cholesterol	1X				X	
Serum glucose	Daily	X				
Serum lactate	1X			X		
Serum transferrin	1X				X	
Serum triglycerides	1X				X	
Total lymphocytes	2X				X	
Urinary urea nitrogen	1X				X	
Vitamin and trace elements	1X					As needed

and lactate levels reflect carbohydrate metabolism with a measure of liver enzymes and carbon dioxide production indicating glucose tolerance.[18]

Serum cholesterol and triglyceride levels indicate adequacy of lipid metabolism. Protein metabolism is followed by observing changes in visceral protein or albumin and transferrin. Monitoring these serum levels means acknowledging the half-life of albumin at 20 days and transferrin at 8 to 10 days. Somatic proteins are tracked by nitrogen balance.

Nitrogen balance can be monitored as frequently as urinary urea nitrogen is measured since urinary urea nitrogen is the most complete measure of daily nitrogen loss. Minimal nitrogen loss occurs from skin and feces. When nitrogen balance is positive, the anabolic state exists and more nitrogen is taken in than is excreted. Conversely, a negative balance or catabolic state exists when more nitrogen is excreted than ingested. Nitrogen balance is calculated as follows:

$$\text{Nitrogen balance} = (\text{protein intake} \div 6.25) - (24 \text{ hr UUN} + 4)$$

The proportion of BUN to creatinine should not exceed 20:1 by 20 percent. This measure provides a check on prerenal azotemia and excessive protein intake, possibly warranting reformulation of the care plan.[18]

Fluids should be checked daily, with particular attention given to fluid losses from fistula drainage and diarrhea.[52] Vitamins and trace elements should be measured as needed. Normal adult blood levels of chromium, copper, manganese, and zinc should be achieved—for example, chromium, 1.5 μg per L; copper, 80 to 163 μg per L; manganese, 6 to 12 μg per L; and zinc, 10 to 12 μg per L.[8]

A few other variables to monitor pertain to the type of feeding. Hyperkalemia is common with enteral therapy.[31] Therefore, if banana flakes are included in the enteral feeding to lower the risk of diarrhea, then serum potassium levels should be monitored.

During parenteral nutritional therapy, daily body weight and periodic laboratory values such as electrolytes, glucose, BUN, creatinine, liver enzymes, and blood counts are essential. Hypophosphatemia, elevated glucose, and decreased hemoglobin due to anemia are commonly observed in the patient receiving parenteral therapy. Baseline measures of magnesium, zinc, and copper should be obtained. Magnesium can be monitored on a weekly basis, but glucose, electrolytes, and BUN should be measured every third day thereafter. Urinary glucose may need to be monitored three to four times a day at the beginning of therapy until the patient is stabilized.[39]

The adequacy of nutritional support may also be monitored by a skin test for cell-mediated immunity although there is some difference of opinion among the medical community about validity of this measure. When a skin test is administered, if there is no response to the antigens, then the body's defense system fails to recognize and to fight infection.[53] A 74.4 percent mortality rate was observed among patients whose skin tests did not improve with nutritional support compared with a 5.1 percent mortality rate for patients with improved immune status.[54]

Caution should be taken with interpretation of the skin test results. A skin test result can be negative among many cancer patients; elderly patients; immobilized patients; and those with uremia, liver disease, and sepsis.[53]

To integrate several parameters, a prognostic nutritional index (PNI) has been devised and tested with high-risk surgical patients. The risk for postoperative morbidity and mortality ranges from low, less than 30 percent PNI; to intermediate, between 30 to 59 percent PNI; and high, greater than 59 percent PNI.[55] The four parameters constituting the PNI are serum albumin (ALB [g/100 ml]), transferrin (TFN [mg/100 ml]), triceps skinfold (TSF [mm]), and delayed hypersensitivity (DH) testing. The formula requires the multiplication of constants times the actual parameter of the patient. The formula is as follows:

$$\text{PNI (percent)} = 158 - 16.6\ (\text{ALB}) - 0.78\ (\text{TSF}) - 0.20\ (\text{TFN}) - 5.8\ (\text{DH})$$

An eightfold increase in complications, a sevenfold increase in major sepsis, and a 30-fold increase in mortality were noted for patients as they move from a low to a high risk according to the PNI.[55]

Step 10 involves discharge and home care instructions. Teaching patients and their families how to continue sound nutritional feedings when the patient is at home should begin at least a week before discharge. Concomitant teaching can occur as the patient receives various forms of nutritional support in the hospital. In particular, information regarding tube-feeding techniques, tube preparation and cleaning, the monitoring of problems, and the reason for such therapies should be clear and consistent. If a certain family member is selected to assume the nutritional care of the patient, then this individual should be allowed to implement all activities under the supervision of the nutrition and nursing staff while the patient is hospitalized.

Written and verbal instruction should accompany the patient, particularly if a home health agency will provide intermittent care. Likewise, the patient and family should receive the telephone numbers and names of the visiting nurses, the primary physician, and the hospital staff attending the patient. Having this information is a reassurance that continuity of care will exist and questions can be answered when the need arises. The location for securing nutritional products, if needed, should be identified for the patient and family. If possible, several day's supply should accompany the patient upon discharge. The Social Services Department of the hospital should be involved with the patient discharge to arrange financial support for supplies and supplements if the patient is in need and to set up home nursing care.

The patient and family should not be overloaded with untimely detail. For example, patients get confused if given instructions for a future eating pattern, when in fact that pattern may not occur for several weeks. If it is anticipated that the patient will progress to solid food after discharge, then tentative plans for return clinic visits should be identified during discharge instruction. Staff names, location and phone numbers should be provided regarding return visits. General follow-up visits should be tentatively arranged to provide the physical and emotional support needed and the nutritional care essential for chronic wound healing.

CLINICAL DECISION MAKING

The following abbreviated case studies apply information outlined in the chapter and should strengthen the reader's skill in developing and implementing a nutritional care plan.

Case A

Mrs. Y is a 64-year-old woman with diabetes controlled by Glucotrol and diet. She is 5'5" tall, weighs 179 pounds, and lives alone in the country about 22 miles from town. She had experienced several days of dark stools and a persistent infection in her large toe on the left foot. In fact, an ulcer had developed on the bottom of her foot and she was now unable to walk with shoes. She had waited until her usual appointment with her physician since she does not drive and depends on a neighbor to take her. She has now been feeling weak for over a week, eating only soup, jello, and crackers. At the physician's office, Mrs. Y's laboratory tests revealed a fasting blood glucose level of 210 mg%, an albumin concentration of 4.0 g per dl, and electrolytes in normal range, but a total urinary nitrogen of 16 per 100 ml. The physician admits Mrs. Y to the hospital. Determine the caloric requirements and outline the immediate nutritional care plan appropriate for this patient.

SOLUTION

The energy (caloric) requirement of Mrs. Y is calculated as follows:

BEE female = 655.0955 + [9.5634 × (wt in kg)] +
[1.8496 × (ht in cm)] − [4.6756 × (age in yrs)]

Substituting 165.1 cm for 65 inches and 81.4 kg for 179 pounds, the BEE becomes 1440 kcal.

Using the Long formula,[19] which includes activity and injury, the total energy needs per 24 hours is determined as BEE × 1.3 × 1.2 = 2246 kcal. The registered dietitian recommends a 2250 kcal diet with 309 g carbohydrate (55 percent), 101 g protein (18 percent: 1.24 g per kg of body weight), and 68 g fat (27 percent).

The goal of the nutritional care plan is to create an anabolic state for wound healing and to return Mrs. Y to independent living with normal blood chemistries. The immediate care plan responds to several factors: the energy and protein needs of the patient; infection of the foot due to the high blood sugar; the need for tissue repair with adequate ascorbic acid from food and supplement (250 to 500 mg); dark stools, which immediately imply internal blood loss; an albumin level of 4.0 g per dl, which is low but higher than the 3.5 g per dl that produces a 1.8 times greater risk of developing complications; a fasting blood sugar of 210 mg%, which is very high and warrants insulin use and/or weight loss.

The patient can ingest food by mouth, has dentures, and enjoys eating so the nutritional substrate is prescribed as solid food and calorie-controlled beverages. The physician places the patient on NPO for about 12 hours, however, due to the reported dark stool and further testing.

Important questions assess whether the soup regimen at home was due to preference, difficulty swallowing, or lack of money. One should determine if the current body weight is the usual body weight. After interview, it was learned that Mrs. Y had not had more than a 2- to 5-pound weight change in the past 6 months and that she "just didn't feel like cooking" and preferred the soup for ease. She did not eat much meat as it was too expensive for her. She was taking several self-prescribed iron tablets to "fight the weakness," which, after other laboratory tests, proved to be the primary cause of the dark stools.

From a 24-hour recall it was learned that Mrs. Y was drinking 5 to 8 cups of hot tea each day with regular sugar and making puddings and regular jello to "give her energy." These, of course, compounded the problem by keeping the blood sugar high and spilling into the urine. She was averaging about 1750 kcal a day distributed as 60 percent carbohydrate, 30 percent fat, and 10 percent protein. She is classified as a high-risk patient, as her protein intake of 44 g is less than 85 percent of the recommended amount (approximately 55 g) for her age and sex; furthermore, the catabolic index is calculated and determined to be +5 or moderate risk, but branched-chain amino acids are not deemed necessary.

Blood counts are observed closely, blood sugar levels are determined before each meal, and both regular and NPH insulin are begun. Anthropometric measures of triceps, arm circumference, and arm muscle circumference are determined. The ability of the patient to provide the type of food, nursing care, and medical care needed when living alone is now investigated.

Mrs. Y's acceptance of the 2250-kcal diet with insulin therapy is followed closely. Mrs. Y's progress is monitored with routine glucose, insulin, and urinary nitrogen and lactate levels. Nitrogen balance is calculated daily for 3 days. Weight is measured daily and thorough diet instruction with a weekly planned home visit by both a registered nurse and a registered dietitian is recommended for the first month after discharge.

Case B

Mr. H is a 69-year-old man who has had a recent hip fracture due to a fall. He has been bedridden for several weeks. At a recent visit to his physician, a large sacral pressure ulceration at stage III was observed. He was admitted to the hospital for surgical debridement of the ulceration and evaluation of nutritional status. What should be the nutritional care plan for this patient?

SOLUTION

Several values are checked: urinary urea nitrogen (UUN), albumin, hemoglobin, hematocrit, and serum protein. UUN excretion was 11 g per day. Since surgical debridement of the ulceration was required and strong chemical agents were used, additional tissue damage occurred and healing was slow. Because the wound was open, extra protein was lost. The patient was in a negative nitrogen balance. The catabolic index was +2 denoting moderate stress.

The patient was given a high-protein diet, with 25 percent of total calories derived from protein. Total calories was calculated at 1.5 times the BEE, and 500 mg of ascorbic acid supplement was added to aid wound healing. Solid foods were used, as Mr. H had no impairment of his gastrointestinal tract. Laboratory values were repeated routinely until the patient was in a normal range and the healing was evident.

Mr. H was kept mobile and good skin care was begun. A pressure-relieving mattress was placed on his bed. Nursing care used topical agents to cleanse and aid wound healing—in particular, enzymes, antiseptics, ointments, and sterile gauze.

SUMMARY

Energy and protein metabolism are altered proportional to the level of stress for the individual experiencing cellular injury. The immediate response is a circulatory insufficiency of protein and energy followed by an increased metabolic state when body protein can become depleted rapidly. When suboptimal nutritional status exists, the individual's recovery rate is compromised. Determining the appropriate nutritional care plan for the patient is demanding and complex but essential for daily improvement.

In this chapter, 10 steps were outlined for developing a program of tailored nutritional care. The steps were presented as four stages of program development: planning, assessing, implementing and monitoring. These steps are logical and direct because they establish the parameters to measure and the decisions to be made for optimal nutritional care of the patient.

Although registered dietitians skilled in critical-care nutrition are essential to the evaluation and assurance of quality nutritional care, multiple health-care professionals interact daily. This cadre of medical and allied health-care practitioners are needed to implement the total nutritional care plan for the patient.

Logically, readjustment and recalculation of nutritional therapy complements the daily response of the parameters monitored. The process of monitoring and tailoring must remain interactive throughout the patient's care. The purpose is to create and to maintain an anabolic state for wound healing and to return the patient to good health.

GLOSSARY

Anabolic: metabolic state in which compounds are combined for tissue repair or growth; opposite of catabolic

Adrenocorticotropic hormone (ACTH): pituitary gland hormone that stimulates adrenal cortex to secrete hormones, which promote gluconeogenesis

Antidiuretic hormone (ADH): pituitary gland hormone that stimulates water reabsorption in the kidney and reduced urine formation

Catabolic: metabolic state in which compounds are broken down into simpler parts; opposite of anabolic

Catecholamines: adrenal medulla hormones, including epinephrine and norepinephrine, which affect fat and carbohydrate metabolism

Enteral Nutrition: nutrients provided through the gastrointestinal tract

Glucagon: pancreatic hormone that increases blood glucose concentration

Homeostasis: the body's tendency to maintain a state of equilibrium when nutrients are removed and replenished at an equivalent rate and amount

Hyperalimentation: ingestion or administration of a greater than normal amount of nutrients; may be either enteral or parenteral

Hypermetabolic: functioning at an accelerated rate of metabolism

Immunocompetency: pertaining to the body's ability to resist harmful substances with an antigen-antibody response

Lipolysis: the catabolism of lipids

Metabolism: the series of processes needed for building cells and tissues and maintaining their continuous functioning

Parenteral nutrition: supply of any nutrient to body cells bypassing the alimentary canal

Protein-sparing therapy: a form of hypocaloric nutrition support that contains amino acids, vitamins, and minerals/electrolytes and that may or may not consist of an isotonic dextrose solution

Somatic protein: protein mass contained in muscle—primarily skeletal muscle

Substrate: a substance transformed by an enzyme

Total parenteral nutrition: supply of all nutrients intravenously or intramuscularly

Visceral protein: protein mass contained in body organs, as measured by lymphocytes, transferrin, albumin, and other serum proteins

REFERENCES

1. Randall, HT: Surgical nutrition: Parenteral and oral. In Committee on Pre and Postoperative Care, American College of Surgeons (eds): Manual of Preoperative and Postoperative Care. WB Saunders, Philadelphia, 1971.
2. Cuthbertson, DP: Post-shock metabolic response. Lancet 1:433, 1942.
3. Blackburn, GL and Moldawer, LL: Amino acid metabolism after injury. In The Catabolic Phase—Proceedings from the Metabolic and Nutrition Support for Trauma and Burn Patients Symposium. Mead Johnson and Company, Evansville, IN, 1982, p 37.
4. Agriesti-Johnson, C: Nutrition-support team survey. In Training for Dietitians Working in Critical Care. Report of the Sixth Ross Roundtable on Medical Issues. Ross Laboratories, Columbus, OH, 1985, p 7.
5. Hooley, RA: The role of the registered dietitian on a nutrition support team. Nutritional Support Services 1:52, 1981.
6. American Dietetic Association Study Commission: A new look at the profession of dietetics. Final report of the 1984 Study Commission Dietetic. American Dietetic Association, Chicago, 1984.
7. Steinbaugh, M: Training for Dietitians Working in Critical Care. Report of the Sixth Ross Roundtable on Medical Issues. Ross Laboratories, Columbus, OH, 1985, p 47.
8. Suggested Guidelines for Nutritional Management of the Critically Ill Patient. The Quality Assurance Committee, Dietitians in Critical Care Dietetic Practice Group. American Dietetic Association, Chicago, 1984, p 99.
9. Gussler, J (ed): Nutritional Screening and Assessment as Components of Hospital Admission. Ross Laboratories, Columbus, OH, 1988, p 53.
10. Seltzer, MH, et al: Instant nutritional assessment. JPEN 3:157, 1979.
11. Faintuch, J, et al: Anthropometric assessment of nutrition depletion after surgical injury. JPEN 3(5):369, 1979.
12. Blackburn, GL, et al: Nutritional and metabolic assessment of the hospitalized patient. JPEN 1:11, 1977.

13. Frisancho, AR: Triceps skinfold and upper arm muscle size norms for assessment of nutritional status. Am J Clin Nutr 27:1052, 1974.
14. Bistrian, BR: A simple technique to estimate the severity of stress. Surg Gynecol Obstet 148:675, 1979.
15. Custer, PB and Grant JP: A nutritional assessment manual for adults. Duke University Medical Center, Durham, NC, 1979.
16. Grant, JP, Custer, PB, and Thurlow, J: Current techniques of nutritional assessment. Surg Clin North Am 61:437, 1981.
17. Moldawer, LL, Echenique, MM, and Bistrian, BR: The importance of study design to the demonstration of efficacy with branched chain amino acid enriched solutions. Second Bermuda Symposium on Total Parenteral Nutrition. Plenum Press, New York, 1982.
18. Konstantinidis, NN, et al: Nutritional requirements of the hypermetabolic patient. Nutritional Support Services 4(2):41, 1984.
19. Harris, JA, and Benedict, FG: A Biometric Study of Basal Metabolism in Man. Carnegie Institute, Washington, DC, 1919.
20. Lang, CE and Schulte CV: The adult patient. In Lang, CE (ed): Nutritional Support in Critical Care. Aspen Publishers, Rockville, MD, 1987, p 61.
21. DuBois, D and DuBois, EF: A formula to estimate the approximate surface area if height and weight be known. Arch Int Med 17:863, 1916.
22. Long, C, et al: Metabolic response to injury and illness: Estimation of energy and protein needs from indirect calorimetry and nitrogen balance. JPEN 3:452, 1979.
23. Cerra, FB, et al: Branched chains support postoperative protein synthesis. Surgery 92:192, 1982.
24. Nutrition Advisory Group: Multivitamin preparations for parenteral use: A statement by the Nutrition Advisory Group. JPEN 3:258, 1979.
25. Standards for Nutrition Support: Hospitalized Patients. American Society for Parenteral and Enteral Nutrition, Washington, DC, 1984.
26. Allardyce, DB and Groves, AC: A comparison of nutritional gains resulting from intravenous and enteral feeding. Surg Gynecol Obstet 139:179, 1974.
27. Grant, JP: Handbook of Total Parenteral Nutrition. WB Saunders, Philadelphia, 1980, pp 47–69, 125–194.
28. Rombeau, JL, and Barot, LR: Enteral nutritional therapy. Surg Clin North Am 61:605, 1981.
29. Alverdy, J, Chi, HS, and Sheldon, GF: The effect of parenteral nutrition on gastrointestinal immunity: The importance of enteral stimulation. Ann Surg 202:681, 1985.
30. Pingleton, SK and Hadzima, SK: Enteral alimentation and gastrointestinal bleeding in mechanically ventilated patients. Crit Care Med 11:13, 1983.
31. Cataldi-Betcher, EL, et al: Complications occurring during enteral nutrition support: A prospective study. JPEN 7:546, 1983.
32. Schwartz, DB: Enteral therapy. In Lang, ED (ed): Nutritional Support in Critical Care. Aspen Publishers, Rockville, MD, 1987, p 61.
33. Askanazi, J, et al: Nutrition and the respiratory system. Crit Care Med 10:163, 1982.
34. Vanlandingham, S, et al: Metabolic abnormalities in patients supported with enteral tube feeding. JPEN 5:322, 1981.
35. Heimburger, DC and Weinsier, RL: Guidelines for evaluating and categorizing enteral formulas according to therapeutic equivalency. JPEN 9:61, 1985.
36. Groziak, P: Modular feeding—an overview. Dietitians in Nutrition Support 9:6, 1987.
37. Principles of enteral tube feeding. Part 2: Administration and Monitoring. Ross Laboratories, Columbus, 1982, p 1–10.
38. Hooley, RA: Parenteral nutrition—general concepts, part I. Nutritional Support Services 1:36, 1981.
39. Parrish, G, Gibney, AM, and Lugene, E: Total parenteral nutrition—an update. Nutritional Support Services 2:9, 1982.
40. Maintenance Peripheral Nutrition (MPN). Travenol Laboratories, Deerfield, IL, 1979.
41. Hooley, RA: Parenteral nutrition—general concepts, part II. Nutritional Support Services 1:41, 1981.
42. Hooley, RA: Parenteral nutrition—general concepts, part III. Nutritional Support Services 1:41, 1981.
43. Segar, WE: Parenteral fluid therapy. Curr Prob Pediatr 3:3, 1972.
44. Madan, PL, Madan, KD, and Palumbo, JF: Total parenteral nutrition. Drug Intell Clin Pharm 10:684, 1976.
45. American Medical Association: Department of Foods and Nutrition. Guidelines for essential trace element preparations for parenteral use. JPEN 2:263, 1979.
46. Robinson, CH and Lawler, MR: Normal and Therapeutic Nutrition, ed 15. Macmillan, New York, 1977, p 739.
47. Statement by an Expert Panel: Essential trace element preparations for parenteral use. JAMA 1a:241, 1979.
48. American Medical Association, Department of Foods and Nutrition: Multivitamin preparations for parenteral use. JPEN 3:258, 1979.
49. Butterworth, CE: The skeleton in the hospital closet. Nutrition Today 9(2):4, 1974.
50. Maillet, JO: Calculating parenteral feedings: A programmed instruction. JADA 84:1312, 1984.
51. Andrassy, R: Controversies in enteral nutrition. Nutritional Support Services 5(5), 1985, pp 11–12.

52. Just, PM: Total parenteral nutrition. In Wellcome Program in Pharmacy. Park Row Publishers, Educational Services, Raliegh, NC, 1985, pp 1–9.
53. Decker, EL: Skin testing for anergy: A review with proposed guidelines. Hospital Formulary 15(5):368, 1980.
54. Meakins, JL, et al: Delayed hypersensitivity—indicator of acquired failure of host defenses in sepsis and trauma. Ann Surg 186(3):241, 1977.
55. Mullen, JL: Prediction of operative morbidity and mortality by preoperative nutritional assessment. Surg For 30:80, 1979.

Part II

EVALUATION

CHAPTER 7

Evaluation of Patients with Open Wounds

Joseph M. McCulloch, Ph.D., P.T.
Luther C. Kloth, M.S., P.T.

HISTORY AND SUBJECTIVE EXAMINATION

In examining any patient, the lesion or pathology in question and the entire anatomic make-up and physiologic functioning of the patient must be considered. No less important in this scrutiny is the history and subjective findings, which provide the examiner with a more complete picture of the patient. Information gathered during this process not only helps to clarify the primary problem but also provides the rehabilitation specialist with valuable information relating to how the condition affects the patient's functional independence. The end result of this process should be the beginning of a therapeutic plan that is practical and followed by the patient.

The History

The first step in any patient examination is the gathering of a complete history. Although much information may have been previously obtained by another health-care practitioner and may be totally accurate, a great deal can be gained by repeating parts of the process and obtaining current information.

Two major benefits come readily to mind. One relates to the fact that humans communicate differently. The way one examiner might interpret a patient's response to a question may differ significantly from another's interpretation. This reality does not mean that one answer is right and the other wrong, but more likely that the question may have been asked in a different context.

A second benefit relates to the examiner-patient relationship. History taking should provide an opportunity for the patient to become at ease with the examiner. This rapport and confidence is important to establish before beginning the process of physically examining the patient. If a complete history has been taken previously, the

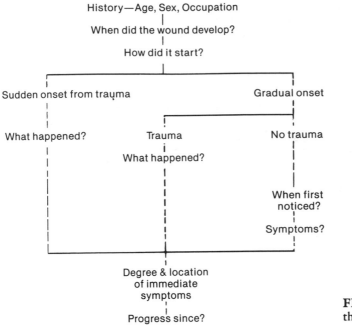

FIGURE 7–1. Schematic of the history taking process.

examiner may wish to compare the information obtained by the other practitioner with what he or she has obtained. Careful attention should be given to any aspects of the histories that do not correlate.

The first step in the history-gathering process is to obtain information concerning the patient's age, sex, and occupation. While age and sex may be more significant in differentiating other disease processes from open wounds, this information is of great importance when demographic data are desired for research purposes. Moreover, age is an important factor in wound healing and is addressed in Chapter 4. The patient's occupation or daily activities may be one of the first pieces of information to indicate a possible cause for the wound being examined. Venous pooling encountered by individuals whose jobs require them to spend long periods on their feet exemplifies a situation in which an occupation might predispose someone to tissue breakdown.

Once baseline information has been obtained, the examiner may inquire about the events that led to the development of the wound. This process should include inquiring about the mechanism of injury, if any, that caused the wound, and the series of events that led up to the present examination. The flow chart presented in Figure 7–1 is offered as a guide to the history-taking process.

PREVIOUS HISTORY

The examiner should inquire about aspects of the patient's history that the patient may not offer voluntarily because of not understanding the possible relationship between the current symptoms and other medical problems. Some specific areas that may be relevant to wound pathogenesis and that should be addressed are discussed in this section.

Is the Patient a Diabetic?

Whereas patients may understand the importance of diet and insulin in controlling their diabetes, they may be currently unaware of the neuropathic processes that may accompany the disease and lead to cutaneous insensitivity. This insensitivity, often more pronounced in the feet, may predispose the patient to the development of pressure ulcerations.

Determining the patient's age at the onset of diabetes, as well as the method and quantity of insulin required, may provide the examiner with insight into the extent and relative severity of secondary neuropathic and vascular changes that have occurred over time.

Is There a History of Peripheral Vascular Disease, Hypertension, or Congestive Heart Failure?

Affirmative indications from the patient in response to questions related to coldness of the hands or feet may suggest existence of a pathologic condition that causes arterial insufficiency and tissue hypoxia. Patients who report having chronic swelling of the feet and ankles may have venous or lymphatic insufficiency. Further objective examination may corroborate the patient's complaints and help to establish the etiology of the wound.

A majority of the chronic problem wounds seen in an outpatient setting result from a dysfunctional vascular system. This dysfunction can be manifested by poor arterial supply or inadequate venous and lymphatic drainage. Appreciating where in the circulatory or lymphatic system the problem lies may help the clinician plan for the objective examination.

What Medications Is the Patient Currently Taking?

Frequently the only information the examiner can obtain about a patient's medical problems is a list of oral and topically applied medications the person currently uses or has used in the immediate past. Once provided with this list, the examiner can then more closely investigate the pharmacologic actions of the drugs as well as the adverse reactions that might be expected. Examples include the retarding effects of steroids on wound healing and the irritating effects of residues from heavy metals contained in antimicrobial agents that may be mobilized by therapeutic treatment methods.[1]

Does the Patient Have Any Allergies?

The response to this question may provide several important pieces of information. The first could be that a contact dermatitis or pruritus could have been the causative factor for the extremity wound. Possibly of greater importance is the need to understand whether the patient may be allergic to certain agents that might be applied in treatment.

Has the Patient Had Previous Treatment for this Condition? If So, What Was the Treatment and What Were the Results?

As noted earlier, one reason for taking a history is to develop rapport and allow the patient to gain confidence in the practitioner's abilities. This confidence can fade quickly if the examiner elects to treat a patient with the same techniques that were previously used without success. Identifying previous treatments can prevent this situation from occurring. If the examiner feels that the previous treatment was beneficial but perhaps not performed in an appropriate manner, this can be explained to the patient. Involving the patient in this decision-making process will help later in obtaining compliance with therapy.

SOCIAL HISTORY

The primary information to be gathered from questioning in this area relates to the use of tobacco. One must ascertain whether the patient is a smoker and, if so, how many packs of cigarettes are smoked per day. Cigarette smoking can be a significant factor in preventing an arterial ulcer from healing. The negative effects of tobacco on the arterial system are twofold. One is the immediate vasoconstriction of the arteries, caused by the nicotine, and the other is a more long-term effect on the vessel wall leading to arterial insufficiency.[2] In chronically ill individuals, information relative to dietary intake and the degree of alcohol ingestion should be obtained. The reader is referred to Chapter 6 for an in-depth discussion of this subject.

The Subjective Examination

The subjective examination is the portion of the evaluation during which the patient is asked to describe his or her current symptoms. Questioning in this area is designed to provide the examiner with information concerning how the symptoms change in varying situations.

What Are the Symptoms?

Many symptoms can indicate that the patient should seek medical attention. With respect to wounds, usually pain or impending cutaneous ulceration actually convinces the patient to seek help. The degree and localization of the symptoms help the examiner determine the severity of the problem.

Where Are the Symptoms Located?

As was stated, pain is often the presenting symptom. The patient should be questioned about where the pain is located. Is the pain located within or around the lesion, or in other areas? Is there an associated paresthesia which could be indicative of initial nerve pathogenesis? In situations when the presenting sign is an ulceration, the clinician must determine whether the area is truly anesthetic. Such a condition may indicate a condition such as diabetes or a peripheral neuropathic process.

How Do the Symptoms Behave?

When pain is a presenting complaint, the clinician must determine how the pain is affected by different body positions. For example, when dealing with lower extremity ulcerations caused by venous insufficiency, the patient often notes that the pain is relieved by elevation and aggravated by exercise and the gravity-dependent position. Arterial problems, on the other hand, tend to be aggravated by elevation of the extremity and relieved or lessened by placing the extremity in the gravity-dependent position.[3]

The behavior of the symptoms, combined with location and appearance, helps to determine the type of ulceration involved. The schematic presented in Figure 7–2 is provided as a guide to the questioning of patients relative to their symptomatology.

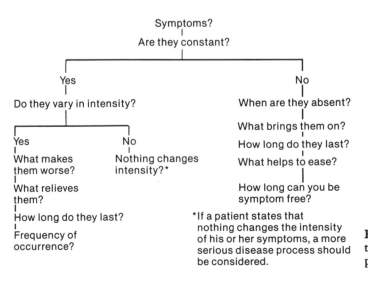

FIGURE 7–2. Schematic of the subjective examination process.

As previously mentioned, improper nutrition may be associated with many wounds. In this regard, weight loss becomes an important consideration. Although weight change is objective and is therefore more appropriately termed a sign, it is mentioned here as a finding the patient may report that cannot be immediately confirmed by the examiner. Weight loss can be caused not only by decreased intake as a result of anorexia, dysphagia, and vomiting but also by metabolic disorders such as diabetes mellitus and nutrient loss through the feces or urine. Symptoms of malnutrition, weakness, easy fatigability, cold intolerance, flaky dermatitis, and ankle edema should be noted, and if present a nutritional consult should be initiated.[4]

THE OBJECTIVE EXAMINATION

> *When you can measure what you are speaking about and express it in*
> *numbers, you know something about it, but when you cannot measure*
> *it, when you cannot express it in numbers, your knowledge is of a*
> *meager kind.*

> Lord Kelvin

As this quote indicates, objective tests and measures are of utmost importance in medicine. The following section will provide the examiner with information about numerous objective tests that are useful in evaluating patients with dermal ulcerations. For the most part, these tests are designed to be used on all patients with ulcerations. The examiner may not believe, however, that the present complaints and symptoms require all of the tests to be performed at this time.

Planning the Examination

The evaluation should be planned before starting the examination, in order to help ensure that the procedure is performed efficiently and smoothly and that no important information is overlooked. The objective examination will look not only at the wound itself, but also at other signs. These signs may relate to problems that caused the ulceration or to problems that developed as a result of it.

Observation

Although an assessment of the patient's general health is important, the reader should consult a more comprehensive text on physical examination for additional insight. This section will focus primarily on techniques designed to assess the status of the patient's wound, in addition to findings in the vascular system and other associated systems.

The examiner should begin by observing the lesion, noting its location and characteristics. The location of an ulcer can be one of the first indicators of its cause. Venous ulcers, for example, are most commonly found over the area of the medial malleoli. Only rarely do these ulcers appear over the anterior or lateral aspect of the shin, in contrast to the findings in individuals with ischemic ulcers secondary to chronic arterial disease. Ischemic ulcers occur most frequently above the lateral malleoli or in small infarcted areas of the toes.[5] The reason for these findings is discussed in Chapter 10.

A sign frequently associated with skin lesions is edema. Edema may be divided by cause into one of two categories. *General or systemic edema* is caused by such conditions as congestive heart failure, hypoalbuminemia, and excessive retention of salt and water by the kidneys. Such edema tends to be bilateral and is usually more pronounced in the distal lower extremities. *Localized edema*, on the other hand, is associated with conditions such as venous insufficiency, lymphatic stasis, and prolonged dependency, and it tends to occur in discrete areas of the body.

Lesions can be classified by type into one of two major categories—primary or secondary. *Primary lesions* include macules, papules, and vesicles and usually arise from previously normal skin. *Secondary lesions*, however, usually occur as a result of changes in primary lesions. Ulcers fall into this category. In addition to this system of classification, ulcers are frequently categorized by depth of tissue involvement (partial or full thickness) or according to a four-stage system that describes levels of destruction from the epidermis inward.[6-8] A *Stage I* lesion is limited to the epidermis and presents as an ill-defined area of erythema and edema (Fig. 7–3). If pressure is not relieved, the lesion advances to *Stage II* (Fig. 7–4). At this stage, epidermis, dermis, and subcutaneous fat become involved and discontinuity of the skin occurs. Stage I and II lesions fall into the category of partial-thickness wounds. *Stage III* lesions are full-thickness wounds, and often result in undermining deeper tissues (Fig. 7–5). *Stage IV* lesions are also full thickness but penetrate the fascia, with frequent involvement of muscle and bone (Fig. 7–6). Some individuals classify an ulcer as *Stage V* if bony erosion occurs.[9] Stage I and II ulcers are reversible if pressure is removed and preventive measures are intensified. Stage III and IV lesions are not reversible, however, and must heal via epithelialization. Frequently, Stage III and IV lesions are covered with a thick eschar, which masks deeper destruction.

The degree of hydration of a wound also provides information about the nature of the problem. The intact skin normally serves as a barrier to the outside world. As such, skin is impermeable to most substances, including water. Whereas water is lost transepidermally by insensible perspiration, there is no appreciable passage of water in the opposite direction.[10] When the epidermis is disrupted, permeability changes greatly. The

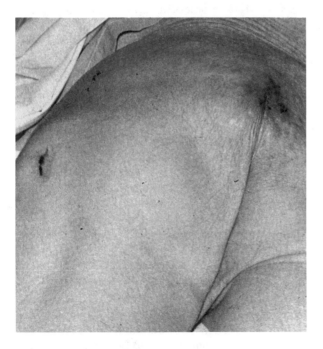

FIGURE 7–3. A stage I lesion demonstrating ill-defined erythema and edema (From Reddy,[9] p. 60, with permission).

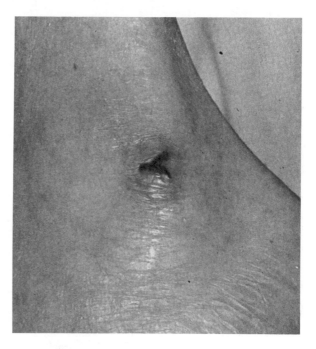

FIGURE 7–4. A stage II lesion demonstrating involvement of the epidermis, dermis, and subcutaneous fat (From Reddy,[9] p. 60, with permission).

dermis is now exposed to the outside environment and many substances are allowed free passage in and out of the body. In this regard, the relative extent of wound hydration serves as an indicator of fluid loss from the body or the development of an inflammatory process, possibly secondary to infection. In like manner, a dry lesion can indicate poor vascular supply to the area or a wound that has been poorly protected from the drying effects of the surrounding milieu.

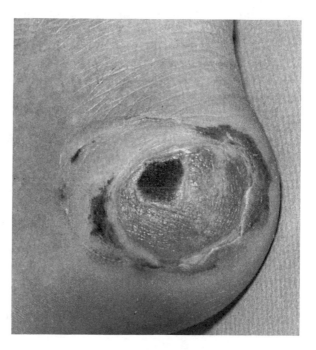

FIGURE 7–5. A stage III lesion demonstrating a full-thickness involvement of the dermis (From Reddy,[9] p. 60, with permission).

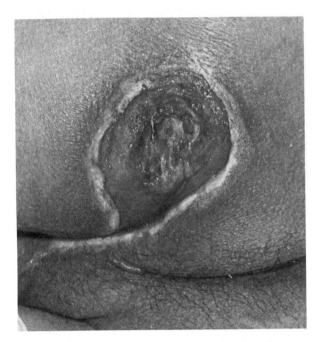

FIGURE 7-6. A stage IV lesion demonstrating involvement of muscle and bone (From Reddy,[9] p. 60, with permission).

Hydration also plays a role in turgor and mobility of the skin. The examiner should lift a fold of skin and note how easily it is moved (mobility) and how quickly it returns to the resting position (turgor). Conditions such as scleroderma or clinical manifestations of edema restrict skin mobility. Dehydration can result in decreased turgor.

If inflammation is present, the examiner should observe the degree of the inflammatory reaction, documenting the presence and extent of pain, swelling, redness, and increased temperature. Many of these factors will be measured objectively later in the examination. If the redness in the surrounding tissues is significant and extends a distance from the wound edges, cellulitis should be considered. Cellulitis may indicate the need to refer the patient to a physician so that antibiotic therapy can be initiated.

Drainage from a wound should be examined noting its amount, color, odor, and consistency. An increase in the amount of wound drainage may indicate a worsening condition or represent the recent opening of an abscess. Color and odor provide useful information about infection. Anyone who has seen the greenish-blue drainage of Pseudomonas and has smelled its characteristic sweet aroma cannot mistake it. In addition, the consistency of wound drainage can provide information relative to the source of the drainage and the degree of irrigation or debridement that might be needed to cleanse the wound. Chapter 5 provides further discussion of drainage and infection.

Structures in the tissues adjacent to the wound should also be examined. Trophic changes in the skin, manifested by changes in skin texture, may provide information about the relative nutritional status of the area. In the healthy state, the skin should be soft and moist. The degree to which these findings are present obviously depends on the patient's age and sex and the regions of the body being examined. In situations when blood flow is inadequate, the skin may become dry and scaly, hair loss may occur readily, and nails may thicken.

Skin color should also be noted, because additional information, relative to the patient's problem, can be gained. In addition to the redness of inflammation, a cyanotic blue area of skin may be indicative of venous obstruction. Patients with venous insufficiency may also demonstrate characteristic brownish discoloration of the skin due to deposition of hemosiderin. Arterial insufficiency may be manifested by either a cyanotic appearance or pallor caused by low partial pressure of oxygen. The appearance of fingernails, lips, and mucous membranes of the mouth provides the most information regarding oxyhemoglobin concentration.

Swelling, temperature, wound size, and wound shape definitely need to be evaluated and will be addressed in the clinical measurements section that follows. Before concluding the discussion of observation, the reader should examine Table 7–1, wherein some of the more commonly encountered ulcerations have been classified by the characteristics discussed here.

Clinical Measurements

CULTURE

If a culture has not been previously taken, one should be obtained before beginning any therapy. Doing so helps to provide baseline information. If topical antibiotic therapy is required, the physician will be able to make a better choice of topical agents based on the culture report (see Chapter 5 for information on taking and interpreting the results of cultures.)

DETERMINING SIZE, DEPTH, AND SHAPE OF AN ULCER

Wounds frequently heal at a slow rate, making documentation of their changes difficult. One means of objectively documenting wound size is to use a piece of sterile acetate or exposed radiographic film and a permanent marking pen. The clear film is superimposed on the wound and the borders of the wound traced (see Chapter 11, Fig. 11–8). A tape measure can then be used to measure the vertical and horizontal dimensions of the wound. Alternatively, the tracing can be transposed onto metric graph paper to allow the surface area of the wound to be measured in square centimeters. Computer technology also permits these tracings to be copied and the information digitized so that surface area can be computed. The equipment necessary for such measures is costly, however, and not readily available in most clinics.

A quick method of assessing wound size is to use a piece of acetate that contains a calibrated grid. This device (Fig. 7–7) can often be obtained from pharmaceutical representatives.

Frequently, the wound is not a broad, shallow lesion but rather a deep tracking one. In these instances, measuring the wound depth is very important, as this may be the only indication that a wound is closing prematurely. This measurement is made easily by placing a sterile cotton-tipped applicator to the depth of the wound, and then withdrawing it. The depth of penetration is then measured (Fig. 7–8).

Another technique for measuring wound size involves the use of Jeltrate,* an alginate hydrocolloid used by dentists. This rapidly setting plastic, when poured into the wound, provides a positive mold of the area. This mold is then volumetrically measured by means of a standard volumeter and graduated cylinder. The Jeltrate is reportedly well tolerated by granulating wounds and does not cause patient discomfort.[11]

When the wound cavity can be positioned perpendicular to the line of gravity, a

---

*Jeltrate, L.D. Caulk Company, Milford, DE 19963.

TABLE 7–1. Classification of Ulcers Via Various Characteristics

Ulcer Type	Primary Cause	Typical Location	Other Characteristics
Venous	Venous insufficiency	Lower one third of leg, medial aspect	Irregular shape Pinkish-red base Surrounding area of pigmentation Mild pain
Arterial	Arterial insufficiency	Toes, feet, and lower one third of leg	Irregular shape Pale base Poor granulation Severe pain
Neurotropic	Insensitivity	Plantar surface of foot	Circular lesions Indolent Often deep

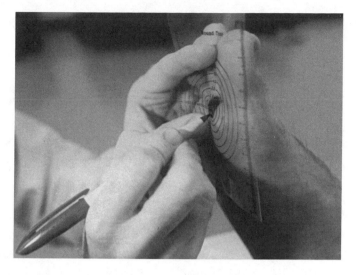

FIGURE 7–7. A calibrated grid for tracing wound size.

simple technique may be used to measure wound volume. A syringe is filled to a specific level with water, which is then injected into the wound cavity until the cavity is filled. The amount of water remaining in the syringe is subtracted from the starting amount, to indicate the volume in cubic centimeters required to fill the wound.

TEMPERATURE

Temperature measurements are of value in determining the severity and limits of the inflammation. Baseline measurements provide information that is useful when following the response to therapy. Several commercial instruments are available for measuring temperature. The least expensive of all the devices is a thermistor. The device consists of a temperature probe that measures temperature by surface contact (Fig. 7–9). A radiometer, on the other hand, measures infrared radiations from the body, does not require surface contact, and can be used directly over an open wound. The radiometer

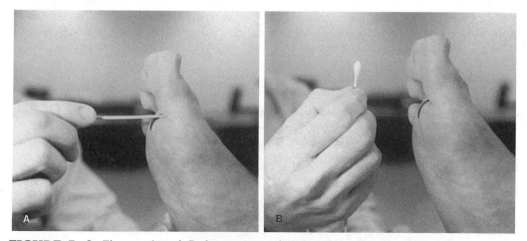

FIGURE 7–8. Figures *A* and *B* demonstrate the use of a cotton-tipped applicator in the measurement of the depth of a tracking lesion.

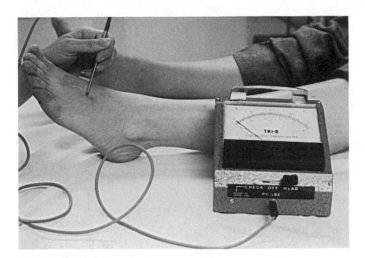

FIGURE 7–9. Thermistor used for surface temperature measurement (From McCulloch,[3] p. 375, with permission).

has the added advantage of scanning an area adjacent to a wound to obtain a quick indication of temperature variations (Fig. 7–10). Much more costly and sophisticated thermographs are also available but are not readily used in routine clinical settings. These thermographic devices provide a multicolor picture of the area studied, with each color representing a gradient change in temperature (Fig. 7–11).

GIRTH

If swelling or atrophy is evident, baseline girth measurements are made simply by obtaining circumferential measurements of the extremity with a tape measure (Fig. 7–12). Care should be taken to measure girth with reference to bony landmarks to ensure that the measurement is reproducible and that future measurements will be of comparative significance. When measuring the size of an irregular body part, such as the foot, the examiner may wish to perform a volumetric measurement. To do so, a volumeter is required (Fig. 7–13). These devices come in a variety of designs, the least costly of which is a plexiglass container equipped with an overflow spout. The container is filled to overflowing, with tap water. When all water flow ceases, the extremity is

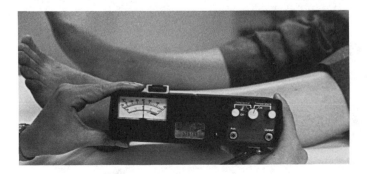

FIGURE 7–10. Radiometer used to measure surface temperature by infrared radiation (From McCulloch,[3] p. 376 with permission).

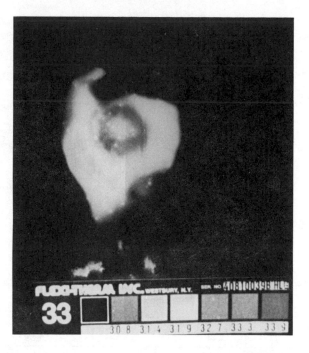

FIGURE 7–11. Liquid crystal thermography used in surface temperature measurement.

placed into the tank and all displaced water is collected and measured in a graduated cylinder. The water collected represents the volume of the body part. Some care should be taken to ensure that the temperature of the water is consistent from one examination to the next because the volume occupied by water changes with temperature; this change is probably not of major clinical significance, however.[12]

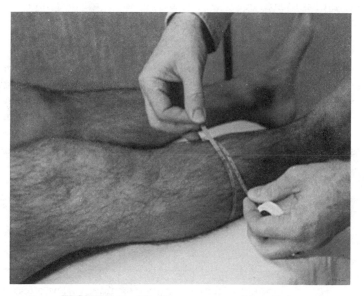

FIGURE 7–12. Measurement of leg girth.

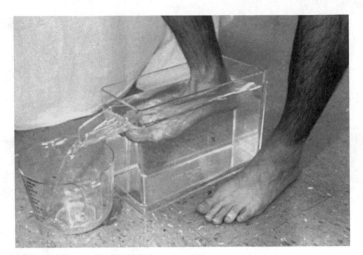

FIGURE 7–13. Volumetric measurement of the lower extremity.

VASCULAR AND NEUROLOGIC EXAMINATIONS

Patients who present with ulcerations should be screened for vascular and neurologic conditions, in addition to the previously discussed assessment of the skin. The pathophysiologic factors related to findings in these systems are discussed in other chapters of this text. This section focuses more directly on specific tests and their significance.

Pulses

The quality and presence of pulses should be noted for all patients. Although the radial and carotid pulses are most frequently palpated, those of the lower extremity (common iliac, femoral, popliteal, dorsalis pedis, and posterior tibial) are of much greater importance in patients with lower extremity ulcerations. To properly examine lower extremity pulses, the patient should be positioned supine and draped so the legs are completely exposed. One should *never* attempt to assess pulses through clothing. A significant decrease or absence of an arterial pulse is most frequently related to arteriosclerosis. Commonly, arteries tend to develop occlusion from atherosclerotic deposits at points where the vessels bifurcate or split. Most pulses in the lower extremity are reasonably easy to palpate. The primary exception is the popliteal artery, which, because of its deep placement, is often more difficult to detect. Strong pulsations in the more distal arteries (posterior tibial and dorsalis pedis) are indicative of good flow through the popliteal area. Pulses can be graded as $2+$ = normal, $1+$ = diminished, and 0 = absent.

Auscultation

Blood flow is usually laminar in nature. If the examiner listens over a normal artery with the assistance of a stethoscope, there are no audible signs of blood flow. When the motion becomes turbulent, however, as occurs in the presence of any situation that narrows the arterial lumen, a swishing sound may be noted. This sound, known as a *bruit*, is much like that heard during a blood pressure measurement. The examiner should assess all large arteries in the neck, abdomen, and limbs for the presence of bruits. If a bruit is detected, the primary care physician should be notified. The examiner should also listen over all large scars, because arteriovenous fistulas may develop, which require medical attention.

Blood Pressure

Blood pressure should be checked routinely on all patients. The test is simple and quick and provides the clinician with important information on the current status of the cardiovascular system. Patients can develop hypertensive ulcers. Although rare, such ulcers are preventable, and can be treated through antihypertensive therapy. The patient should be placed in a comfortable position and all clothing removed from the arm. A properly fitting cuff is placed around the upper arm, with the lower edge of the cuff resting approximately 1 inch above the elbow. A properly fitting cuff is of utmost importance; cuffs that fit improperly may cause erroneous readings. Appropriate cuff selection is satisfied when the width of the bladder, with the cuff applied to the arm, is approximately 40 percent of the circumference of the arm, and the bladder length is approximately 80 percent of this circumference.[4]

Three recordings of blood pressure measurements should be made from patients with vascular conditions.[13] This procedure helps to avoid confusion when individuals use different criteria for determining diastolic pressures. Some individuals record the muffling of the sound as the diastolic reading, while others use the disappearance of the sound. Using all three measures, so that both "diastolic" readings are noted (e.g., 120/80/70), helps to avoid confusion.

Tests of Peripheral Arterial Circulation

RUBOR OF DEPENDENCY

This test of the arterial system determines the adequacy of flow by evaluating color changes in the skin during elevation and dependency. To perform the test, the patient is positioned supine and the leg is elevated approximately 60 degrees for about 1 minute. Normally, there is no significant change in skin color on the plantar aspect of the foot. When arterial insufficiency is present, pallor develops owing to the inadequate pressure and compromised blood flow. The leg is then placed in a dependent position. In individuals with uncompromised circulation, no significant change in color is noted. Those with arterial insufficiency, however, develop a reactive hyperemia (rubor of dependency) in an attempt to compensate for tissue hypoxia (Fig. 7–14).[14] Another variable considered is the length of time necessary for the color change to occur. If the arterial circulation is impaired, the color change may take longer than 30 seconds to occur. The accuracy of this test is diminished in the presence of venous insufficiency.

VENOUS FILLING TIME

The time necessary for veins to refill after emptying is an indication of the patency of the arterial system. This test, like that of rubor of dependency, is only of value in persons with a competent venous system because retrograde flow would invalidate the results. With the patient in the supine position, the leg is once again elevated about 60

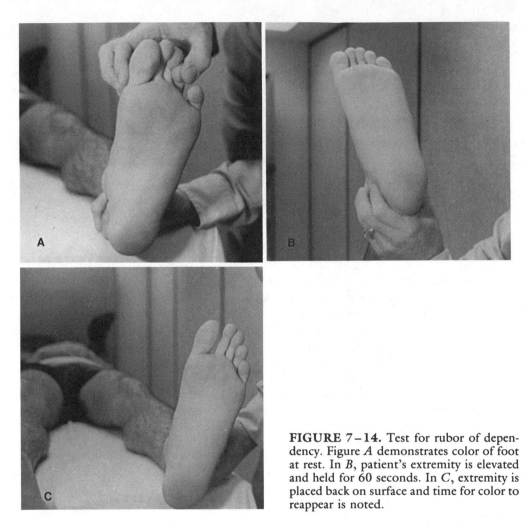

FIGURE 7–14. Test for rubor of dependency. Figure *A* demonstrates color of foot at rest. In *B*, patient's extremity is elevated and held for 60 seconds. In *C*, extremity is placed back on surface and time for color to reappear is noted.

degrees for approximately 1 minute. The leg is then placed into a dependent position and the time necessary for the veins to refill is noted. A filling time greater than 10 to 15 seconds indicates arterial insufficiency.

CLAUDICATION TIME

Intermittent claudication, a muscular distress due to ischemia, is a fairly subjective yet valuable source of information when assessing a patient's response to therapy. Because the distress is directly related to the demand for blood, attempting to objectify this information is important. One means of doing so is to have the patient walk on a treadmill at 1 mile per hour on a level grade. When claudicatory pain stops the test, the elapsed time is noted. Because the environment is controlled, the test can be repeated as a means of monitoring changes in the patient's functional status.

Tests of Peripheral Venous Circulation

PERCUSSION TEST

When patients present with a dilated saphenous vein, the percussion test is useful in assessing the patency of the venous valves. The patient is asked to stand so the varicosities fill with blood. The examiner palpates one segment of the vein while percussing the vein approximately 20 cm higher in the leg. If the impulse is transmitted to the lower hand, the intervening valves are incompetent. Competent valves should block the transmission of the impulses.

TRENDELENBURG TEST

The Trendelenburg test, also known as the retrograde filling test, assists in the assessment of valvular competence in the communicating veins and the saphenous system. The patient is positioned supine and the leg elevated to 90 degrees, allowing it to empty of venous blood. A tourniquet is then placed around the proximal thigh to occlude venous flow. The patient is asked to stand as the examiner notes the manner in which the veins fill. The veins should fill via the normal pathway, taking approximately 30 seconds. Should the superficial veins fill rapidly with the tourniquet in place, the valves in the communicating veins are incompetent. After observing this response, the examiner should release the tourniquet. If sudden additional filling occurs, the valves of the saphenous vein are incompetent.

TEST FOR DEEP VEIN THROMBOPHLEBITIS (HOMANS' SIGN)

In the test for deep vein thrombophlebitis, the examiner squeezes the patient's gastrocnemius while forcefully dorsiflexing the patient's ankle. Tenderness associated with increased firmness suggests a deep vein thrombophlebitis. This test obviously lends itself to a rather subjective interpretation. One way to add some degree of objectivity is to apply a blood pressure cuff around the calf, and then inflate it to see if the patient experiences discomfort. Normally, individuals with deep vein thrombophlebitis cannot tolerate pressures greater than 40 mmHg.

Other Tests

DOPPLER ULTRASOUND

Doppler ultrasound provides a simple method of determining ankle systolic pressure in individuals with arterial insufficiency and is also of value in assessing deep vein thrombosis. The instruments necessary for this test are relatively inexpensive and easy to use. Because of the importance of this tool in evaluation, an entire chapter is devoted to it (see Chapter 8 for a comprehensive discussion of the theory and application of this method of measurement).

IMPEDANCE PLETHYSMOGRAPHY

While venography is the most accurate method of diagnosing deep vein thrombosis, impedance plethysmography has been demonstrated to be reliable in detecting most thrombi that occur proximally in the leg.[15] The test is based on Ohm's law (Voltage =

Intensity × Resistance) and the fact that blood is the preferred path of electrical conductance in the body. Because of this fact, voltage changes become a reflection of blood volume of the limb. To properly perform the test, the examiner must acquire specific knowledge that is not within the scope of this text.

TEST OF CUTANEOUS SENSIBILITY

Loss of sensation, especially in the feet, can have serious consequences because foreign bodies and/or pressure undetected by the patient rapidly lead to skin erosion. An assessment of the patient's sensory status must be made. This evaluation can be performed very quickly by assessing the individual's perception of being touched lightly with a fine wisp of cotton and making a comparison with the contralateral side. For a much more objective assessment, one may elect to use Semmes-Weinstein monofilaments. The graded nylon filaments are engineered to bow when specific forces are applied and thereby give an indication of the cutaneous sensibility of the area tested.[16]

ASSESSMENT

At this point in the examination, the examiner should assimilate all of the subjective and objective data to ensure that all of the findings correlate. Discrepancies should be noted in the assessment area of the progress note. An example of such an incompatibility might be a patient who complains of pain in the area of an ulcer while sensory examination reveals the area to be anesthetic.

Based on all information obtained, short- and long-term goals of treatment should be established. Once these goals have been determined, the clinician can then be very logical in the selection of treatment techniques to achieve these goals and guarantee that inappropriate treatments are not given.

CLINICAL DECISION MAKING

In this section, information on two clinical cases is provided. After reading the cases, the reader should decide what type of ulceration is present. The explanation of the cases may be found at the end of the section.

Case A

Mr. Jones enters your clinic with a draining wound over the medial aspect of his right ankle. The wound is small and quite painful. On examination, you note that the patient has some trophic changes in his nails and that he has decreased pulses in his feet. The ulcer has an irregular margin and is surrounded by a reactive hyperemia. The base of the ulcer appears pale. There is minimal swelling in the feet.

What is the most likely cause of this ulceration?

SOLUTION

Signs such as these are most indicative of arterial insufficiency. Although arterial ulcers tend to occur more in the toes and lateral aspects of the ankle, they can occur anywhere and are sometimes seen over the medial aspect of the ankle. The trophic changes in the nails and decreased pulses in the feet are also suggestive of arterial involvement. The minimal swelling in the feet could contribute to the inability to palpate pulses. Swelling is not an uncommon finding in arterial insufficiency and often results from vasodilation of more competent arteries. A Doppler examination would be helpful to further evaluate this patient. In addition to aiding in the detection of pulses, Doppler pressures would provide a good indication of arterial flow in the extremity. Some of the best information about this patient comes from the description of the ulcer and the degree of pain associated with it. Arterial ulcers are typically small with irregular margins and have a pale granulation base. In addition, such ulcers tend to be quite painful.

Case B

Mr. Conrad has come to see you as an outpatient with a referral that reads: "Chronic venous insufficiency with ulceration. Please evaluate and treat as indicated." On examination, you find that Mr. Conrad has a grossly edematous right lower extremity with an ulceration over the mid-calf of the right leg just above the medial malleolus. The ulcer measures 6 × 4 cm. The patient does not have any major complaints of pain; his primary complaint is of the drainage. Peripheral pulses are good. Some brownish discoloration is present around the wound, and the wound margin is somewhat irregular. The wound is covered with a necrotic debris, but there appears to be a good granulation base beneath the debris.

What is the most likely cause of this ulceration?

SOLUTION

This patient presents with classic signs of venous insufficiency. Venous ulcers tend to be irregular in shape with a necrotic base. While the ulcers are often quite large, they do not tend to be very painful. Edema, excessive drainage, and hemosiderin deposits in the surrounding skin are also frequently noted. Although peripheral pulses are good in this individual, it should be noted that patients can and often do have concurrent arterial problems. For this reason, the patient's arterial system should be evaluated.

SUMMARY

This chapter has provided the basic components of the examination of any patient who presents with an ulceration. Emphasis throughout the chapter has been on the use of clinical decision making in the development and implementation of the patient examination. The importance of the patient history and subjective information in conjunction with objective tests in determining the cause of various lesions was stressed. Although numerous objective tests are available, as presented in this chapter, the objective examination should be planned in the same manner in which a treatment program is planned, by selecting the tests that should provide the most valuable information. The examination process ends with all information being drawn together and conclusions being formed that are the basis for the treatment that is to follow. Several examination techniques that were discussed only briefly here will be handled in greater depth in subsequent chapters.

REFERENCES

1. Hunt, TK: Fundamentals of Wound Management in Surgery; Wound Healing: Disorders of Repair. Chirurgecom, Southfield, NJ, 1976, p 76.
2. Correlli, F: Buerger's disease: Cigarette smoker disease may always be cured by medical therapy. J Cardiovasc Surg 14:28, 1973.
3. McCulloch, J: Peripheral vascular disease. In O'Sullivan, SB and Schmitz, TJ (eds): Physical Rehabilitation: Assessment and Treatment. FA Davis, Philadelphia, 1988, p 375.
4. Bates, B: A Guide to Physical Examination and History Taking. JB Lippincott, Philadelphia, 1987, pp 130–131.
5. Lazarus, GS and Goldsmith, LA: Diagnosis of Skin Disease. FA Davis, Philadelphia, 1980, pp 314–315.
6. Shea, D: Pressure sores: Classification and management. Clin Orthop 112:100, 1975.
7. Thompson, GT: Moist wound healing combined with localized pressure relief—A new dressing. Ostomy/Wound Management, Spring 1987.
8. Cooper, DM, Watt, RC, and Alterescu, V: Guide to Wound Care. Holliser, Libertyville, IL, 1983.
9. Reddy, MP: Decubitus ulcers: Principles of presentation and management. Geriatrics 38:7, 1983.
10. Pillsbury, DM and Heaton, CL: A Manual of Dermatology. WB Saunders, Philadelphia, 1980, p 29.
11. Pories, WJ, et al: The management of human wound healing. Surgery 59(5):821, 1966.
12. Beach, RB: Measurement of extremity volume by water displacement. Phys Ther 57:286, 1977.
13. DeGowin, EL and DeGowin, RL: Bedside Diagnostic Examination, ed 3. Macmillan, New York, 1976, p 387.
14. Spittell, JA: Clinical Vascular Disease. FA Davis, Philadelphia, 1983.
15. Barnes, RW: Current status of noninvasive tests in the diagnosis of venous disease. Surg Clin North Am 62:3, 1982.
16. Bell, JA: Semmes-Weinstein Monofilament Testing for Determining Cutaneous Light Touch/Deep Pressure Sensation. The Star, National Hansen's Disease Center, Carville, LA, Nov/Dec, 1984.

CHAPTER 8

Doppler Ultrasound Assessment in Peripheral Vascular Disease*

Joyce MacKinnon, Ed.D., P.T.

The Doppler ultrasound assessment is an effective diagnostic technique for determining peripheral vascular status.[1] Unlike arteriograms and venograms, the Doppler ultrasound assessment is a noninvasive procedure, while still providing information concerning the status of the arterial and venous systems. The equipment can also be used to detect changes in blood flow in the carotid arteries, but because the focus of this chapter is on the evaluation of the peripheral vascular system, this technique is not discussed.

DOPPLER PRINCIPLE

Doppler ultrasonic evaluation of the peripheral vascular system was developed in the mid-1960s.[2] The assessment uses the Doppler principle to determine the relative velocity of blood flow in the major arteries and veins in the arms and legs. An oscillator in the Doppler equipment vibrates at a frequency of 5 to 10 MHz, which causes a piezoelectric crystal in the instrument to emit an ultrasound beam. The beam is directed transcutaneously over an artery or vein. As blood cells move through the blood vessel, their movements cause a shift in the frequency of the ultrasound beam. This shift is known as the Doppler effect. The reflected sound waves are received by a second crystal in the Doppler instrument. If the blood is motionless, then the reflected sound waves have the same frequency as the transmitted waves, and there is transmission silence. Any shift in frequency that occurs between the time the ultrasound beam is emitted and the time the reflected sound waves are received produces an audible signal.[1-4] This

---

*Readers interested in pursuing Doppler ultrasound assessment in depth should review the programmed text, which also includes an audible component, by Barnes and colleagues, 1975.[4]

signal can be analyzed in its auditory form, or can be transposed into a visual readout. Through the analysis of this signal, a person who is skilled in performing Doppler examinations can determine the presence of arterial disease, arterial or venous obstruction, and valvular competency.

EQUIPMENT

The Doppler ultrasonic equipment found in most clinics can take one of two forms. Equipment can consist of a handheld ultrasound probe that contains the oscillator and crystals previously described (Fig. 8–1), or it can be more stationary with the oscillator and crystals being housed in a box-like casing (Fig. 8–2). A pencil probe is attached to the casing by means of a jack. The probe is the part of the equipment that actually transmits the sound waves to the artery or vein being examined. The advantage of using the handheld Doppler is that its portability allows easy transportation to a patient's room or from one part of a clinic to another. The more stationary Doppler equipment permits an operator to choose settings appropriate for listening to arterial or venous blood flow. The stationary equipment may also have an attachment that allows a visual readout to be produced from the audible signal received. As with other ultrasound devices, the Doppler requires a medium for sound-wave transmission. Therefore, an ultrasound gel must be applied to the skin surface over which the probe will be located, or to the tip of the probe itself. The audible signal is heard through either an attached stethoscope or a head-set. The former is used with the handheld probe, and the latter with the stationary equipment. An aneroid sphygmomanometer is a necessary piece of equipment to have when performing arterial examinations.

ASSESSMENT OF THE PERIPHERAL ARTERIAL SYSTEM

An arterial Doppler ultrasound examination may be indicated when a patient complains of intermittent claudication or rest pain in a limb, or when tissue necrosis is present. When the Doppler ultrasound is used to assess the peripheral arterial system,

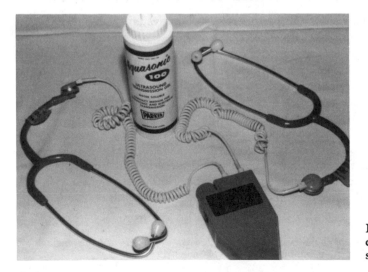

FIGURE 8–1. Doppler equipment—hand-held ultrasound probe.

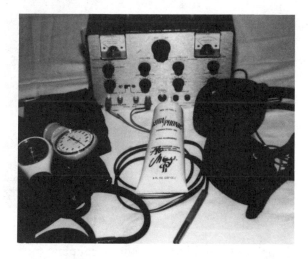

FIGURE   8–2.   Doppler
equipment.

two measurements are performed. An ankle-arm index ratio is the first measurement
obtained in an arterial examination. Segmental blood pressure readings constitute the
second measurement (see Arterial Doppler Ultrasound Evaluation form at the end of
this chapter). The ankle-arm index ratio is used to detect and quantify arterial vascular
disease, whereas the segmental blood pressure readings are used to locate obstructions.
The ankle-arm index ratio is calculated by comparing the systolic blood pressure in the
brachial artery with the systolic blood pressure in the posterior tibial artery. The patient
is placed in a supine position with hips in slight external rotation, knees slightly flexed,
and the lateral borders of the foot in contact with the table or bed (Fig. 8–3). This
position permits the examiner to accurately place the ultrasound probe and ensures that
the patient's position will not occlude the blood flow to the limb, as might occur with a
position of complete knee extension. A sphygmomanometer cuff is placed around the
upper arm. The brachial artery is located by manual palpation, and then the Doppler
ultrasound probe with a coupling medium is placed over the artery. The probe is held at
a 45-degree angle in relation to the artery, and is moved until the audible signal is at its
strongest (Fig. 8–4). The examiner must not exert a heavy pressure with the probe to
avoid compressing the artery externally and cutting off the audible signal.

The sphygmomanometer cuff is placed around the leg just above the malleoli, and
the posterior tibial artery is located by manual palpation. Once the artery is located, the

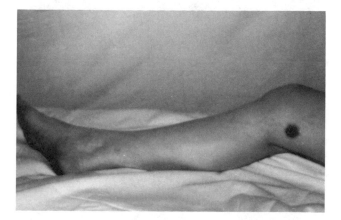

FIGURE 8–3. Limb position
for Doppler ultrasound assessment.

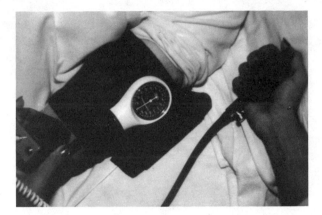

FIGURE 8–4. Systolic blood pressure—brachial artery.

Doppler ultrasound probe with a coupling medium is placed over the artery (Fig. 8–5). Again, the probe is held at a 45-degree angle in relation to the blood vessel, and is moved until the audible signal is at its strongest. The sphygmomanometer cuff is inflated until the sound is no longer heard, at which point it is slowly deflated and the systolic blood pressure is recorded when the sound first reappears.

The ankle-arm index ratio is the number obtained when the systolic blood pressure recorded from the posterior artery is divided by the systolic pressure recorded from the brachial artery.[4,5] For example, 120 mmHg (the systolic blood pressure recorded at the ankle) divided by 120 mmHg (the systolic blood pressure recorded at the arm) would be recorded as an ankle-arm index ratio of 1.0. A ratio of 1.0 or greater is considered normal; there is no indication of arterial vascular disease. A reading of 0.9 or 0.8 correlates with the symptoms of intermittent claudication. A reading of 0.7 to 0.5 is usually correlated with rest pain, and a reading of 0.4 or less usually indicates tissue necrosis.

Segmental blood pressure readings are obtained at the ankle, below the knee (Fig. 8–6), above the knee (Fig. 8–7), and high up on the thigh (Fig. 8–8). The sphygmomanometer cuff is moved to each of these regions for the reading of interest, while the Doppler probe remains constant at the posterior tibial artery.[6] Actually, any artery

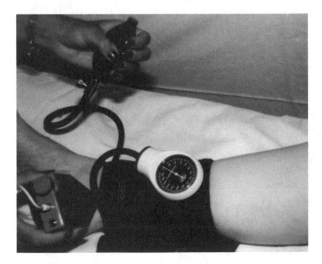

FIGURE 8–5. Systolic blood pressure-ankle.

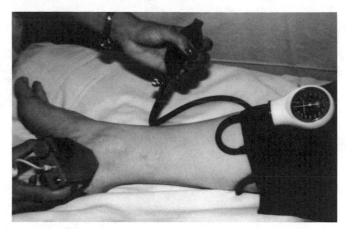

FIGURE 8–6. Systolic blood pressure—below knee.

below the placement of the sphygmomanometer cuff can be used to measure the blood pressure at the area where the cuff is placed. Use of the posterior tibial artery throughout the entire testing sequence is more efficient. Adjoining segmental readings should not vary by more than 30 mmHg. For example, if the segmental blood pressure reading at the ankle is 120 mmHg, the reading below the knee should be less than 150 mmHg. A greater difference between blood pressure in adjoining segments is indicative of an obstruction between those two segments, although an abnormal reading may also be obtained if the arterial system is calcified. However, if the arterial system is calcified, the readings are usually quite high; sometimes the blood flow cannot be occluded at all and often a reading greater than 200 mmHg is obtained. The anatomic reason for these results is that the blood vessels have become so rigid that an external force, such as an inflated sphygmomanometer cuff, is unable to compress the arterial walls enough to occlude the flow of blood. Although it is usually the lower limbs that are evaluated by Doppler ultrasound assessment, the technique can be used to detect arterial obstructions in the arm as well as in the leg.

Arterial Doppler ultrasound assessments can also be used to assist a surgeon in determining the level of a lower limb amputation.[7] For example, if the ankle-arm index ratio demonstrates that tissue is not viable below the ankle, then a surgeon may choose

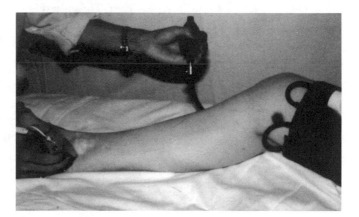

FIGURE 8–7. Systolic blood pressure—above knee.

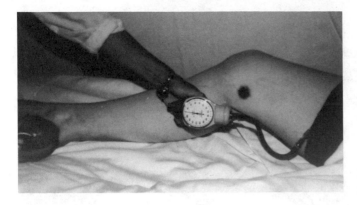

FIGURE 8–8. Systolic blood pressure—high thigh.

to plan a higher level of amputation to ensure healing and reduce the chances of having to revise an amputation based on inadequate blood flow to the remaining limb segment.

A Doppler ultrasound evaluation can be used as part of a walking test to determine the presence of intermittent claudication.[4] Using the Doppler equipment and a sphygmomanometer, blood pressure is taken below the knee or at the ankle. The patient is instructed to walk at a specific pace or is placed on a treadmill set at a 12-degree angle at a pace of 2 miles per hour. When the patient begins to complain of calf pain or at the end of 5 minutes, whichever comes first, arterial blood pressure is taken again and is compared with the first reading.

ASSESSMENT OF THE PERIPHERAL VENOUS SYSTEM

A venous Doppler ultrasound examination may be indicated in patients who have localized limb pain (especially upon deep pressure or palpation) or whose limb is warm to the touch or edematous. A Doppler ultrasound evaluation of the peripheral venous system is a more subjective test than an arterial evaluation because the audible signal produced during the test must be interpreted by the examiner rather than being quantified into a systolic blood pressure reading, as is the case with an arterial evaluation.[4,8] The Doppler probe is placed over the posterior tibial (Fig. 8–9), common femoral (Fig. 8–10), superficial femoral (Fig. 8–11), and popliteal (Fig. 8–12) veins in turn, and the audible signal is analyzed at each of the four locations. Some examiners have likened the sound to that of a phasic windstorm. The signal is noted as spontaneous, augmentable, at an appropriate pitch, cycling with respiration, and compressible (see Venous Doppler Ultrasound Evaluation form at the end of this chapter). As part of the assessment, the examiner should compare the normal limb with the limb whose venous system is in question, to detect variations in individual patients. When assessing the posterior tibial, common femoral, and superficial femoral veins, the patient is positioned with the hips in slight external rotation, the knees slightly flexed, and the medial border of the foot exposed. The legs should not be elevated, as this will lead to venous pooling and an inaudible signal. When assessing the popliteal vein, the patient should be prone with the knees slightly flexed and the feet resting on a pillow.

To assess a venous signal's spontaneity, the Doppler probe is placed over the posterior tibial vein, and an audible signal is either present or absent. This signal is recorded as being either spontaneous or not spontaneous. Even in a person with no

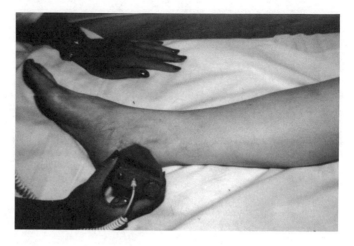

FIGURE 8–9. Doppler ultrasound assessment — posterior tibial vein.

venous problems, sometimes the posterior tibial venous sound is not spontaneous. This occurrence is usually caused by blood flow too slow for an appreciable shift to occur. However, the signal at the other three sites should be spontaneous; if it is not, then an obstruction is probably present.

Of the four veins, the popliteal is the most difficult to localize; an inexperienced examiner might locate the saphenous vein by mistake. Also, if a patient has a large thigh circumference, it may be difficult to accurately assess the superficial femoral vein.[4]

All signals, spontaneous or not, are tested for augmentation.[9] In this technique, pressure in the form of a quick, manual squeeze is applied distal to the probe to enhance the audible signal (Fig. 8–13). All locations should be augmentable. If a signal does not augment at all, a complete obstruction is suspected between the area where the examiner is augmenting and the location of the Doppler probe. If a signal is poorly augmentable, the examiner should suspect a partial obstruction.

The audible signal has an associated definite pitch. A pitch that is higher than expected usually means that the blood is flowing through a channel that is smaller than normal, indicating that there is probably a partial obstruction of this vessel. However, another explanation for the higher pitch may be that the patient has had a previous episode of obstruction, and that either collateral vessels have formed or recanalization

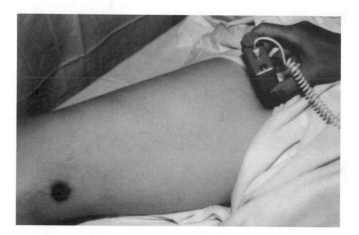

FIGURE 8–10. Doppler ultrasound assessment — common femoral vein.

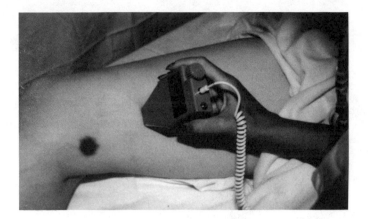

FIGURE 8–11. Doppler ultrasound assessment—superficial femoral vein.

has occurred. This event means that the blood is now flowing in a narrower channel and has bypassed the area of obstruction. To differentiate between the normal route of the vein and a new route, the examiner should use the adjacent arterial sound as an anatomic landmark, and listen particularly closely for phasicity. Often, blood flowing in collateral vessels is continuous rather than phasic.

The venous signal should also be in phase with the patient's respiratory cycle. In contrast, the arterial signal is in phase with the patient's cardiac cycle.

Finally, valvular competency is assessed by using a technique called *compression*.[4,9] The examiner manually compresses the limb proximal to the location of the Doppler probe (Fig. 8–14). If the venous valves are competent, sound should cease with compression and resume with release of compression. A sound heard when compression is being performed is an indication that the valves are allowing a backflow of blood and are therefore not competent. This technique is modified for the common femoral vein; the patient is asked to perform a Valsalva's maneuver to compress the vein proximal to the Doppler probe.

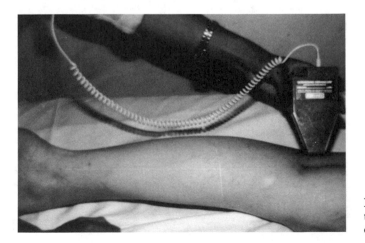

FIGURE 8–12. Doppler ultrasound assessment—popliteal vein.

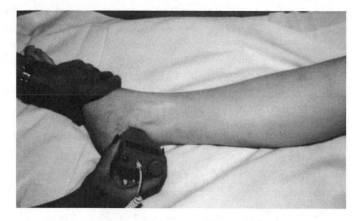

FIGURE 8–13. Augmentation of the posterior tibial vein.

COMPARISON OF DOPPLER ULTRASOUND ASSESSMENT WITH OTHER METHODS

Many studies have been performed to compare the results of Doppler ultrasound assessments of peripheral vascular disease with results of invasive tests such as arteriograms and venograms.[1,3,5,8–17] Most of these studies were undertaken in the mid-1960s to early 1970s, and the majority of them focused on venous Doppler examinations, since these are more subjective than arterial Doppler examinations. The measure of accuracy used in most of the studies was the detection of an obstruction in the vein when Doppler assessment results were compared with venogram results. Accuracy ranged from 76 to 94 percent, depending on such factors as the experience of the examiner, the examiner's knowledge of vascular anatomy, previous patient history of peripheral vascular disease, the cooperation of the patient, the presence of an incomplete obstruction, and the presence of other medical conditions.

Impedance plethysmography is another method used to detect peripheral vascular disease.[18] Like Doppler ultrasound, this technique is noninvasive and requires placing circumferential electrodes at four sites on the leg, inducing a low-voltage, high-frequency current through the two outer electrodes, and then detecting changes in voltage as the current passes through the electrodes. Given the amount of current applied and the voltage produced, the impedance can be calculated using Ohm's law $(I = \dfrac{V}{R})$. The

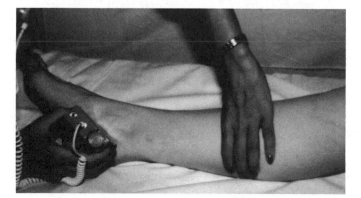

FIGURE 8–14. Compression to assess valvular competency of the posterior tibial vein.

technique can be used to calculate arterial blood flow and thus to detect arterial vascular disease or to screen for venous obstructions and incompetent valves. As with Doppler ultrasound assessments, results obtained from the use of impedance plethysmography correlate well with those obtained from invasive tests. Impedance plethysmography may be more accurate than Doppler ultrasound assessment in detecting changes in the deep calf veins, but the techniques are equally reliable for all other peripheral vascular assessments.

CLINICAL DECISION MAKING

1. You are performing a venous Doppler ultrasound assessment of the left leg and record the following results:

Vein	Spontaneous	Augmentable	Competent	Phasic
Posterior tibial	No	Yes	Yes	Yes
Common femoral	Yes	Yes	Yes	Yes
Superficial femoral	Yes	Yes	Yes	Yes
Popliteal	Yes	No	Yes	Yes

Does the patient have a problem in the venous peripheral system, and if so, what is the apparent nature of the problem? What information led to your decision?

The patient appears to have an obstruction in the left calf. While it is not necessarily an abnormality for the posterior tibial vein to be spontaneously inaudible, it is abnormal for the popliteal vein not to augment. This finding would suggest an obstruction in the calf.

2. You are performing a venous Doppler assessment. While listening to the blood flow in the superficial femoral vein, and comparing the sound in the right leg to that in the left leg, you notice that the audible signal in the left leg is at a higher pitch compared with the signal from the right leg. What is an interpretation of this difference?

There is a partial obstruction in the left superficial femoral vein.

3. You are performing an arterial Doppler assessment. Systolic arterial blood pressure readings in the right limbs are as follows:

Brachial	120 mmHg
Ankle	100 mmHg
Below knee	120 mmHg
Above knee	160 mmHg
High thigh	170 mmHg

What is your impression of the patient's arterial peripheral vascular status, considering the ankle-arm index ratio and the segmental blood pressure readings?

The ankle-arm index ratio is 0.83, which is indicative of intermittent claudication. The 40 mmHg difference in adjacent blood pressure readings between the below-knee and above-knee sites is indicative of an obstruction between the two sites.

4. You are performing an arterial Doppler assessment. Systolic arterial blood pressure readings in the right limb are as follows:

Brachial	160 mmHg
Ankle	180 mmHg
Below knee	210 mmHg
Above knee	225 mmHg
High thigh	Unable to obliterate the audible signal

What is your impression of the patient's arterial vascular status, considering the ankle-arm index ratio and the segmental blood pressure readings?

The ankle-arm index ratio is 1.13, which is a normal reading. However, it appears as though the patient might have some calcification in the lower limb venous system based on the high blood pressure readings in the four leg sites.

SUMMARY

Doppler ultrasound assessments constitute an evaluative technique that may be used to detect abnormalities in the peripheral vascular system. The technique is noninvasive and, due to the portability of the handheld Doppler ultrasound equipment, is readily offered in a variety of situations. To perform the assessments successfully, an examiner should gain experience in a supervised setting, be knowledgeable about vascular anatomy, and have access to a patient's history to determine if the patient has documented vascular disease, previous obstruction in the peripheral vascular system, or any other medical condition that might affect the test results. If the results of a Doppler ultrasound evaluation are equivocal, then an invasive test might be indicated.

ARTERIAL DOPPLER ULTRASOUND EVALUATION

Patient Name: _____ Date: _____
Pre-Test Comments: _____
_____

Pressure At Rest (mmHg)

Brachial Artery   R   L

Right Extremity

Ankle

Below the Knee

Above the Knee

High Thigh

Left Extremity

Ankle

Below the Knee

Above the Knee

High Thigh

ARTERIAL DOPPLER ULTRASOUND EVALUATION—Continued

Ankle/Arm Index Ratio

Right Extremity:

Left Extremity:

Post-Test Comments:

_____

_____

_____

_____

_____

Signature: _____

VENOUS DOPPLER ULTRASOUND EVALUATION

Patient Name: _____ Date: _____

Pre-Test Comments: _____

_____

NOTE: A false-negative response may be obtained in the presence of an isolated calf thrombosis or if compensatory channels have developed.

	Spontaneous	Augmentive	Compressible	Comments
Right Extremity				
Posterior tibial v				
Popliteal v				
Superficial femoral v				
Common femoral v				
Left Extremity				
Posterior tibial v				
Popliteal v				
Superficial femoral v				
Common femoral v				

Post-Test Comments:

_____

_____

_____

_____

_____

Signature: _____

REFERENCES

1. MacKinnon, JL: A Study of Doppler ultrasonic peripheral vascular evaluations performed by physical therapists. Phys Ther 63(1):30, 1983.
2. Rushmer, R, Baker, D, and Stegal, H: Transcutaneous Doppler flow detection as a nondestructive technique. J Appl Physiol 21(2):554, 1965.
3. Holmes, MCG: Deep venous thrombosis of the lower limbs diagnosed by ultrasound. Med J Aust 1:427, 1973.
4. Barnes, RW, Russell, HE, and Wilson, MR: Doppler Ultrasonic Evaluation of Venous Disease/Doppler Ultrasonic Evaluation of Peripheral Vascular Disease. University of Iowa, Iowa City, 1975.
5. Yao, JST: New techniques in objective arterial evaluation. Arch Surg 106:600, 1973.
6. Barker, WF: Diagnostic methods in peripheral arterial disease. Am Surg 543, 1973.
7. Bell, G, et al: Measurements of systolic pressure in the limbs of patients with arterial occlusive disease. Surg Gynecol Obstet 136(2):177, 1973.
8. Strandess, DE and Sumner, DS: Ultrasonic velocity detector in the diagnosis of thrombophlebitis. Arch Surg 104:180, 1972.
9. Sigelk, B, et al: A Doppler ultrasound method for diagnosing lower extremity venous diseases. Surg Gynecol Obstet 127:339, 1968.
10. Barnes, RW, Russell, HE, Wu, KK, and Hoak, JC: Accuracy of Doppler ultrasound in clinically suspected venous thrombosis of the calf. Surg Gynecol Obstet 143:425, 1976.
11. Sumner, DS and Strandess, DE: The relationship between calf blood flow and ankle blood pressure in patients with intermittent claudication. Surgery 65:763, 1969.
12. Sumner, DS, Baker, DW, and Strandess, DE: The ultrasonic velocity detector in a clinical study of venous disease. Arch Surg 97:75, 1968.
13. Strandess, DE, McCutcheon, EP, and Rushmer, RF: Application of a transcutaneous Doppler flowmeter in evaluation of occlusive arterial disease. Surg Gynecol Obstet 122:1039, 1966.
14. Strandess, DE, et al: Ultrasonic flow detection: A useful technique in the evaluation of peripheral vascular disease. Am J Surg 113:320, 1967.
15. Evans, DS: The early diagnosis of deep vein thrombosis by ultrasound. Br J Surg 57:726, 1970.
16. Yao, JST, Gourmos, C, and Hobbs, JT: Detection of proximal vein thrombosis by Doppler ultrasound flow-detection method. Lancet 1:1, 1972.
17. Yao, JST, Henkin, RE, and Bergan, JJ: Venous thromboembolitic disease: Evaluation of new methodology in treatment. Arch Surg 104: 664, 1974.
18. Golden, JC and Miles, DS: Assessment of peripheral hemodynamics using impedance plethysmography. Phys Ther 66(10):1544, 1986.

Part III

PRINCIPLES AND METHODS OF TREATMENT

CHAPTER 9

Conservative Management of Chronic Wounds

Jeffrey A. Feedar, P.T.
Luther C. Kloth, M.S., P.T.

Indolent, nonhealing wounds may arise from many causes including infection, persistent foreign bodies, the presence of toxic irritants, burns, prolonged cutaneously applied pressure, and poor blood supply secondary to compromised venous or arterial circulation. Various diagnoses of chronic wounds include sepsis, chemical toxicity, pressure ulcers, venous insufficiency ulcers, and atherosclerotic ulcers. In each case, tissue homeostasis and the wound environment is compromised so that either healing fails to occur or healing begins but progression is subsequently halted. Some factors that may interfere with homeostasis and the healing environment include tissue necrosis, dehydration, chronic wound edema, fibrotic induration, and small blood vessel disease.

Many commercial wound care products are available, which may be used appropriately in the conservative management of chronic wounds to restore normal tissue homeostasis, facilitate healing, and eliminate the need for surgical intervention.

The objectives of this chapter are (1) to identify factors that interfere with wound tissue homeostasis; (2) to discuss the appropriate selection and application of wound care products; (3) to provide guidelines for wound debridement; (4) to discuss other conservative techniques of wound management; (5) to challenge the reader with thought-provoking questions that encourage clinical decision-making processes in determining when a particular wound care product should be used; and (6) to provide the reader with a list of wound care product manufacturers and their products.

WOUND ENVIRONMENT (HOMEOSTASIS)

Uncompromised cellular homeostasis is essential for expeditious wound healing and wound repair. Within the healing tissue microenvironment, certain conditions are required for optimizing the concomitant development of granulation tissue and epithelial budding. These homeostatic conditions include but are not limited to (1) the degree

135

of hydration; (2) sufficient blood perfusion; (3) availability of various growth factors; (4) an appropriate partial pressure of oxygen; (5) acceptable levels of endogenous nonpathogenic microflora; and (6) maintenance of voltage gradients between the wound and adjacent normal skin. Protection of this environment from exogenous pathogens and selection of the most appropriate wound care products are also essential for healing.

Wound Moisture

In a homeostatic environment, cells are bathed in body fluids that allow for normal growth and repair processes. Within the confines of a wound, tissue fluids accumulate and create an environment for angiogenesis and the desirable formation of granulation tissue on which re-epithelialization may occur. In a moist environment, favorable microflora may be found, which stimulates epidermal cell migration and healing.[1] In a wound where the moist state is maintained, the epidermal cell migration takes place over a moist tissue layer (Fig. 9–1). For example, healing of wounds in the oral mucosa is well known to proceed more rapidly than healing in skin.[2] Certainly, the higher metabolic rate, higher temperature, and better blood supply are also important factors that contribute to the faster healing rate of the mucosa. Perhaps equally important is the fact that migrating epithelial cells in the moist oral cavity do not meet the resistance offered by a crusty, dehydrated scab that characteristically develops after skin wounds.

Secretory enzyme activity may also affect migratory cells during wound healing. Enzymes such as collagenases[3,4] and proteinases[5] apparently enable cells to migrate across a wound in moist areas where fibrin is deposited beneath the dessicated superficial crust covering the wound. However, when exposure to air results in excessive dehydration of damaged tissues, efficiency of migratory cell movement is reduced owing to the prolonged route of travel and the need for additional secretion of collagenase enzymes. Additionally, a drying out of wound tissue may dampen the lateral voltage gradient thought to control the direction of epidermal cells in their migration across the wound. A discussion of these gradients is presented in Chapter 12.

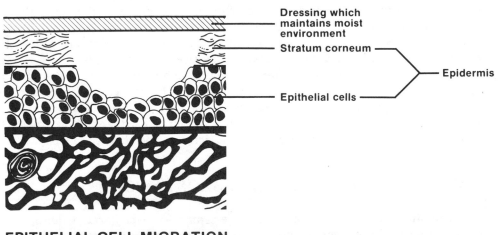

EPITHELIAL CELL MIGRATION UNDER MOISTENED ENVIRONMENT

FIGURE 9–1. Epidermal cell migration in a moist wound environment.

SCAB FORMATION AND FUNCTION

Within hours after a wound occurs, the surface of the tissue defect loses moisture and begins to dry partially from the influences of coagulated blood containing red cells, the presence of fibrinogen molecules, and evaporation. Normally, a wound, if left to run its course, will form a scab. In this environment, where a relative loss of hydration occurs, there is increased resistance to epidermal cell migration, owing to obstruction by dead and crusty tissue. In experiments on domestic pigs, Winter[6] found that immediate drying of exposed dermal tissue occurred after removal of the epidermis. Pollack[1] has suggested that as this drying occurs, a "water table" forms below the wound surface. This underlying moist environment may allow for more efficient epidermal migration. Thus, if the surface tissue is excessively dehydrated and thick wound crust (scab or eschar) is present, epidermal cells may have to burrow to a deeper plane beneath the scab to reach moist, live cells where they can migrate and perform their function[7] (Fig. 9-2). This route of migration is less efficient because of random probing by cells for the path of least resistance. Rovee and associates[8] have shown that a hydrophobic dressing maintains wound moisture which, in turn, prevents scab formation and decreases the path of resistance to migrating cells, thereby augmenting the rate of epithelialization. Thus, the presence of a scab or of leathery, necrotic eschar may serve as the body's natural hydrophobic "dressing" to keep moisture in the wound. However, in chronic wounds like decubitus ulcers, the efficiency of epithelial cell migration, which occurs inward from the wound periphery, may be diminished considerably by eschar, resulting in delayed healing.

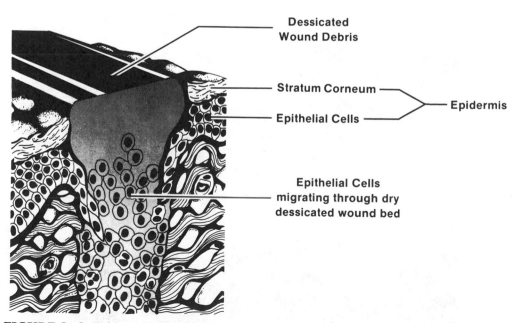

FIGURE 9-2. Epidermal cell migration beneath a desiccated wound environment. Re-epithelialization is less efficient because of impedance of epithelial cells by encrusted necrotic tissue.

EPITHELIALIZATION

The processes of epithelialization and the development of granulation tissue formation, as discussed in Chapters 2 and 3, occur concomitantly. They are presented separately here to provide the reader with information on how tissues respond in desiccated and moist wound environments.

In superficial wounds of the epidermis such as abrasions, re-epithelialization occurs from the epidermal appendages (hair follicles and sweat glands). This process proceeds rapidly, since epidermal cells only migrate the short distances between appendages. Generally, epidermal cell migration occurs via laminated sheets of cells which close the wound when sheets from opposite sides of the wound meet[9] (Fig. 9–3). In deeper wounds of the dermis and in Stage III or IV wounds such as decubitus ulcers, epithelialization develops from the wound periphery and takes much longer.[1] In chronic dermal and indolent ulcers, cell migration from the wound periphery may not occur if necrotic, desiccated tissue is obstructing it, or if repeated applications of pressure causing ischemia are applied. Thus, a clean, moist wound environment with an ample blood supply facilitates tissue repair.

GRANULATION TISSUE

Tissue destruction resulting in a wound that has extended through the dermis or deeper is considered a full-thickness lesion. Before re-epithelialization and healing, this type of wound fills with collagenous scar tissue. Vascularization of collagen takes on a beefy-red, granular appearance created by projecting ends of endothelial sprouts that form perfused capillary arcades[10] (Fig. 9–4). Before epidermal cells will migrate across a Stage II or IV ulcer, as described in Chapter 7, a base of well-hydrated granulation tissue must be present.[11] When a wound surface has dried, epidermal cells inefficiently migrate down into the desiccated scab and will not penetrate through as easily. The epithelium, therefore, will be inhibited from migrating across the surface or cutting

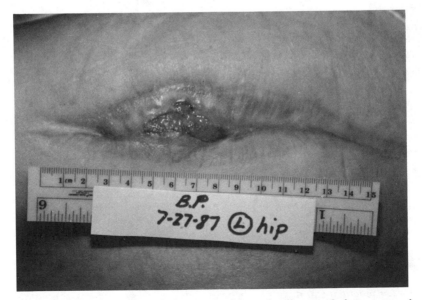

FIGURE 9–3. Laminated sheets of epidermal cells resurfacing a wound.

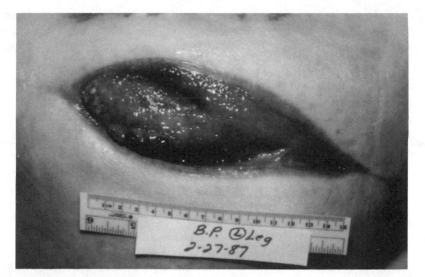

FIGURE 9–4. Wound bed filled with well-vascularized tissue. Beefy-red appearance indicates good endothelial growth and capillary perfusion.

through beneath the scab.[10] Thus, the importance of maintaining a moist environment during the entire process of wound healing must be remembered.

Infection Vulnerability

Moist wounds have been thought of as environments that are highly conducive to supporting bacterial overgrowth. Wound sepsis caused by bacterial overgrowth is defined by the United States Institute of Surgical Research as a bacterial contamination exceeding 10^5 organisms per gram of tissue.[12] If a wound biopsy reveals a bacterial concentration greater than 10^5 organisms per gram of tissue, the Institute recommends that the wound be left open to heal by secondary intention. Secondary intention involves both granulation tissue formation and re-epithelialization. Healing by secondary intention may reduce the bacterial count; however, necrosis of viable tissue may still occur if the wound environment is allowed to dry out. Wound pathogens may accompany necrotic tissue as it is sloughed off and, therefore, sloughing may be facilitated by gentle whirlpool jet agitation directed at the wound.

In contrast to decontaminating wounds by air exposure or water turbulence, both of which promote tissue erosion, another approach is to cover the wound with an occlusive dressing designed to keep the wound moist without causing tissue erosion. Although advantages of healing wounds (with or without minimal amounts of necrotic tissue) beneath occlusive dressings have been recognized for more than two decades, clinicians feared that these dressings promoted wound infection. Some of the reasons for this fear may be attributed to the following observations: (1) proliferation of microorganisms has been shown to increase on normal skin beneath occlusive coverings;[13,14] (2) tissue desiccation retards microbial overgrowth (occlusive dressings prevent tissue desiccation);[15,16] and (3) many white blood cells appear in serous wound fluid to form pus,[16] which may appear after an occlusive dressing is applied. Despite these observations, a paucity of reports exists in which wound infections occurred beneath occlusive dressings.[17-19] Not only have wound infections beneath occlusive dressings been rare, but in one study of chronic ulcers treated with an occlusive dressing, healing occurred despite gross bacterial overgrowth.[20] In addition, occlusive dressings may reduce infection vulnerability by excluding bacteria from the wound.[16]

Wound Edema

The development of edema in a chronic wound often follows debridement of necrotic tissue. If debridement is performed with a scalpel, the degree of trauma, bleeding, and tissue irritation may be considerable. If debridement is performed by enzymes, there is much less trauma and little or no bleeding, but irritation of delicate tissues still occurs. Regardless of the method used to debride, the resulting trauma and/or tissue irritation lead to increased permeability of capillary walls and the outpouring of exudate. Usually the exudate is watery and may be absorbed from the wound by saline-moistened gauze dressings reapplied as needed. If the exudate is clear and watery but excessive, or if it is purulent and excessive, cleansing and absorption may be done with a hydrophilic material like dextranomer. Dextranomer is a high molecular weight dextran derivative manufactured as dry, insoluble spherical beads. Each gram of dextranomer can absorb 4 g of fluid.

Wound edema occurs when an excessive amount of hydrophilic plasma protein leaks out of damaged or irritated capillaries allowing mositure to accumulate with subsequent formation of an opaque, gelatinous covering in the base of the wound (Fig. 9–5). This edematous mass contains proteolytic enzymes and other elements like bacteria, bacterial toxins, prostaglandins, and necrotic debris, all of which contribute to sustaining and perpetuating a chronic inflammatory state. Unlike the homeostatic moist wound environment previously described, the edematous wound environment suppresses proliferation of granulation tissue.[21] In addition, epithelial cells must have a compact fibrin, collagenous, connective tissue surface to which they can adhere and advance by ameboid action (Fig. 9–6). Cleaning gelatinous edema from the wound may be achieved by whirlpool jet agitation followed by applications of dextranomer for a few days, or by using dextranomer alone. To avoid tissue dehydration and to allow establishment of a granulation base, dextranomer should be discontinued immediately when exudate or wound edema is no longer present. Furthermore, if the wound is located on the distal aspect of an extremity and wound edema continues to develop, the limb should be elevated to reduce capillary filtration pressure, which is potentiated by gravity and increased hydrostatic pressure.

Factors Influencing Capillary Blood Flow

The most superficial capillary loops that extend into the dermis are very delicate and thin walled. These capillaries provide oxygen and nutrients to the integument, and the flow of blood through them is affected by external pressures and temperatures applied to the skin. Hydrostatic pressure in the subepidermal capillary loops averages 25 to 35 mmHg but is reduced in debilitated individuals. When local outside pressures greater than 80 mmHg are applied to the skin, the capillaries will collapse and thrombose if the pressure is applied for a few hours.[22] In fact, pressures of 70 mmHg applied to healthy tissue for only 2 hours will cause irreversible tissue damage.[23] When high pressures (exceeding 150 mmHg) are applied to the skin and maintained for a shorter

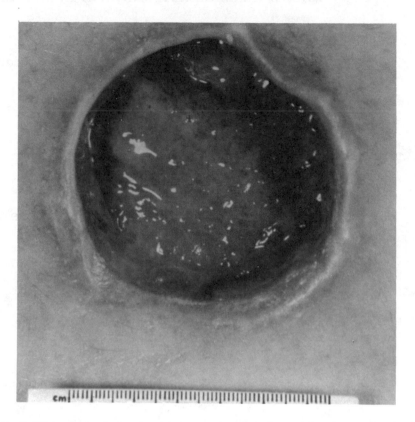

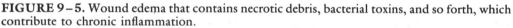

FIGURE 9–5. Wound edema that contains necrotic debris, bacterial toxins, and so forth, which contribute to chronic inflammation.

period of time, local capillaries collapse, tissue hypoxia develops, and tissue destruction begins.[24] Once tissue damage with capillary thrombosis, anoxia, and a reduced nutritional state has occurred, the physiologic response is inflammation. The inflammatory state elevates local tissue metabolism, causing local tissue temperature to rise, which further increases local metabolism. This vicious cycle ultimately leads to tissue necrosis and cell death.

Pressure sores caused by pressure alone are often the size of the underlying bony prominence on which pressure is exerted in the recumbent individual. With aging, capillary fragility increases, which increases the vulnerability of dermal vessels to the deleterious effects of pressure.

Another factor that increases the risk of skin breakdown is the shear force of bony prominences over subcutaneous tissue, which can cause ischemia, metabolite accumulation, and cell death (Fig. 9–7). Friction can denude the epidermis by disrupting the rete pegs and epidermal attachments that bind the epidermis to the dermis. Prolonged moisture accumulation from lying on a water vapor–impermeable mattress and/or moisture from incontinence can macerate the epidermis and lead to tissue necrosis. Factors influencing capillary blood flow will be discussed in greater detail later in this chapter.

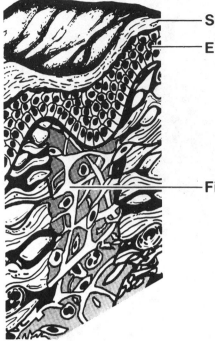
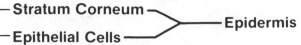

FIGURE 9–6. Desirable connective tissue surface on which epithelial cells can adhere and cover the wound defect.

DEBRIDEMENT

Debridement is the removal of necrotic and devitalized tissue from a wound. During the inflammatory phase following injury and during the development of a pressure sore, migrating leukocytes and polymorphonuclear leukocytes are found in exudate within 6 to 12 hours after wounding. These phagocytes debride the wound by ingesting bacteria. Within a few days, the remnants of these cells are incorporated into the wound crust that forms from evaporation at the surface.[1] Four or five days after wounding, assuming a normal inflammatory response, macrophages derived from monocytes and

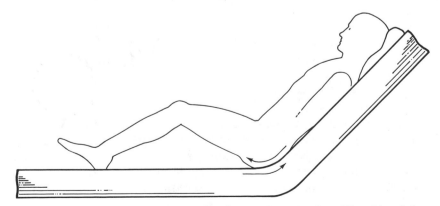

FIGURE 9–7. Shear forces contributing to decreasaed capillary blood flow.

phagocytic white blood cells (neutrophils) arrive at the wound site below the desiccated crust to complete the clean-up process. Macrophages that secrete proteolytic enzymes play a major role in phagocytic debridement of necrotic tissue, foreign matter, and dead cells. They achieve maximal phagocytic efficiency in an oxygen-rich environment.[25] As macrophage debridement proceeds, they release chemotactic factors that attract more macrophages into the wound environment along with stimulatory agents, which in turn increase fibroblastic proliferation and neoangiogenesis, leading to enhancement of the healing process.[26]

Unlike the normal inflammatory response discussed in Chapter 1, in the chronic wound, obstructive necrotic tissue impedes the formation of granulation tissue and prevents epithelial cells from migrating across the wound. In wounds of this type, debridement not only removes dead tissue on which bacteria survive, but also removes many of the microorganisms that may be present. Bacteria and debris may be washed out by saline irrigation or by the gentle force of water agitation from a whirlpool jet directed at the wound. When large amounts of necrotic tissue are present in a wound, other methods may be used to speed up the debridement process and facilitate wound repair.

Types of Debridement

There are two types of debridement: selective and nonselective. Selective debridement removes only necrotic tissue whereas nonselective debridement indiscriminately removes both nonviable and viable tissue from the wound.

SELECTIVE DEBRIDEMENT

Selective debridement may be performed in one of three ways: (1) with topical application of enzymes; (2) by facilitating autolysis with synthetic dressings; or (3) by surgical excision. Surgical debridement is the fastest way to selectively debride and the most efficient method as long as only devitalized tissue is removed. Although selective debridement is the intent of the surgical approach, this method poses risks of sepsis and bleeding, owing to the inadvertent trauma inflicted on healthy tissues. Surgical debridement should be used with caution on patients who have low platelet counts or who are taking anticoagulants. Debridement with topical enzymes is also selective because enzymes only digest necrotic tissue. When an excess quantity of desiccated eschar is present, proteolytic enzymes such as fibrinolysin and deoxyribonuclease, combined into the commercial product known as Elase,* debride denatured proteins slowly but most efficaciously, usually in less than 15 days by attacking DNA, as well as the fibrin of clots and fibrinous exudates. The proteolytic enzymes elaborated by Bacillus subtilis form the active ingredient of another commercial product known as Travase,† which also effectively debrides necrotic protein. Other proteolytic enzyme preparations such as papain, streptodornase, streptokinase, and sutilains may also be used to dissolve necrotic tissue. Although proteolytic enzymes are often able to debride heavy eschar and denatured proteins, Howes and associates[27] showed that stubborn necrotic tissue may be anchored to the wound surface by strands of undenatured collagen. Howes and coworkers[27] and Boxer and colleagues[28] have demonstrated that the enzyme collagenase can hydrolyze

*Parke-Davis, Division of Warner Lambert Co., Morris Plains, NJ 07950.
†Travenol Laboratories, Inc., Flint Laboratories Division, Deerfield, IL 60015.

undenatured collagen and facilitate debridement of stubborn necrotic collagen tissue. Examples of commercial collagenase debridement products are Biozyme-C‡ and Santyl.§ Enzymatic ointments should be applied to the necrotic tissue every 3 to 5 hours in very thin layers and then covered with saline-moistened gauze packing to absorb the liquified slough.[29] When an excessive quantity of eschar is present, the crust should be cross-hatched with a scalpel to allow the proteolytic enzyme to permeate into it.

Autolysis is self-digestion of necrotic tissue leading to the process of eschar liquification by enzymes that are naturally present in wound fluids. Many health professionals involved in the care of existing wounds now believe that fluids seeping from noninfected wounds should be sequestered by trapping the fluids over the wound, enabling macrophages to digest necrotic debris. This closed, moist wound environment may be compared with a watery blister with its skin covering substituted either by synthetic dressings or saline-moistened gauze as discussed later in this chapter. This concept of maintaining a closed, moist wound environment, combined with the growing belief that atmospheric oxygen may be of less value in the healing of wounds than was formerly believed,[30,31] has led to the development of synthetic dressings that, in addition to providing autolytic debriding action,[32-34] also encourage granulation development, cell migration, and healing.[35] Autolytic debridement facilitated by occlusive dressings relies upon normal phagocytic activity of white blood cells and is therefore the most selective form of debridement.

NONSELECTIVE DEBRIDEMENT

The nonselective forms of debridement include the use of wet-to-dry, wet-to-wet, and dry-to-dry gauze dressings; vigorous whirlpool jet agitation and/or wound irrigation; Dakin's solution; and hydrogen peroxide applications.[36] The various gauze dressings should be used only on necrotic wounds, and care must be taken when they are removed because not only does necrotic tissue cling to the dressing, but delicate epithelium and granulation tissue may also be removed in the process, sometimes intentionally to speed up debridement. Likewise, vigorous wound cleansing by whirlpool or saline irrigation and the foaming action of hydrogen peroxide should also be used only on necrotic wounds because the mechanical action created by water turbulence and foaming effervescence will wash away healthy tissue along with necrotic tissue. Caution must be used when debriding deep tunneling wounds with hydrogen peroxide because it may cause tissue trauma when it bubbles in the tunnels.[36] Hydrogen peroxide has been shown to oxidize wound debris as well as healthy tissue protein. Because this compound may also cause blisters of new tissue, sources have suggested that hydrogen peroxide should not be used when healthy granulation tissue is present.[37,38] Generally, nonselective debridement is chosen for wounds containing extensive necrotic tissue and debris that may be promoting an infectious process.

Once debrided, a wound will normally undergo granulation, contraction, and epithelialization. Thus, debridement of necrotic wound tissue must be performed to allow the healing processes of granulation development and fibroblastic deposition of collagen upon which epidermal cells can migrate and close the wound. Patients should be informed that necrotic tissue retards the healing process and that they should not be alarmed by the observable increase in the dimensions of their wound following removal of nonviable tissue. Often patients consider crusty eschar to represent a favorable scabbing over and progress toward healing, especially if the wound has been draining

---

‡Armour Pharmaceutical Co., P.O. Box 511, Kankakee, IL 60190.
§Knoll Pharmaceutical Co., Whippany, NJ 07981.

previously. To not forewarn the patient that debridement will temporarily increase the wound size may cause them unnecessary emotional suffering.

HYDROTHERAPY

One of the oldest therapeutic methods used for treating chronic open wounds is hydrotherapy.[39] Today, the primary method used to administer hydrotherapy to wounds is the whirlpool, which may be used to debride necrotic tissue[40,41] for soaking off adherent, wet-to-dry dressings that are too painful to remove and for cleansing wounds of dirt,[42] foreign contaminants,[43] and toxic residues from various topical agents. In addition, various antimicrobial agents may be added to the water of a whirlpool bath to kill bacteria present in infected wounds.[44,45]

Although a whirlpool may be used to produce a moist tissue environment for wound healing, one must use it with discretion to avoid harmful effects to regenerating wound tissues, skin grafts, and tissue flaps caused by excessively high turbulence and water temperatures.

In dermal ulcers, hydrotherapy is most appropriately used twice daily (BID) following incomplete surgical debridement to facilitate softening and separation of eschar and other necrotic tissue. In this case, whirlpool is most effective when used in conjunction with interim wound dressings. In this regard, whirlpool should be administered daily or BID in conjunction with wet-to-dry saline gauze dressings or synthetic dressings intended to facilitate debridement of wounds covered with a yellow fibrous debris or gelatinous surface exudate.[46] Both the water turbulence and removal of the wet-to-dry dressing help to remove surface debris and/or viscous exudate.

In wounds that have a beefy-red appearance owing to the presence of granulation tissue and migrating epidermal cells, a whirlpool with even moderate water agitation may mechanically damage vulnerable endothelial and epithelial cells, which are best treated by protecting them with an appropriate dressing.

Various antibacterial agents may be added to the whirlpool water to help reduce wound infection. Even though all open wounds contain microflora, some of which may be pathogenic, this does not necessarily mean the wound is infected. Therefore, one must weigh the alleged benefit of such agents in preventing infection against the possibility of suppressing tissue repair secondary to cytotoxic effects, especially in wounds that are exposed daily to recommended dilutions of commonly used agents such as povidone-iodine and sodium hypochlorite solutions. Povidone-iodine diluted to 4 parts per million in whirlpool water has been reported to reduce whirlpool bacterial colony counts by more than 90 percent.[44] Sodium hypochlorite (household bleach) has been shown to be effective against resistant burn wound microorganisms in dilutions of 1:160,[45] but dilutions of 1:60 or 1:120 are recommended. A more detailed discussion of these and other topical agents follows.

TOPICAL AGENTS

Topical agents can have a profound effect on the rate of wound healing and, in some cases, may even retard healing. Topical antimicrobials and cleansers have frequently been overused in wound therapy, resulting in harmful cytotoxic effects and minimal antimicrobial and cleansing effectiveness. Antiseptic agents act to destroy bacteria. Various antiseptic solutions are often used to irrigate wounds and are also traditionally applied to dressings to prevent or rid a wound of bacterial invasion. The concentration of an antiseptic solution used in wound care should not exceed that required to maintain its bactericidal effectiveness and should be noncytotoxic to regenerating tissues. Solutions and ointments are frequently prescribed based on tradition rather than on evidence from scientific studies. This section will cover some commonly used topical agents and solutions and examine the decision-making process behind selecting, not selecting, or changing the use of these agents during the healing process.

Povidone-Iodine Solution

Free iodine, although useful as an antimicrobial agent,[47] is toxic to skin and mucosal membranes. Free iodine also has a low water-solubility ratio and therefore is complexed with the polymer polyvinyl-pyrrolidone, making the solution water soluble and stable and less toxic to viable tissues. When iodine is complexed in such a solution, it is referred to as an *iodophor*. The iodophor, although stabilized, still contains a small amount of free iodine, which, in appropriate dilutions, may be an effective antimicrobial without being cytotoxic to healing tissues. Lineaweaver and coworkers,[48] found that povidone-iodine diluted to a 0.001 percent concentration is bactericidal to Staphylococcus aureus, yet is noncytotoxic to cultured human fibroblasts. Additionally, they reported that concentrations of povidone-iodine at 1 percent were 100 percent cytotoxic, and concentrations at 0.05 percent were 50 percent ± 25 percent cytotoxic. Moreover, the tensile strength of wounds in rats irrigated with 1 percent povidone-iodine 4 days after wounding was only 21 percent that of control wounds. There were no significant differences at 8, 12, or 16 days. Wound epithelialization was also significantly reduced at 4 and 8 days by exposure to 1 percent povidone-iodine.[48] Lineaweaver's study demonstrates that there is an appropriate dilution of povidone-iodine that is bactericidal to Staphylococcus aureus and noncytotoxic to cultured human fibroblasts. These findings argue against the use of povidone-iodine at concentrations greater than 0.001 percent and should caution the clinician against using povidone-iodine and other topical agents for extended periods based only upon manufacturer's claims. This caution suggests that more accurate clinical guidelines could be formulated for the use of povidone-iodine solution in whirlpool baths and on gauze dressings.

There are other conflicting reports on the use of povidone-iodine. Clinical studies have reported decreased[49] and unchanged[50,51] rates of wound complication following its use. Povidone-iodine may not produce the same effect(s) on human, chronic full-thickness wounds as in animal model partial-thickness wounds or in in vitro or in situ studies. Although povidone-iodine may[48] or may not[52] retard epithelialization and decrease wound tensile strength, its antimicrobial action may be desirable. Determining the effects of povidone-iodine use in whirlpool baths would seem beneficial for bacterial toxicity, for epithelialization, and for rate of healing of chronic Stage III and IV ulcers at concentrations reported by Lineaweaver.[48] Those results could then be compared with the results of wounds treated in whirlpool baths, with povidone-iodine guidelines reported by Simonette and colleagues.[44] Serial dilutions of povidone-iodine could also be used in gauze-packed chronic wounds to determine its effects on various wound-healing events. The proposed studies would allow clinicians to determine the usefulness of povidone-iodine and possibly to eliminate its habitual use if proven detrimental to wound healing. In addition, clinicians must be aware of the possible long-term effects of topical povidone-iodine solutions that may occur through systemic absorption of iodine with repeated use.[53]

Another clinical consideration that should be kept in mind when using povidone-iodine is that iodine is the active antiseptic agent released from the solution and is readily inactivated by binding to serum proteins.[54] If povidone-iodine is used in exudating wounds, the solution will have weakened antiseptic effects. Hugo and Newton[55] found that in cultures of Staphylococcus aureus, the addition of serum abolished the antiseptic activity of iodine in 2 minutes. After 24 hours, they found increased numbers of Staphylococcus aureus in cultures treated with iodine in the presence of serum, and therefore have questioned the value of povidone-iodine as an antimicrobial in the presence of organic wound fluid and debris. Kucan and coworkers[54] reported that the application of 10 percent povidone-iodine to chronic human pressure sores every 6 hours was no more effective than saline washes in reducing bacterial counts. Rodeheaver and associates[56] reported that povidone-iodine solution afforded no therapeutic benefit because wounds contaminated with Staphylococcus aureus and treated with iodine solution had the same level of viable bacteria as those that received only saline solution. Other research studies have reported that povidone-iodine is ineffective if applied to a wound colonized with greater than 10^5 organisms per gram of tissue.[57-59] Therefore, the question to be answered is: When does the clinician use povidone-iodine in the treatment of chronic wounds?

Evidence suggests that until more research is performed, the use of povidone-iodine solution is at best limited to noninfected wounds that are free of necrotic tissue and exudate. Even then, these superficial, clean wounds appear to do better with just saline flushes, or, as discussed in a later section, they may be treated most expeditiously with microenvironmental dressings. Thus, the addition of povidone-iodine to whirlpool water is more useful for antiseptic action applied to the tank and drains to prevent cross-contamination than for treatment of the wound.

Sodium Hypochlorite Solution (Household Bleach)

The effectiveness of sodium hypochlorite (in a 0.25 percent to 0.5 percent solution) as an antimicrobial agent in controlling sepsis is attributed to the release of chlorine when this compound is placed into solution such as when used in a whirlpool bath. Labarraque[60] introduced the use of this solution to prevent the decomposition of corpses. Later, Dakin[61] suggested that the antiseptic action of sodium hypochlorite might be beneficial to infected surgical wounds irrigated with the solution. Although the antimicrobial effectiveness of this chlorine-liberating compound has been demonstrated, such compounds may be cytotoxic. Lineaweaver and associates[48] have demonstrated that 0.5 percent sodium hypochlorite is cytotoxic to cultured human fibroblasts and adversely affects wound healing in an animal model. On serial dilution studies, they have further shown that a 0.005 percent solution is bactericidal in vitro but is noncytotoxic to fibroblasts.

To minimize toxic effects, the chlorine molecule can be linked to a hydrogen-nitrogen bond forming an amine known as chloramine-T (chlorazene).* Although considered to be a potent germicidal agent when used in whirlpool baths at a concentration of 200 parts per million (a 1:5000 dilution), chlorazene is reported to be less irritating and cytotoxic than sodium hypochlorite. When the chlorine molecule is linked to a hydrogen-nitrogen bond, the release of free chlorine is controlled by formation of hypochlo-

---

*Badger Pharmacal, Inc., New Berlin, WI 53151.

rous acid, which reduces the irritating qualities of chlorine.[45] According to Steve and coworkers,[45] 50 g of chlorazene is optimum for a 60-gallon leg or hip whirlpool tank, and 320 g for a Hubbard tank.

Dakin's Solution

In 1915, during World War I, Henry D. Dakin, an American chemist, developed this very dilute neutral solution consisting of 0.45 to 0.5 percent sodium hypochlorite and 0.4 percent boric acid for cleansing wounds.[62] This solution is known to be bactericidal against streptococci, staphylococci, and pyocyaneus microorganisms. When a full-strength solution is applied to an open wound, the formation of free alkali may cause local irritation to the skin immediately surrounding the wound border. The repeated exposure of the skin to dilute bleach (sodium hypochlorite solution) may cause the same effect. To avoid these adverse effects, Dakin's solution is frequently applied to wounds in 0.25 to 0.5 percent dilution and rarely as a full-strength solution.

Acetic Acid Solution

Weak acetic acid applied as a 0.5 percent solution to irrigate wounds may help to remove select pathogens such as Pseudomonas aeruginosa.[63] Acetic acid solution has been shown to be effective against both gram-positive and gram-negative microorganisms[64] but has not been shown to significantly enhance the healing process.

Hydrogen Peroxide

As previously mentioned, hydrogen peroxide (H_2O_2), because of its effervescent action, is a mechanical cleansing agent and a nonselective debriding agent. Hydrogen peroxide has little bactericidal action in wounds. When it contacts wound tissue, the enzyme catalase, found in blood and most tissues, rapidly decomposes hydrogen peroxide to oxygen and water.[65] Because this results in foaming effervescence, hydrogen peroxide is primarily indicated to help loosen dried exudate or debris on the wound surface. A 3 percent solution is often used for cleansing wound debris and skin immediately adjacent to the wound perimeter. This agent should not be used after crust separation has occurred and new granulation tissue is developing. Furthermore, because hydrogen peroxide is rapidly decomposed to oxygen and water, this compound should not be applied to closed wounds. The resulting gas build-up may cause trauma secondary to tissue expansion or may be released into the vascular system and result in embolism.

Neosporin Ointment, Silvadene, and Furacin

In the healing of superficial wounds, topical bactericidal agents are widely used to prevent excessive bacterial contamination and infection of wounds. The literature contains numerous reports that support the claims that certain agents are very effective in their antimicrobial activity.[66-70] Ideally, a topical antimicrobial agent should inhibit pathogenic microorganisms in wounds without retarding the normal rate of tissue repair. However, a few published reports indicate that some antimicrobials promote the rate of epidermal repair, while others retard repair.

Geronemus and associates[51] studied the effects of selected commonly used topical antimicrobial agents on the rate of re-epithelialization of clean wounds in white domestic pigs. One agent studied, Neosporin ointment,* is known to cover a wide spectrum of bactericidal activity, including most gram-positive and gram-negative bacteria found in the skin of pigs and humans. One of the three antibacterial components of this agent, zinc bacitracin, was found to promote epidermal healing by 25 percent compared with untreated control subjects. Interestingly, the isolated, inert petrolatum base of Neosporin ointment showed a slight, but statistically nonsignificant, increase in healing time. This finding is in conflict with a significant reduction in the rate of epidermal healing of 17 percent with USP petrolatum previously reported by others.[71]

Another commonly used antibacterial agent, 1 percent Silvadene† cream (silver sulfadiazine), which acts upon a wide range of gram-negative and gram-positive bacteria as well as fungi, was found to promote re-epithelialization 28 percent faster than untreated control wounds.[51] The healing effects of Neosporin and Silvadene are not related to their antimicrobial activity.[72]

A third agent, Furacin‡ (nitrofurazone), has an antibacterial range comparable to those of Neosporin ointment and Silvadene cream. However, Furacin was the only topical antibacterial agent of the three studied that significantly retarded the rate of re-epithelialization, suggesting that the agent may be cytotoxic to epidermal cells.[51,72]

Despite the fact that some antibacterial agents have been shown to promote healing of normal wounds in animal models, others may retard it. Both the active and inert substances in topical agents may affect healing. Since these results were reported from studies on induced animal wounds, the clinician should be cautioned not to make direct correlations as to how these topical agents would retard or enhance chronic wound healing in humans.

Zinc Applications

In 1883, Unna[73] is reported to have wrapped leg ulcers with rolled gauze impregnated with zinc oxide, calamine, and gelatin. The Unna boot is a semiocclusive dressing that, when used on a swollen extremity, may help to reduce edema and keep the wound moist. Harnar[73] has demonstrated that the Unna boot is a very beneficial dressing for skin graft–recipient sites on the lower extremity.

The effect of topically administered zinc oxide to incised human wounds[74] and to granulating wounds in normal animals[75] and in zinc-deficient animals[76] has been studied by various investigators. No beneficial effects of zinc were observed in any of these studies. In zinc-deficient humans and animals, wound healing is impaired. If zinc is administered orally to zinc-deficient humans, wound healing is accelerated.[77,78] However, the role of oral zinc therapy in the treatment of chronic venous leg ulceration is uncertain, since a number of reports with confusing and contradictory results appear in the literature.[79-81]

*Burroughs Wellcome Co., 3030 Cornwallis Road, Research Triangle Park, NC 27709.
†Marion Laboratories, 10236 Bunker Ridge Road, Kansas City, MO 64137.
‡Norwich Eaton Pharmaceutical, 1327 Eaton Avenue, Norwich, NY 43815.

WOUND DRESSINGS

Conventional Gauze Dressings

Traditional wound coverings usually consist of permeable, absorbent materials that often reduce moisture content in the wound by absorbing exudate and allowing for its evaporation. Because these dressings are composed primarily of gauze, upon removal from the wound, secondary trauma occurs by their adherence to the desiccated tissues. Frequent gauze dressing changes can cause additional necrosis of epithelial cells by removing important exudate and allowing for continued wound dehydration and additional trauma to new growth. This destruction of new tissue growth usually leads to the development of crust formation in and around the wound. As discussed earlier, the lack of moisture and the development of crust formation in the wound may inhibit re-epithelialization because new cells have a difficult time migrating from the periphery of the wound over a dry surface. In addition, epidermal cells may have to burrow deeper under the crust formation and migrate a longer distance to reach a moist environment where they can bridge the wound's gap.[82-84] The wound in the dehydrated state may also cause unnecessary prolongation of inflammatory responses as neutrophils and macrophages invade in their attempt to rid the body of desiccated tissues. Evidence suggests that the electrical conductivity that is normally present in a moist wound is decreased if the wound is allowed to dry out.[85] Therefore, the use of gauze as a dressing may indirectly inhibit the normal bioelectric signals found in a moist wound that may be necessary for the regeneration of tissues.

In addition to being permeable to air and possessing the potential to dry out new epithelial cell growth, gauze is also permeable to bacteria, and its use may increase the opportunity for wound sepsis. Using gauze may also cause foreign debris particles to be left behind in the wound, especially if the gauze is cut to approximate the wound's dimensions. Gauze fibers may become embedded, causing inflammation and a delay in healing. Pain at the wound site may also be greater with gauze coverings than with other dressings, presumably because cutaneous nerve endings may dry out as moisture evaporates.

Additional problems occur with gauze dressings because they are traditionally used as a "coverall" dressing, during the entire management of many or all types of wounds throughout their course of treatment. For example, gauze continues to be used as a dressing during the treatment of pressure ulcers, venous insufficiency ulcers, diabetic neurotrophic ulcers and many others, with little or no attention given to whether they are necrotic and dry, beefy-red and moist, or heavily exudating. Using gauze as a wound dressing may also require extra personnel time required to perform dressing changes, and gauze inhibits the visual monitoring of the wound's status without dressing removal.

Gauze, however, can be the material of choice during the initial treatment of some wounds when infection may be present, when other dressings are contraindicated, and/or when rapid debridement is indicated. Wounds requiring frequent dressing changes because of excessive exudate may benefit temporarily from utilizing gauze dressings by absorbing exudate and allowing for evaporation. Continued use of gauze by itself, however, is not advised to control copious amounts of drainage. Exudate-absorbing products and dressings and their indications will be discussed in later sections of this chapter. Some wounds with necrotic tissue may be treated beneficially from the use of wet-to-dry gauze dressings during debridement. When using wet-to-dry dressings, there is, however, destruction of new epithelial growth upon the removal of the gauze from the wound, and this must be evaluated when gauze dressings are being considered for debridement.

Conventional gauze, when saturated by saline and covered by plastic wrap, has been demonstrated to be an acceptable wound dressing in the absence of anaerobic infections.[86,87] However, in one study[88] a similar non–vapor permeable dressing was used to produce a moist environment, resulting in a 100 percent growth rate of pseudomonal infection, presumably because the characteristics of the occlusive dressing produced an anaerobic environment favorable to pseudomonal growth.[89] Therefore, great care should be taken by the clinician when using a totally occlusive wound covering such as plastic wrap.

Gauze used alone without the plastic wrap was successfully used by Barnett and colleagues[90] on one patient who previously suffered pseudomona infection three times while using a synthetic dressing. Dressing wounds with saline-moistened gauze and covering them with plastic wrap may be indicated for wounds undergoing enzymatic debridement and/or other treatment such as electrical stimulation, as a cost-effective method to absorb slough during debridement protocols requiring twice daily treatment applications and dressing changes.

After debridement, saline-saturated gauze covered by plastic wrap may be used to promote granulation tissue formation by supplying the wound with readily available moisture. When choosing gauze in these treatment situations, fine mesh gauze such as 44/36 weave may be more conducive to healing than regular gauze, by allowing epithelial growth to occur, with less chance for the new growth to be entrapped in the weave of the gauze upon removal of the dressing. Iatrogenic ulcerations can occur with this technique if the periwound tissue is covered with the plastic wrap and insensible perspiration or wound exudate is not controlled. Therefore, when selecting plastic wrap and moistened gauze, care should be taken to approximate the gauze dressing to the wound size and to prevent the gauze from covering the surrounding skin. One way to accomplish this task is to place a plastic transparency over the wound and trace the wounds inside the perimeter with a fine-point transparency marker. Cutting out the tracing, placing it over the gauze, and cutting out a supply of gauze that will last for 1 week is advisable. This procedure should be repeated when the wound's dimensions decrease. When cutting gauze for this purpose, there is a chance for gauze debris particles to be left in the wound and cause undesirable irritation; therefore, before each subsequent treatment and/or covering of the wound, the wound should be flushed with normal saline to get rid of any remaining gauze particles.

The plastic wrap cover applied over the gauze need not be cut as precisely as the gauze. A large piece of plastic wrap can be folded by hand and pressed together and continually be refolded to approximate the wound's dressing size. After the piece of plastic wrap is in place over the dressing, it can be taped to the skin. The tape should be placed with half of its width on the plastic wrap and the other half on the skin.

Microenvironmental (Occlusive) Dressings

During the last decade, many new wound dressings have been developed and marketed for wound-care management. Improved technology, research, and design of these dressings using synthetic and semisynthetic materials have yielded a variety of impermeable and semipermeable dressings with characteristics both different and similar. These dressings can aid in producing a microenvironment that is conducive and supportive to the body's own healing mechanisms, which enable wound repair to occur more efficiently. By knowing and understanding the different characteristics of these microenvironmental dressings and of their effects on wound healing, clinicians can choose an appropriate dressing for various types of wounds and thereby be better able to manage wounds during healing. Some of the effects produced by these dressings have been known for more than 25 years[82,91] and include rapid re-epithelialization of acute wounds and an enhanced rate of healing of chronic wounds.[92] One characteristic of all microenvironmental dressings is their impermeability to water, although some are permeable to water vapors. All of these dressings allow a wound to retain sufficient moisture[93] and to heal at accelerated rates,[83,90,91,94] when compared with wounds covered by gauze[90] or left open to dehydrate.[95]

Initially, clinicians feared that moist wounds that were not permitted to "breathe" would become infected, but the use of these dressings has proved so successful that there is now an accepted philosophy in the health field that "a moist wound is a healing wound." Because these dressings all maintain tissue hydration,[92] they are also referred to as *occlusive dressings*. In the following sections, these dressings will be classified according to their degree of permeability to water vapor and the specific characteristics they possess (see Fig. 9–8).

In addition to their effects on tissue hydration, different occlusive dressings have different biologic effects on the wound's environment and adjacent tissue, related to the following:

1. Permeability or impermeability to oxygen, carbon dioxide, and other gases, and bacteria transmission
2. Adhesion to periwound and healing tissues and subsequent ability or inability to allow removal of the dressing without causing secondary trauma to new tissues
3. Ability or inability to absorb exudate when excessive; difference in water vapor transmission; ability to retain and control exudate, which contains important electrolytes, metabolites, and cells necessary for tissue regeneration
4. Ability to maintain a constant temperature that is closer to body temperature when compared with conventional cotton dressings
5. Ability to be free of particulates and toxic contaminants
6. Mechanical properties including flexibility and contourability to the wound's surface
7. Overall biocompatibility to healing and surrounding cells to allow for favorable healing rates
8. Effect on the wound's pH

Additional benefits using occlusive dressings include increased angiogenesis under certain conditions; more efficient epidermal cell migration through the wound's own exudate;[83] maintenance of voltage gradients;[96] better visual monitoring with transparent films; and fewer dressing changes and therefore improved cost efficiency.[97,98] Occlusive dressings can also help produce and maintain a favorable microenvironment where normal microflora are allowed to exist.[99,100] These microflora may conceivably stimulate epidermal cell production[101] and therefore provide a better opportunity for the wound to perform the biologic act of healing.

Additional clinical advantages using occlusive dressings may include increased patient compliance with any wound-healing protocol due to the relative ease of application of these dressings; the functional ability to shower or bathe[102] without changing the dressing; a decrease in odor from the wound, as its exudate is managed better; and an overall decrease in pain[90,102–103] at the wound site.

The following section will identify, classify, compare, and contrast the characteristics, composition, and properties of occlusive dressings. By using different dressings on

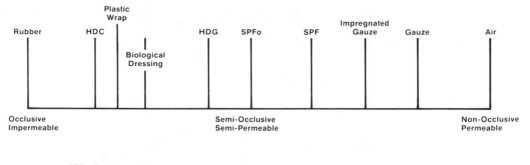

FIGURE 9–8. Water vapor permeability range of dressings.

different wound types, events within the wound can be altered.[92,104,105] The reader should use this knowledge when treating wounds and when engaged in clinical decision making (CDM) to select the appropriate occlusive dressing(s) for a given wound during its particular course of healing.

Occlusive dressings can be classified according to their degree of permeability or impermeability, with the term *occlusive* being synonymous with *impermeable*, and *semiocclusive* with *semipermeable* (see Fig. 9–8).

SEMIPERMEABLE FILMS

Moisture vapor–permeable (MVP) dressings, vapor-permeable membranes (VPM), transparent film dressings (TDF), synthetic adhesive moisture vapor–permeable (SAM) dressings, and polyurethane films (PUF) are all acronyms for semipermeable films (SPFs). SPFs are constructed from transparent polyurethane or similar synthetic films, coated on one surface with a water-resistant hypoallergenic adhesive. SPFs are highly elastic, conform easily to body parts, and are generally resistant to shear and tear. SPFs are permeable to moisture vapor and oxygen but impermeable to water and bacteria.[106,107] Examples of SPFs include Op-Site, Bio-occlusive, Tegaderm, and Polyskin, as listed in Table 9–1.

Studies show that moisture vapor transmission through SPFs ranges from approximately 2500 g/m²/24 hours[108] to 35 g/100 inches²/24 hours.[109] Interestingly, water vapor loss from uncovered granulating wounds has been calculated by Turner[108] to be as high as 7000 g/m²/24 hours; therefore SPFs may be used to control and prevent wound dehydration while maintaining the moist environment[110-113] needed to maximize the wound's internal optimal rate of healing. These films are for the most part able to balance properly the state of hydration in wounds with normal to no exudate without macerating the periwound skin. Moderate or heavily exudating wounds, whose exudate exceeds the moisture vapor transmission capabilities of the SPF, can be aspirated and patched with another piece of the film in order to maintain the moist environment without excessively stretching the film. Excessive exudate may, however, become unmanageable while using an SPF, resulting in leaking and nonadherence of the dressing. When copious amounts of exudate are present, management may be simplified by using a pouch dressing, such as Tegaderm Pouch Dressing, composed of the same type of SPF yet having the additional capability for exudate to collect in a pouch. If exudate is still

TABLE 9–1. Semipermeable Film (SPF) Dressings

SPF Dressings	Advantages	Disadvantages
Op-Site Bio-occlusive Tegaderm Polyskin	Moist wound environment Faster healing Cost effective in long run Good visual monitoring Conforms well Good on superficial wounds Good permeability to oxygen Fair moisture vapor transmission Does not dissolve into wound Fair biocompatibility to periwound tissue Decreases pain at wound site Waterproof Minimal irritation to healing tissues with removal vs gauze Cost effective Autolytic debridement—minimal necrotic film	Cannot absorb copious amounts of exudate Easily displaced by mechanical forces Can be difficult to apply Does not maintain body temperature in wound Poor adherence in high-moisture states Adhesive in most SPFs Can pull on epidermal cells More expensive than gauze

unmanageable while using these dressings, the clinician should consider using a dressing that has an absorbent mechanism (as discussed in subsequent sections) or to use a hydrophilic product such as dextranomer.

The rate of oxygen transfer in one SPF was calculated to be 6.48×10^{-3} cc/hr/cm^2 and seems to mimic the gaseous exchange properties of skin.[109,114,115] This gas exchange of oxygen between the wound bed and the atmosphere may facilitate healing, but if copious amounts of exudate are present between the wound bed and its covering, there is a decrease in oxygen accessibility to the wound and the use of an oxygen-permeable SPF is likely to have little influence on conditions at the wound surface. Therefore, for exudating wounds, the clinician may elect to use a dressing that, in addition to being permeable to oxygen, will be able to absorb moderate to heavy exudate. These dressings are discussed in late sections. Another important feature of SPFs may be that they inhibit the formation of anaerobic pathogens during the healing process, which may otherwise occur with the use of a totally occlusive dressing.

Other SPFs that function similarly to the aforementioned SPF but are composed of polyester instead of polyurethane include Blister Film and Co-Film. Although Co-Film has adhesive over the entire surface of the film, Blister Film has adhesive around the perimeter of the film only. This adhesive was designed to reduce trauma to newly formed epithelium upon dressing removal, which can occur with other totally adhesive-backed SPFs. Advantages and disadvantages of the various SPFs can be found in Table 9–1.

SEMIPERMEABLE FOAMS

Semipermeable foams (SPFos) have hydrophilic properties on the wound side of the dressing and hydrophobic characteristics on the other. SPFos allow for absorption of the wound's exudate throughout the hydrophilic side and into the inner foam layers of the dressing. Because evaporation of exudate is controlled, the dressing provides the moist environment for healing to occur without maceration to periwound tissue.

SPFos are better able to manage wounds with moderate to high exudate than SPFs because of their absorbent capabilities. SPFos also provide cushioning and protection to the wound. The foams also act as an insulator, and body temperature is maintained at the wound and dressing interface, allowing for more optimal cellular activity. These and other characteristics of dressings discussed in subsequent sections will be important in deciding which dressing to use for a given wound type during a course of healing. Advantages and disadvantages for SPFos are listed in Table 9–2.

SEMIPERMEABLE HYDROGELS

As discussed earlier, one of the shortcomings associated with using SPFs is their ineffectiveness in controlling copious amounts of exudate when the rate of wound exudate exceeds the moisture vapor permeability of the dressing. SPFs do not possess an absorbent mechanism and may result in the accumulation of unwanted fluid beneath the dressing. Hydrogels (HDGs) are capable of absorbing moderate to maximal amounts of exudate while coincidentally providing a suitable wound microenvironment much like that of the SPFs. HDG dressings are three-dimensional networks of hydrophilic polymers prepared from gelatin, polysaccharides, cross-linked polyacrylamide polymers, polyelectrolyte complexes, and polymers or copolymers derived from methoacrylic esters. These water polymer gels are composed of approximately 96% water and 4% polyethylene oxide in a colloidal suspension on a polyethylene mesh support between two polyethylene films. HDGs are oxygen permeable (Fig. 9–9).

TABLE 9–2. Semipermeable Foam (SPFo) Dressings: Advantages and Disadvantages

SPFos	Advantages	Disadvantages
Primaderm	Moist wound environment	Nonadhesive
Synthaderm	Faster healing	Clinician must supply tape or covering
LyoFoam	Good exudate absorption	Easily displaced by mechanical forces
	Fair moisture vapor transmission	More expensive than SPFs, but still cost effective vs gauze
	Fair oxygen permeability	No visual monitoring of wound
	Maintains body temperature in wound	
	Waterproof	
	Minimal to no irritation to healing tissues with removal	
	Decreases pain at wound site	
	Good biocompatibility to periwound tissues	
	Autolytic debridement — minimal film	

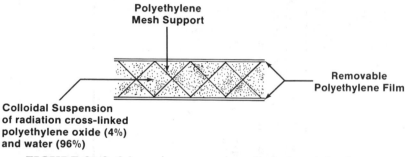

FIGURE 9–9. Schematic cross section of a hydrogel dressing.

To apply the HDG, the polyethelene film is removed on one side, allowing the gel to come into contact with the wound and periwound tissue, providing for a moist wound cover without macerating surrounding tissues. Adherence to the wound is by contact with the gel, but the film also must be kept in place with tape or another covering.

The vapor transmission rate may be increased[116] by removing the outer polyethylene film, resulting in a cooling effect because of evaporative water loss. When used this way, an outer absorbent dressing will be required to control the exudate. This high moisture vapor transmission capability allows for oxygen permeability equal to or greater than that found with SPFos. This transmission will allow the continuation of aerobic function within the wound and may have an effect upon bacterial type and growth, and subsequent epidermal[117] and connective tissue healing rates. HDGs may also influence the inflammatory response and angiogenesis in wounds.

HDGs are flexible, conforming easily to body parts, and they provide some cushioning to the wound. The composition of most HDGs provides very minimal mechanical irritation to healing and surrounding tissues with use and removal.

Commonly available HDG dressings come in sheets, and some of the trade names, along with advantages and disadvantages, can be found on Table 9–3. Other characteristics of HDGs include their safe application over topical antibacterial agents. Unlike the sheet dressings, Debrisan is an HDG packaged as dry, sphere-shaped hydrophilic beads composed of dextranomer, designed to be poured into highly edematous or exudating wounds with or without necrotic tissue; its use as a topical agent has been described previously in this chapter. As an HDG, its function is to absorb the exudate and form a gelatinous mass that should be flushed from the wound daily.

IMPERMEABLE HYDROCOLLOIDS

Hydrocolloids (HDCs) are compound formulations containing not only hydrogels but also elastomeric and adhesive components. The wound contact surface of the HDC is coated with an adhesive, while the inner layer is the primary exudate-absorbing element composed of carboxymethylcellulose (CMC). There may also be varying amounts of pectin and gelatin present. The outer layer is water and bacteria impermeable. HDCs are also impermeable to oxygen and gas and therefore provide an anaerobic wound environment. HDCs, like HDGs, swell as they imbibe wound exudate and are effective in controlling moderate to high levels of exudate. The result of HDC swelling, however, unlike HDG swelling, is that the HDC will expand into the wound with continued support and pressure from the rest of the dressing. The HDC will continue to

TABLE 9–3. Hydrogel (HDG) Dressings: Advantages and Disadvantages

HDG Dressings	Advantages	Disadvantages
Vigilon Spenco 2nd Skin	Moist wound environment Faster healing Good exudate absorption Good moisture vapor transmission Good oxygen permeability Does not dissolve into wound Decreases pain at wound site Cools wound temperature Good biocompatibility to periwound tissue No irritation to healing tissues with removal Visual monitoring of wound Autolytic debridement—minimal necrotic film to moderate/maximal necrotic tissue Nonadherent	Clinician must supply adhesive tape or covering Unable to keep out bacteria by themselves Dehydrates easily Difficult to keep in place More expensive than SPFs

absorb exudate and expand into the wound, conforming to the wound's contours, until the HDC reaches its saturation point. The advantage of this action is its compression to the floor of the ulcer, limiting the amount of water content in the granulating tissue, which aids in maintaining the wound's contents below its edges. Clinically, some HDC are better than others at absorbing exudate without dissolving into the wound bed or onto periwound tissue. This feature is important to consider, because there is no need to flush the wound to possible harmful dressing residues left behind, which may cause harm to healing tissues, as do some HDCs. Clinical studies are needed to compare absorptive capacities of HDCs and to determine the effects of HDC residues, if any.

Like other microenvironmental dressings, HDCs speed the rate of healing, decrease pain at the wound site, and provide minimal to no irritation to healing tissues upon removal. Some HDCs have better contourability and better adhesiveness than others.

There are contradictory reports on re-epithelialization rates under occlusive dressings. Silver[116] reported greater re-epithelialization rates under occlusive dressings that were more permeable to oxygen, while Alvarez and coworkers[95] found more rapid re-epithelialization under a relatively oxygen-impermeable HDC. Many factors may account for these differing findings, including the amount of wound exudate found pooling under the dressing and whether or not any oxygen perfusion took place among the atmosphere, the exudate, and the wound bed when using an SPF. There is also evidence that wound hypoxia may enhance angiogenesis[118,119] and result in increased re-epithelialization rates; therefore, clinicians may sometime dress a wound with an oxygen-impermeable membrane, while at other times using an oxygen-permeable dressing. More information on the role of oxygen in wound healing may be found in Chapters 1, 2, and 15. Additional advantages and disadvantages of HDC can be found in Table 9–4.

HYDROCOLLOID ABSORPTION POWDERS, PASTES, AND GRANULES

These hydrophilic products help absorb excessive wound exudate,[120] control bacteria,[121] and offer other advantages in wound management. They assist in wound cleansing and odor reduction,[122] and they help to decrease dressing changes, which saves staff time and decreases the cost of wound care.

These absorbing products are similar in function, with contents including a graft copolymer starch provided in dry flake form (Bard absorption dressing); carboxymethylcellulose (CMC) and guar cellulose in a petroleum-base soft paste (Comfeel ulcus paste); and CMC, xanthan cellulose, and guar cellulose in a dry powder (Comfeel ulcus powder). These three similar products are suitable for filling uneven ulcers and controlling heavily exudating ulcers. Bard absorption dressing requires mixing with sterile saline before application, while the other two products can be applied to the wound as they are. After filling the wound half full with Comfeel ulcus powder or paste, or loosely packing with Bard absorption dressing, the ulcer may be covered with an HDC dressing if indicated by the wound type, thereby increasing the life span of the dressing and maximizing its absorbing capacities. Removal of these products is recommended by cleansing with lukewarm water or saline.

Biosynthetic and Biologic Dressings

Biologic dressings are composed of tissue derived from animal or human sources in varying degrees. Biologic dressings have found limited application in conservative chronic wound care, but may be outlined as follows. The *cutaneous autograft* is a graft

TABLE 9-4. Hydrocolloid (HDC) Dressings: Advantages and Disadvantages

HDC Dressings	Advantages	Disadvantages

Duoderm
J & J Ulcer Dressing
Restore
Intact
	Moist wound healing environment
	Faster healing
	Easy to apply
	Fair biocompatibility to periwound tissues
	Occlusive
	Good exudate absorption
	Minimal irritation to healing tissues with removal
	Maintains body temperature in wound
	Decreases pain at wound site
	Autolytic debridement— minimal necrotic film to moderate
	   necrotic tissue
		Maceration of periwound tissues may occur with excessive
		   wound exudate
		Dressing residues sometimes left behind in wound or on
		   patient or clothes
		Poor conformity on irregular surfaces
		More expensive than SPFs
		No visual monitoring of wound

from one part of the body to another part of the same person. An *isograft* is a graft from one genetically identical twin to another; whereas an *allograft* is a graft from one person to another who is genetically different. A *zenograft* is a graft from an animal to a human, or vice versa. One biosynthetic dressing (Biobrane) is a biocomposite of an ultra-thin, semipermeable silicone membrane, bonded to a flexible, knitted nylon fabric. A non-toxic, hypoallergenic mixture of highly purified peptides derived from porcine dermal collagen is bonded to the elastic membrane providing a hydrophilic, biocompatible surface.[123] This dressing is semipermeable, allowing water vapor loss at rates comparable to those of normal skin. Applications[124] are primarily intended for use on freshly debrided, excised, or meshed autograft wounds containing less than 10^5 bacteria per gram of tissue. In addition, the manufacturer cautions that all debridement or excision must be done thoroughly to remove all coagulation or eschar. Applications have been mainly limited to dressing wounds following dermabrasion;[123] or burns,[125] and as a dressing for autograft donor sites.[126] Its use in the chronic wound-care setting has been virtually nonexistent, but is presented here for clinicians using this text as a reference in burns or acute care. The clinician who wishes to know more about these dressings should contact the biosynthetic and biologic dressing manufacturers listed in the Appendix at the end of the chapter.

Microenvironmental Dressing Indications and Contraindications

The occlusive dressings discussed in the sections covering SPFs, SPFos, HDGs, and HDCs come with information on specific descriptions, precautions, warnings, and guidelines for intended use in their product literature. The clinician is urged to read this literature before using these dressings. Common contraindications include the use of these dressings over infected wounds; ischemic ulcers; wounds associated with osteomyelitis; active vasculitis; wounds with edge-to-edge eschar; third-degree burns; and ulcers eroded into muscle, tendon, or bone. In addition SPFs should not be used over heavily exudating wounds. Again, the manufacturer's product insert for each dressing should be reviewed by the clinician periodically to determine whether there have been changes issued by the manufacturer.

PRESSURE SORES: CAUSES, TREATMENT, AND PREVENTION

Perhaps the most common of chronic wounds is the decubitus ulcer or pressure sore. The etiology of these wounds is generally attributed to local tissue ischemia from direct mechanical destruction of tissues,[127] pressure,[128-131] and small vessel distortion owing to friction.[132,133] In addition, compounding factors such as nutritional deficiencies[134,135] and immunity[136,137] increase the vulnerability of tissues to destruction from ischemia caused by prolonged application of external forces against the skin.

When pressure is applied to skin for a prolonged time, there is a critical period after which local changes in more vulnerable tissues prohibit new blood from perfusing through those tissues. This irreversible ischemic response is referred to as the "no reflow" phenomenon.[138] The subsequent cessation of blood flow caused by sustained pressure on skin, fat, and muscle usually occurs over bony prominences in the elderly, paralyzed, comatose, or sensory-impaired patient.

Apparently, tissues differ in their abilities to tolerate periods of ischemia. One study of the "no reflow" phenomenon in skin reported that the dermis is capable of tolerating ischemia for between 2 and 6 hours, but that after 8 hours of ischemia, necrotic changes occur, followed by tissue sloughing. Interestingly, muscle and connective tissue subjected to sustained pressure superimposed on the overlying skin may undergo destruction from ischemia after only 2 hours.[139] Seemingly, this fact may account for the commonly held belief that sinuses and fistulas may develop in muscle and subcutaneous tissue before ulceration occurs in the overlying skin. As mentioned previously, the single most important factor contributing to the development of pressure sores is prolonged local pressure applied over bony prominences that exceeds average capillary pressure at its arterial inflow.[140] Landis[141] used a microinjection technique for measuring blood pressure in single capillaries of the skin and determined the average pressure at the arterial end of the capillary to be 32 millimeters of mercury (mmHg). At the capillary bed level, the average pressure was calculated at 20 mmHg, and at the venous end of the capillary, the average pressure was 12 mmHg.

A limited number of studies have examined the effects of varying amounts of pressure applied to the skin for variable amounts of time. Orlando[142] has demonstrated that ulceration can develop after 2 hours of pressure applied at 500 mmHg and after 9 hours of pressure applied at 150 mmHg. No histologic changes were noted in subjects exposed to 35 mmHg of continuous pressure for 4 hours,[143] but doubling of the pressure to 70 mmHg applied to healthy tissue for 2 hours results in irreversible tissue damage.[144] Unfortunately, elderly, debilitated patients often have compromised cardiovascular function, which decreases the mean capillary pressure, resulting in lower occlusive pressures and increased risk of ischemia and ulcer formation.

Pressure-Relieving Devices

The commercial market of pressure-relieving devices (PRDs) provides an abundant variety of cushions, mattresses, specialty beds, and so on, some of which are effective in reducing pressure to below 32 mmHg in capillaries that permeate tissues covering some bony prominences. The reporting and subsequent use of pressure interface measurements of PRDs can be misleading in reporting the products' effectiveness for the treatment or prevention of pressure ulcers.

For example, Maklebust and coworkers[145] reported that although a 2-inch convoluted foam, Biogard foam pad, a Sof·Care bed cushion, and a conventional hospital mattress all provided sufficient pressure relief at the sacrum, the test subjects were all healthy persons and the data therefore may not be valid. The authors theorized that good tone in the gluteal musculature of the healthy subject tends to elevate the sacrum from the support surface and therefore results in artificially lower pressures being recorded at the sacrum more, the authors found that when the four previously mentioned support surfaces were evaluated for pressure relief at the greater trochanter, only one PRD (Sof·Care) relieved pressure to less than 32 mmHg, and none of the products were able to reduce the mean pressure at the heels to less than 32 mmHg. Their findings suggested that even though a support surface may provide adequate pressure relief for the sacrum and trochanter, the heels may still be at risk.

Another study found heel pressure readings greater than 32 mmHg even while on air fluidized beds,[146] therefore suggesting alternate methods of pressure relief should be considered when the ulcer is located on the heel. Clark[147] used a hydraulic pressure sensor taped directly to the skin over the sacrum in elderly and young subjects to determine whether pressure readings would be significantly different in either group.

He found pressure measurements among the elderly higher than those in the young subjects. From these findings, Clark questioned the value of conducting evaluations of "pressure-reducing" surfaces using young volunteers and the sacrum as a measurement site.

Since there are no government standards or rating systems that evaluate the effectiveness of PRD, the clinician must be aware of the overall appropriateness of the product, given the situation. The product manufacturers should state clearly in their literature the pressure-relieving capabilities at the heel, sacrum, trochanter, and so on; the method by which these measurements were taken; and information on the test subjects such as age, diagnosis, and the like. Without these data and standardization of measurements, some product manufacturers may be instilling a false sense of security in the clinician, which leads the clinician to believe that the patient is safe from further tissue insult. The more at risk a patient is, or the more serious an existing ulcer may be, the more careful the clinician must be in choosing an appropriate PRD. Finally, the clinician must keep in mind that some products simply cannot relieve pressure or reduce pressures to harmless levels.

FOAM PRD

Foam padding or convoluted foam is relatively inexpensive and has been used indiscriminately primarily because of cost considerations. This type of foam has been shown to reduce pressure at the sacrum in healthy subjects[145] and does not otherwise provide adequate pressure reduction.[148,149] Other drawbacks using foam as a PRD include its tendency to increase local surface temperature,[150] retain moisture from perspiration and incontinence, and become easily contaminated as bacteria flourish in the warm, humid environment. Washing foam PRDs can cause them to lose their flame retardency and can temporarily leave the patient without a PRD. Foam is usually available in 2- and 4-inch heights and should be used only when a patient is minimally at risk or at no risk for developing a pressure sore. The patient should be ambulatory and able to move independently. Foam PRDs should not be used when an ulcer is present. Foam PRDs have very little practical application as an effective tool to combat pressure. If used at all, foam PRDs should be used only on a patient at minimal to no risk.

WATER FLOTATION PRD

Water flotation pads and beds take advantage of water's weight dispersive characteristics and supply significant pressure relief[148,151] if used properly. However, they are very difficult to handle, implement, and monitor. Filling the water pads excessively will cause a convex, hard surface, preventing the patient's body from sinking in, and thus minimizing the weight-dispersive abilities the mattresses possess. Underfilling these pads can lead to a concave surface and "bottoming out" of the flotation device, once again providing inadequate pressure relief. Inadequate pressure relief may also occur at the heels when the patient is supine because the calcaneous supports much of the lower extremity weight. Once again, inadequate pressure relief may occur over the greater trochanter when sidelying, because of the "bottoming out" that can occur when patients put all of their weight on one side. These devices can be used when the patient is at minimal risk of developing an ulcer or has a manageable ulcer located in a site other than at the heel or greater trochanter, and when the patient has independent mobility. Concern should also be given to the patient with intolerance to the cold sensation of the flotation pad and to possible leaks that may occur.

GEL PRDs

These types of PRDs are intended to simulate the mechanical action of human tissues. Gel PRDs do not flow under pressure, but are partially and temporarily displaced under pressure. They do not "bottom out" and, when not under a load, will return to their original shape. Gel PRDs have a good clinical reputation for preventing pressure sores. Some manufacturers claim that gel PRDs work because they eliminate or reduce shear forces on the skin while distributing pressure. Another inherent feature of gel PRDs is their ability to disperse heat. Their disadvantages include cost, weight, poor moisture absorption, and poor aeration. Perhaps better designed covers would improve the overall performance of the cushion. Gel PRDs can be used to equalize pressure on persons minimally to moderately at risk and on persons with manageable ulcers, who still have independent mobility.

STATIC AIR PRDs

Static air PRDs offer some pressure relief[145] and are usually constructed so that as a patient shifts his or her weight, air flows through channels present between two layers of air cushions and assists in redistributing the weight over the cushion.

Some static air PRDs for wheelchairs are preinflated, but most for either the wheelchair or the bed are not. Disadvantages include fatigue at the seams, a relatively short product life span, and the tendency to overinflate or underinflate the product; considerations given water mattresses apply here also. Repair of the PRD after accidental puncture is rather easy when the device includes a repair kit. There are various manufacturers of static air PRDs, and they can be used on persons minimally to moderately at risk and on persons with manageable ulcers, who still have independent mobility. Static PRDs are easily transported and cleaned.

DYNAMIC AIR PRDs

The principle behind dynamic alternating air PRDs is a shortened time span during which tissues are subjected to constant pressure. These PRDs are composed of compartments that are alternately inflated and deflated by an air pump that cycles repeatedly. As the air flows in and out of these adjacent air compartments, the patient is supported on half the air compartments at any one time. Some pumps will fill the second set of air compartments before deflating the first set. In either case, the time the body rests on either set of inflated compartments is short, and this higher pressure is relieved with the next cycle which completely releases the air, thereby allowing for the manual assistance of circulation and alternation of pressure against the capillaries.

These air PRDs can be used on a moderate at risk person who is mobility dependent and on persons who have manageable ulcers, who are also at minimal to moderate risk of further tissue destruction. These devices must be checked periodically to ensure that the pump is operating properly and the air compartments fully inflate and deflate. Dynamic air PRDs are effective in preventing ulcer occurrence or recurrence and are reasonably priced. There are few disadvantages. All previously mentioned PRDs are placed over standard hospital mattresses or wheelchair seats. The next two sections will address specialty beds.

LOW AIR LOSS PRDs

Low air loss PRDs reduce pressure over bony prominences by placing the patient on air cushions that distribute the weight more uniformly over body surfaces. These air support systems are based on the principle of air support, having the air contained and separated from the patient by a water vapor–permeable membrane. The fabric varies with the manufacturer. The air cushions are segmentally arranged to allow patient movement with a minimum of shear and friction forces to tissues. Configurations of these air cushions vary, depending on the manufacturer. These low air loss PRDs operate on temperature-controlled air, delivered below 100 ft³ per min (2800 1/min) at pressures in the range of 6 to 33 cm (3 to 13 inches) water gauge, and they permit moisture vapor transmission from the skin surface.[152]

The air pressure and air flow can be adjusted in multiple areas of the support surface to allow for body weight and patient comfort, with air entering through multiple inlet manifolds. The temperature of the air ranges from 28 to 31°C. Above those temperatures, patients may have a tendency to perspire. Air pressure is controlled and properly adjusted when the air cushions are depressed to the contour of the body.

Manufacturers differ in component features, with some similar additional characteristics, but the indications for these PRDs are always similar. Low air loss PRDs are indicated for the mobility-dependent patient at moderate to maximal risk of developing an ulcer or the patient who has hard to manage ulcers. Because these beds raise and lower as a unit at the head and foot ends, other indications may include use during rehabilitation programs or when ambulation and transfers are performed frequently. Low air loss PRDs are very expensive and are usually rented.

AIR FLUIDIZED PRDs

These specialty beds are indicated for the patient who is at maximal risk for developing pressure ulcers or the patient with very hard to manage ulcers. Additional indications include the patient on total bed rest or limited to very few weekly transfers out of the bed. Like the low air loss beds, air fluidized PRDs are costly but effective when used appropriately. Air fluidized therapy takes advantage of Archimedes' principle, which states: The buoyant force on a body immersed in a fluid is equal to the weight of the fluid displaced by the object. Therefore, by using Archimedes' principle, air fluidized technology removes pressure by "floating" the patient in a dry environment. This dry environment is achieved by air flow passing through a porous diffuser and rising through a layer of ceramic silicon-coated soda lime beads, which sets the beads in motion, creating a dry fluid one-and-a-half times denser than water. This artificial fluid medium is separated from the patient's skin by a loose-fitting polyester sheet that glides with the patient over the buoyant surface.

This PRD provides low contact pressure and supports the weight of the patient as he or she displaces the fluidized medium. The fluidization tank serves as the container and support surface frame. The loose-fitting sheet is porous and virtually eliminates shear and friction forces. The porous characteristics of the sheet allow for passage of the air flow and eliminate tissue destruction from maceration. Care needs to be taken, however, with use of air fluidized therapy so that the wound bed remains moisturized. The temperature-controlled air flow can be turned off quickly, allowing for total patient stabilization for nursing procedures or emergency care.

OTHER CLINICAL CONSIDERATIONS

Turning schedules are still very important in the overall management of pressure sores. Turning promotes good pulmonary, circulatory, urinary, and other system functions, as well as preventing ulcerations and facilitating healing. Products must be used thoughtfully rather than habitually, even in the patient who is at minimal risk, in order to be effective. The debilitated individual with ulcers can be, and often is, faced with a life-threatening situation. The clinician needs to respond appropriately and quickly with the products best suited to that individual.

No PRD on the market should instill the belief that a patient is no longer at risk or that healing will become automatic. The chance for product failure (or misuse) and wound complication is too great for the clinician to become lax at any time in the treatment and monitoring of all patients who are at risk or have skin breakdown.

CLINICAL DECISION MAKING

Case Histories

1. A 68-year-old woman with a primary diagnosis of Alzheimer's disease has been institutionalized for 10 months. She is disoriented, confused, and confined to her wheelchair and bed 24 hours a day. She cannot ambulate without the maximal assistance of two individuals. Before admission, she was ambulating and did not have ulcers. She now has a Stage IV decubitus ulcer over her right ischial tuberosity (IT) measuring 2.3 cm wide by 3.4 cm long by 4.3 cm deep. The floor of the ulcer contains 50 percent necrotic tissue and 50 percent pale-red granulation tissue. She also has a Stage III decubitus ulcer over her left greater trochanter (GT) measuring 5.6 cm wide by 5.2 cm long by 1.7 cm deep. This ulcer contains 90 percent necrotic tissue and 10 percent granulation tissue. The patient has a history of Pseudomonas aeruginosa infection in the ulcer over her right IT. Both wounds are now contaminated but not infected. The periwound skin of both ulcers is healthy. Both ulcers have remained unchanged the past 3 weeks. Current treatment includes BID hydrogen peroxide flushes followed by dry gauze packings covered by gauze sponges. No other treatment is given. What treatment would you recommend?

2. A 53-year-old obese woman has an 8-month history of a lower leg ulceration secondary to venous insufficiency. The Stage III ulcer measures 4.3 cm wide by 3.1 cm long by 0.4 cm deep. Copious amounts of serosanguineous drainage is present. Half of the wound is covered with necrotic tissue, and the remaining portion is pale pink. Minimal odor is present.

   Her lower extremities do not exhibit pitting edema but swell somewhat when she stands on her feet all day at work. Current treatment includes hydrogen peroxide flushes followed by Neosporin ointment, dry gauze dressings, and Ace wrap. What treatment program would you institute?

Recommended Treatment of Case Histories

1. The patient is nonambulating and is sustaining harmful pressure on her right IT while seated in her wheelchair and on her left GT while sidelying in bed. Treatment priority for this patient includes securing an appropriate pressure-relieving device (PRD) for both wheelchair and bed. The wheelchair PRD must be able to decrease pressure on the IT to below capillary closing pressure or must be able to alternate the pressure. The Action wheelchair pad and Grant alternating air wheelchair pad are good choices. The clinician must also weigh the benefits of complete bed rest for this patient for a short time. The bed PRD is not as critical as that for the wheelchair because the patient appears to have trouble with skin breaking down only when she

is on her left side. Again, the Grant air mattress would be an excellent choice for this person because it is relatively inexpensive. As long as the patient does not remain on her left side, she should do rather well. Her turning schedules should protect her left side.

Treatment of both ulcers should be focused on rapid debridement of the necrotic tissue while protecting the granulating tissue. The Stage IV right IT ulcer could be treated with enzymes in conjunction with saline-moistened large-weave gauze dressings to trap slough while simultaneously being noninjurious (moist) to the granulating tissue. This ulcer could then be covered with plastic wrap to maintain a moist environment. After debridement is complete, the gauze could be changed to fine weave and use of saline and plastic wrap could continue, followed by a switch to Comfeel ulcus paste covered with Comfeel ulcus dressing (hydrocolloid) when wound healing progresses to Stage III. Continuation of saline-moistened fine-weave gauze, however, would remain appropriate if cost is a factor. Once the ulcer is reduced to Stage III/II, the clinician can switch to a semipermeable film or a foam, depending upon the level of exudate.

After debridement, the right IT needs to be monitored closely for possible reinfection by Pseudomonas aeruginosa. Hydrogen peroxide could be used as a nonselective debriding agent, but should be discontinued after granulation tissue is present. Acetic acid may be considered if Pseudomonas develops, but efficient debridement of necrotic tissue should enable the clinician to produce a healthy base of granulation tissue and avoid infection. At no time should the agents be continued once there is 95 to 100 percent beefy-red granulation tissue present. Further treatment may include the use of electrical stimulation and/or ultraviolet, or other modalities, as discussed later in this text.

Because both ulcers have multifactorial etiologies, the patient is at risk for developing additional decubitus ulcers. For example, while confined to her wheelchair, her seated posture may deteriorate and assume more of a slouching position. This approach would increase the pressure on her sacrum and may contribute to the development of an ulcer. An improperly functioning PRD may not provide adequate pressure relief because of a poorly working pump or hole in the alternating air mattress. The clinician must therefore continually re-evaluate product use and function, as well as provide wound evaluation and treatment.

2. The primary reason for this patient's ulcer is her venous insufficiency, followed by incorrect selection of topical agents and dressings. Her new treatment program should focus on techniques covered in Chapter 10, which addresses the use of intermittent compression, compression stockings, and lymphatic exercises designed to help heal ulcers caused by vascular problems. Additionally, the necrotic tissue needs to be debrided as rapidly as possible while controlling the exudate. Lyofoam dressings would be a good choice because they will absorb moderate to maximal amounts of exudate while maintaining the moistened environment needed for autolytic debridement. If drainage remains a problem, exudate-absorbing powders and pastes would be very helpful to control the exudate, and aid in the removal of desiccated tissues. The hydrogen peroxide flushes, Neosporin, and dry gauze should be discontinued. Progress should be noticed quickly. If the autolytic debridement is successful, the patient's ulcer should be clean and beefy-red in 7 to 10 days. If necrotic tissue remains after 2 weeks, enzymatic debridement may be necessary, and modalities covered in later chapters should be considered both for debridement and to accelerate wound healing.

After the exudate flow is substantially reduced, the Lyofoam can be discontinued and semipermeable films can be used. Additional consideration should be given to a vocational change to minimize standing all day at work. Counseling may be required to address the patient's obesity and smoking habits.

SUMMARY

This chapter has presented evidence that favors the maintenance of a moist environment for wound healing. The importance of preventing wound tissue desiccation in relation to granulation tissue formation and re-epithelialization is stressed. Factors that complicate wound repair such as infection, edema, and pressure, as well as remedial treatment interventions for those problems, are discussed. Guidelines for wound debridement and use of several topical chemical substances are presented. Identification and discussion of gauze, synthetic wound dressings, and pressure-relieving devices are discussed. Recommendations for selection in the treatment and prevention of dermal ulcers are made based on clinical studies and research.

REFERENCES

1. Pollack, SV: The wound healing process. Clin Dermatol 2(3):8, 1984.
2. Sciubba, JJ, Waterhouse, JP, and Meyer, J: A fine structural comparison of the healing of incisional wounds of mucosa and skin. J Oral Pathol 7:214, 1978.
3. Grillo, HC and Gross, J: Collagenolytic activity during mammalian wound repair. Dev Biol 15:300, 1967.
4. Brown, SI and Weller, CA: Cell origin or collagenase in normal and wounded corneas. Arch Ophthalmol 83:74, 1970.
5. Im, MJ and Hoopes, JE: Increases in acid proteinase activity during epidermal wound healing. J Surg Res 35:159, 1983.
6. Winter, GD: Epidermal regeneration studies in the domestic pig. In Maibach, HI and Rovee, DT (eds): Epidermal Wound Healing. Year Book Medical Publishers, Chicago, 1972, p 71.
7. Harris, DR: Healing of the surgical wound. J Am Acad Dermatol 1:197, 1979.
8. Rovee, PT, Kurowsky, CA, and Labun, J: Effect of local wound environment in epidermal healing. In Maibach, HI and Rovee, DT (eds): Epidermal Wound Healing. Year Book Medical Publishers, Chicago, 1972, pp 159–181.
9. Martinex, IR: Fine structural studies of migrating epithelial cells following incision wounds. In Maibach, HI and Rovee, DT (eds): Epidermal Wound Healing. Year Book Medical Publishers, Chicago, 1972, p 323.
10. Silver, IA: Cellular microenvironment in healing and non-healing wounds. In Hunt, TK, et al (eds): Soft and Hard Tissue Repair. Draeger Publishers, New York, 1984, p 50.
11. Cooper, AM, Watt, RC, and Alterescu, V: Prevention and treatment of pressure sores. In Guide to Wound Care. Hollister, Inc, Libertyville, IL, 1983, p 56.
12. Robson, M: Management of the contaminated wound aids in diagnosis and treatment. In Krizek, T and Hoopes, J (eds): Symposium on Basic Sciences in Plastic Surgery. CV Mosby, St Louis, 1976, p 50.
13. Leydon, JL, Steward, R, and Kligman, AM: Update in vivo methods for evaluating topical antimicrobial agent on human skin. J Invest Dermatol 72:165, 1979.
14. Aly, R: Effect of occlusion on microbial population and physical skin conditions. Semin Dermatol 1:137, 1982.
15. Mertz, PM, Marshall, DA, and Eaglstein, WH: Occlusive wound dressings to prevent bacterial invasion and wound infection. J Am Acad Dermatol 12(4):662, 1985.
16. Eaglstein, WH and Mertz, PM: Dressings and wound healing. In Hunt, TK, et al (eds): Soft and Hard Tissue Repair. Draeger Publishers, New York, 1984, pp 316–323.
17. Field, LM: Over-sight on Op-site. J Dermatol Surg Oncol 7:597, 1981.
18. Mandy, J: A new primary wound dressing made of polyethylene oxide gel. J Dermatol Surg Oncol 9:2, 1983.
19. Eaton, AC: A controlled trial to evaluate and compare with sutureless skin closure technique (Op-site skin closure) with conventional skin suturing and clipping in abdominal surgery. Br J Surg 67:857, 1980.
20. Alper, JC, et al: Moist wound healing under a vapor permeable membrane. J Am Acad Dermatol 8:837, 1983.
21. Weber, DE, Parish, LC, and Witkowski, JA: Dextranomer in chronic wound healing. Clin Dermatol 2:(3)116, 1984.
22. Trumble, HC: The skin tolerance for pressure and pressure sores. Med J Aust 2:724, 1930.

23. Elliott, RM: Pressure ulcerations. Am Fam Physician 25:171, 1982.
24. Cooper, DM, Watt, RC, and Alterescu, V: Guide to Wound Care. Hollister, Inc, Libertyville, IL, 1983, p 60.
25. Silver, IA: Oxygen and tissue repair. In Ryan, TH (ed): An Environment for Healing: The Role of Occlusion. Royal Society of Medicine, International Congress and Symposium Series, No 88, 1985, pp 15–18.
26. Diegelmann, RF, Cohen, KI, and Kaplan, AM: The role of macrophages in wound repair: A review. Plast Reconstr Surg 68:107, 1981.
27. Howes, EL, et al: The use of Clostridium Histolyticum enzymes in the treatment of experimental third degree burns. Surg Gynecol Obstet 109:177, 1959.
28. Boxer, AM, et al: Debridement of dermal ulcers and decubiti with collagenase. Geriatrics 24:75, 1969.
29. Cassell, BL: Treating pressure sores stage by stage. RN Jan:36, 1986.
30. Alvarez, OM, Mertz, PM, and Eaglstein, WH: The effect of occlusive dressing on re-epithelialization and collagen synthesis. J Surg Res 35:142, 1983.
31. Hunt, TK, Knighton, DR, and Silver, IA: Regulation of wound healing angiogenesis: Effects of oxygen gradients and inspired oxygen concentration. Surgery 80:262, 1981.
32. Winter, GD: Formation of scab and the rate of epithelialization of superficial wounds in the skin of the young domestic pig. Nature 193:293, 1962.
33. Friedman, SJ and Su, PD: Management of leg ulcers. Am Fam Physician 27:219, 1983.
34. Bergman, RB: A new treatment of split-skin graft donor sites. Archiuum Chirurgicum Neerlandkum 29:69, 1977.
35. Tudhope, M: Management of pressure ulcers with a hydrocolloid occlusive dressing: Results in twenty-three patients. Journal of Enterosomal Therapy 11:102, 1984.
36. King, N: Using synthetic autolytic debriding agents for the treatment of full-thickness dermal ulcers. Ostomy/Wound Management 11:51, 1986.
37. Bassen, M, Shalev, O, and Dudai, M: Near fatal oxygen embolism due to wound irrigation with hydrogen peroxide. Postgrad Med J 58:448, 1982.
38. Gruber, R, Vistnes, L, and Pardae, R: The effect of commonly used antiseptics on wound healing. J Plast Reconstr Surg 55(4):472, 1975.
39. Holmes, G: Hydrotherapy as a means of rehabilitation. Br J Phys Med 5:93, 1942.
40. Beasley, R, and Kester, N: Principles of medical-surgical rehabilitation of the hand. Med Clin North Am 53:645, 1969.
41. Koepke, G: The role of physical medicine in the treatment of burns. Surg Clin North Am 50:1385, 1970.
42. Epstein, M: Water immersion: Modern researchers discover the secrets of an old folk remedy. The Sciences, Nov 12, 1979.
43. Mylin, J: The use of water in therapeutics. Arch Phys Med Rehabil 13:261, 1932.
44. Simonette, A, Miller, R, and Gristine, J: Efficacy of povidone-iodine in the disinfection of whirlpool baths and hubbard tanks. Phys Ther 52:450, 1972.
45. Steve, L, Goodhart, P, and Alexander, J: Hydrotherapy burn treatment: Use of chloramine T against resistant microorganisms. Arch Phys Med Rehabil 60:301, 1979.
46. Cuzzell, J: The new RYB color code. Am J Nurs Oct: 1342, 1988.
47. Gershenfeld, L: Iodine. In Reddish, GF (ed): Antiseptics, Disinfectants, Fungicides and chemical and physical sterilization. Lea and Febiger, Philadelphia, 1954, pp 171–211.
48. Lineaweaver, W, et al: Topical antimicrobial toxicity. Arch Surg 120:267, 1985.
49. Sindelove, WF and Mason, GR: Irrigation of subcutaneous tissue with povidone-iodine solution for prevention of surgical wound infection. Surg Gynecol Obstet 148:227, 1979.
50. Rogers, DM, Blouin, GS, and O'Leary, JP: Povidone-iodine wound irrigation and wound sepsis. Surg Gynecol Obstet 157:426, 1983.
51. Geronemus, RG, Mertz, PM, and Eaglstein, WH: The effects of topical antimicrobial agents. Arch Dermatol 115:1311, 1979.
52. Mertz, PM, et al: A new in-vivo model for the evaluation of topical antiseptics on superficial wounds. Arch Dermatol 120:58, 1984.
53. Aronoff, GR, et al: Increased serum iodide concentration from iodine absorption through wounds treated topically with povidone-iodine. Am J Med Sci 279:173, 1980.
54. Kucan, JO, et al: Comparison of silver sulfadiazine, povidone-iodine and physiologic saline in the treatment of chronic pressure ulcers. J Am Geriatr Soc 29:232, 1981.
55. Hugo, WH and Newton, JM: The antibacterial activity of a complex of iodine and a non-ionic surface active agent. J Pharmacol 16:189, 1964.
56. Rodeheaver, G, et al: Bactericidal activity and toxicity of iodine-containing solutions in wounds. Arch Surg 117:181, 1982.
57. Krizek, T and Robson, M: Comparison of topical agents on experimental burn wounds in rats. In Georgedae, J, Boswich, J, and MacMillan, B (eds): Recent Antiseptic Techniques in the Management of the Burn Patient. Purdue Frederick, New York, 1974, p 12.
58. Robson, M, et al: Evaluation of topical povidone: Iodine ointment in experimental wound sepsis. Plas Reconstr Surg 54(3):328, 1974.
59. Tommey, R, Norsberg, H, and Guernsey, J: The use of povidone-iodine in the treatment of burns, a literature review. Oklahoma State Medical Association 73:406, 1980.

60. Esplin, DW: Antiseptics and disinfectants/fungicides; ectoparacitacides. In Goodman, LS, and Gilman, A (eds): Pharmacological Basis of Therapeutics: A Textbook of Pharmacology, Toxicology, and Therapeutics for Physicians and Medical Students. Macmillan, New York, 1970, pp 1032–1066.
61. Dakin, HD: The antiseptic action of hypochlorites. Br Med J, Dec 4, 1915, p 809.
62. Dakin, HD: On the use of certain substances in the treatment of infected wounds. Br Med J, August 28, 1915, p 318.
63. Phillips, I, et al: Acetic acid in the treatment of superficial wounds infected by Pseudomonas aeruginosa. Lancet 1:11, 1968.
64. Avakian, L, Ball, C, and Weiss, E: Wound care and the high risk patient. Life Support Nurs 5:36, 1982.
65. Bennett, RG: Fundamentals of cutaneous surgery. CV Mosby, St Louis, 1988, p 335.
66. Eells, LD, et al: An evaluation of the safety and efficacy of topical antimicrobial therapy for primary skin infections (abstr). J Invest Dermatol 82:404, 1984.
67. Anderson, V: Over-the-counter topical antibiotic products: Date on safety and efficacy. Int J Dermatol 15(Suppl 1 & 2):1, 1976.
68. Physician's Desk Reference, ed 32. Medical Economics Co, Oradell, NJ, 1976, pp 726, 849, 1073, 1333.
69. Leyden, J and Kligman, A: Rationale for topical antibiotics. Cutis 28:515, 1978.
70. Urbach, F: Combined chemotherapy in the treatment of superficial bacterial infections of the skin. Curr Ther Res 8:199, 1966.
71. Eaglstein, WH and Mertz, PM: "Inert" vehicles do affect wound healing. J Invest Dermatol 74:90, 1980.
72. Eaglstein, WH and Mertz, PM: Effect of topical medicaments on the rate of repair of superficial wounds. In Dineen, P (ed): The Surgical Wound. Lea and Febiger, Philadelphia, 1981, p 167.
73. Harnar, T: Dr. Pay Unna's boot and early ambulation after skin grafting the leg: A survey of burn centers and a report of 20 cases. Plast Reconstr Surg 69:359, 1982.
74. Murray, I, and Rosenthal, S: The effect of locally applied zinc and aluminum on healing incised wounds. Surg Gynecol Obstet 126:1298, 1968.
75. Norman, JN, Rahmat, A, and Smith, G: Effect of supplements of zinc salts on the healing of granulating wounds in the rat and guinea pig. J Nutr 105:815, 1975.
76. Hallmang, G: Wound healing with adhesive zinc tape. Scand J Plast Reconstr Surg 10:177, 1976.
77. Hallbook, T, and Lanner, E: Serum zinc and healing of venous leg ulcers. Lancet 2:780, 1972.
78. Haeger, K and Lanner, E: Oral zinc sulfate and ischaemic leg ulcers. VASA: Zeitschrift für Gefaesskrankheiten (Bern) 3:77, 1974.
79. Greaves, MW and Ive, FA: Double-blind trial of zinc sulfate in the treatment of chronic venous leg ulceration. Br J Dermatol 87:632, 1972.
80. Husain, SL: Oral zinc sulfate in leg ulcers. Lancet 1:1069, 1969.
81. Barcia, BJ: Lack of acceleration of healing with zinc sulfate. Ann Surg 172:1048, 1970.
82. Hinman, CC, Maibach, HI, and Winter, GD: Effect of air exposure and occlusion on experimental human skin wounds. Nature 200:377, 1962.
83. Rovee, DT, et al: Effect of local wound environment on epidermal healing. In Maibach, HI: Epidermal wound healing. Year Book Medical Publishers, Chicago, 1972, pp 159–181.
84. Harris, DR and Keefe, RL: A histologic study of gold leaf treated experimental wounds. J Invest Dermatol 52:487, 1969.
85. Alvarez, OM, et al: The healing of superficial skin wounds is stimulated by external electrical current. J Invest Dermatol 81:144, 1983.
86. Bothwell, JW and Rovee, DT: Surgical dressings and wound healing. J & J Research Publication, 1970.
87. Kloth, LC and Feedar, JA: Acceleration of wound healing with high voltage, monophasic, pulsed current. Phys Ther 68:503, 1988.
88. Harris, DR, Filarski, SA, and Hector, RE: The effect of silastic sheet dressing on the healing of split graft donor sites. Plast Reconstr Surg 52:189, 1973.
89. Buchan, IA, et al: Clinical and laboratory investigation of the composition and properties of human skin wound exudate under semipermeable dressings. Burns 7:326, 1980.
90. Barnett, A, et al: Comparison of synthetic adhesive moisture vapor permeable and fine mesh gauze dressings for split-thickness skin graft donor sites. Am J Surg 145:379, 1983.
91. Winter, GD: Formation of the scab and the rate of epithelialization of superficial wounds in the skin of the young, domestic pig. Nature 193:293, 1962.
92. Varghese, MC, et al: Local environment of chronic wounds under synthetic dressings. Arch Dermatol 122:52, 1986.
93. Rovee, DT, Linsky, CB, and Bothwell, JW: Experimental models for the evaluation of wound repair. In Maibach, HI (ed): Animal Models in Dermatology. Churchill-Livingstone, New York, 1975, pp 253–266.
94. Lobe, TE, et al: An improved method of wound management for pediatric patients. J Pediatr Surg 15:886, 1980.
95. Alvarez, OM, Mertz, PM, and Eaglstein, WH: The effect of occlusive dressings on collagen synthesis and re-epithelialization in superficial wounds. J Surg Res 35:142, 1983.
96. Barker, AT, Jaffe, LF, and Vanable, JW, Jr: The glabrous epidermis of cavies contains a powerful battery. Am J Physiol 1982; 242:R348–366.
97. Haessler, RM: Transparent I.V. dressings vs. traditional dressings. J NITA 6(3):169, 1983.
98. Gardezi, SAR, et al: Role of polyurethane membrane in postoperative wound management. Journal of the Pakistan Medical Association 33:219, 1983.

99. Leydon, JL, Steward, R, and Kligman, AM: Update in vivo methods for evaluating topical antimicrobial agents on human skin. J Invest Dermatol 72:165, 1979.
100. Aly, R: Effect of occlusion on microbial population and physical skin conditions. Semin Dermatol 1:137, 1982.
101. Eaglstein, WH: Effect of occlusive dressings on wound healing. Clin Dermatol 2:(15)107, 1984.
102. Moshakis, V, et al: Tegaderm versus gauze dressing in breast surgery. Br J Clin Pract 38:149, 1984.
103. Shell, JA, et al: Comparison of moisture vapor permeable (MVP) dressings to conventional dressings for management of radiation skin reactions. Oncol Nurs Forum 13:11, 1986.
104. Hartwell, SW: The Mechanisms of Healing in Human Wounds. Charles C Thomas, Springfield, IL, 1955, pp 4–5.
105. Eaglstein, WH, et al: Local environment of chronic wounds under synthetic dressings. Arch Dermatol 122:52, 1986.
106. Turner, TD: Semiocclusive and occlusive dressings. In Ryan, TH (ed): An Environment for Healing: The Role of Occlusion. Royal Society of Medicine, International Congress and Symposium Series, No 88, 1985, pp 5–14.
107. McCarthy, DJ and Montgomery, B: Polyurethane in the management of ulcerating lesions of the lower extremities. J Am Podiatr Assoc 7:1, 1983.
108. Turner, TD: Desirable properties of occlusive dressings. J Pharmacol 22:421–422, 1979.
109. Rovee, DT: Personal communication and data on file. Johnson & Johnson Products, New Brunswick, NJ, 1977.
110. Lingner, C, et al: Clinical trial of a moisture vapor permeable dressing on superficial pressure sores. J Ent Ther 2:147, 1984.
111. May, SR: Physiology, immunology, and clinical efficacy of an adherent polyurethane wound dressing: Op-Site®. In Wise, DL (ed): Burn Wound Coverings. Vol II. CRC Press, Boca Raton, FL, 1984, pp 53–78.
112. Tinckler, L: A significant advance. Nursing Mirror, February 16, 1983, p 26.
113. Alper, JC, et al: Moist wound healing under a vapor permeable membrane. J Am Acad Dermatol 8:347, 1983.
114. James, JH and Watson, ACH: The use of Op-Site, a vapor permeable dressing on skin graft donor sites. Br J Plast Surg 28:107, 1975.
115. Miller, TA: The healing of partial-thickness skin injuries. In Hunt, TK (ed): Wound Healing and Wound Infections: Theory and Surgical Practice. Appleton-Century-Crofts, New York, 1980, pp 81–96.
116. Silver, I: Oxygen tension and epithelialization. In Maibach, H and Rovee, D (eds): Epidermal Wound Healing. Year Book Medical Publishers, Chicago, 1972, pp 291–305.
117. Mandy, SH: A new primary wound dressing made of polyethylene oxide gel. J Dermatol Surg Oncol 9:2, 153, 1983.
118. Cherry, GW and Ryan, TJ: Enhanced wound angiogenesis with a new hydrocolloid dressing. In Ryan, TH (ed): An Environment for Healing: The Role of Occlusion. Royal Society of Medicine, International Congress and Symposium Series, No 88, 1985, pp 61–68.
119. Knighton, DR, Silver, IA, and Hunt, TK: Regulation of wound healing angiogenesis—effect of oxygen gradients and inspired oxygen concentration. Surgery 90:262, 1981.
120. Comfeel Ulcus Powder, Technical Handout. Coloplast, Inc, Tampa, FL.
121. Bard Absorption Dressing, Technical Handout. Bard Home Health Division, Berkely Heights, NJ.
122. Jeter, KF, et al: Comprehensive wound management with a starch-based copolymer dressing. J Enterostom Ther 13:217, 1986.
123. Pinski, JB: Dressings for dermabrasion: New aspects. J Dermatol Surg Oncol 13(6):673, 1987.
124. Biobrane, Temporary wound dressing. Technical Handout. Winthrop Pharmaceuticals, New York.
125. Gerding, RL, et al: Biosynthetic skin substitute vs. 1% silver sulfadiazine for treatment of inpatient partial-thickness thermal burns. J Trauma 28(8):1265, 1988.
126. Tavis, MN, et al: A new composite skin prosthesis. Burns 7:123, 1980.
127. Groth, KE: Klonische Beobachtungen und Experimentelle Studien uber die Entstehung des Dekubitus. Acta Chir Scand (Suppl 76)87:1, 1942.
128. Linder, RM and Upton, J: The prevention of pressure sores. Surg Rounds 6:(6)42, 1983.
129. Sacks, AH, et al: Skin deformation and blood flow under external loading. In Rehabilitation Research and Development Progress Report. VA Medical Center, Palo Alto, CA, 1988, p 100.
130. Kosiak, M, et al: Evaluation of pressure as a factor in the production of ischial ulcers. Arch Phys Med Rehabil 39:623, 1959.
131. Kosiak, M: Etiology and pathology of ischemic ulcers. Arch Phys Med Rehabil 40:62, 1959.
132. Dinsdale, SM: Decubitus ulcers: Role of pressure and friction in causation. Arch Phys Med Rehabil 55:147, 1974.
133. Dinsdale, SM: Decubitus ulcers in swine: Light and electron microscopy study of pathogenesis. Arch Phys Med Rehabil 54:51, 1973.
134. Daniel, RK, Priest, DL, and Wheatley, DC: Etiologic factors in pressure sores: An experimental model. Arch Phys Med Rehabil 62:492, 1981.
135. Perkash, A and Brown, M: Anemia in patients with traumatic spinal cord injury. Paraplegia 20:235, 1982.
136. Chandra, KK: Cell mediated immunity in nutritional imbalance. Fed Pract 39:3088, 1980.
137. Lee, BY: Chronic ulcers of the skin. McGraw-Hill, New York, 1985.

138. Ames, A, et al: Cerebral ischemia II, the no reflow phenomenon. Am J Pathol 52:437, 1968.
139. Willms-Kretschmer, K and Majno, G: Ischemia of the skin. Am J Pathol 54:237, 1969.
140. Narsete, TA, Orgel, MG, and Smith, D: Pressure sores. Am Fam Physician 28:135, 1983.
141. Landis, EM: Microinjection studies of capillary blood pressure in human skin. Heart 15:209, 1930.
142. Orlando, JC: Pressure ulcers: Principles of measurement. In Reichel, W (ed): Clinical Aspects of Aging. Williams and Wilkins, Baltimore, 1983 pp 469–478.
143. Kosiak, M: Etiology of decubitus ulcers. Arch Phys Med Rehabil 42:19, 1961.
144. Elliott, RM: Pressure ulcerations. Am Fam Physician 25:171, 1982.
145. Maklebust, J, Mondoux, L, and Sieggreen, M: Pressure relief characteristics of various support surfaces used in prevention and treatment of pressure ulcers. J Enterostom Ther 13:85, 1986.
146. Boorman, JG, Carr, S, and Harvey, KJ: A clinical evaluation of the air fluidized bed in a general plastic surgery unit. Br J Plast Surg 34:165, 1981.
147. Clark, M: Contact pressure measurements between the sacrum of young and elderly subjects lying upon two specialized mattresses. Paper presented at the Second National Symposium—Pressure Sores. Sponsored by the University of Chicago, Oct 22–23, 1988.
148. Souther, SG: Wheelchair cushions to reduce pressure under boney prominences. Arch Phys Med Rehabil 55:460, 1974.
149. Kosiak, M: Evaluation of pressure as a factor in the production of ischemic ulcers. Arch Phys Med Rehabil 39:623, 1958.
150. Fisher, SV: Wheelchair cushion effect on skin temperature. Arch Phys Med Rehabil 59:68, 1978.
151. Weinstein, ID: A fluid support mattress and seat for prevention and treatment of decubitus ulcers. Lancet 2:625, 1965.
152. Kenedi, RM, Cowden, JM, and Scales, JT (eds): Bed Sore Biomechanics. MacMillan Press, New York, 1976, pp 259–267.

Appendix

ENZYMATIC DEBRIDING AGENTS

Biozyme "C"
Armour Pharmaceutical Company
303 South Broadway
Tarrytown, NY 10591

Elase
Parke-Davis
Division of Warner-Lambert Co.
Morris Plains, NJ 07950

Santyl
Knoll Pharmaceutical Co.
Whippany, NJ 07981

Travase
Travenol Laboratories, Inc.
Flint Laboratories Division
Deerfield, IL 60015

TOPICAL BACTERICIDAL AGENTS

Furacin (nitrofurazone)
Norwich-Eaton
Norwich, NY 13815

Neosporin
Burroughs Wellcome
3030 Cornwallis Road
Research Triangle Park, NC 27709

Silver Sulfadiazine Cream
Travenol Laboratories, Inc.
Flint Laboratories Division
Deerfield, IL 60015

Chlorazene
Badger Pharmacal, Inc.
New Berlin, WI 53151

SEMIPERMEABLE FILM (SPF) DRESSINGS

Bio-occlusive Dressing (J & J)
Johnson & Johnson
New Brunswick, NJ 07903

Op-Site dressing (Smith & Nephew)
Acme United Corp.
Bridgeport, CT 06609

Polyskin (Kendall Company)
Kendall
Hospital Products
One Federal Street
Boston, MA 02101
(800) 225-2600
(800) 882-2000—MA only

173

Tegaderm
3M
P.O. Box 33211
Eagen, MN 55133

Blister Film
Chesebrough-Pond's, Inc.
Greenwich, CT 06830

Co-Film
Chesebrough-Pond's, Inc.
Greenwich, CT 06830

SEMIPERMEABLE FOAM DRESSINGS

LyoFoam
Acme United Corporation
Medical Products Division
Fairfield, CT 06430
(203) 255-2744

Primaderm
Absorbent Cotton Co., Inc.
Valley Park, MO 63088

Synthaderm
Calgon Vestal Laboratories
St. Louis, MO 63110

HYDROGEL DRESSINGS

Spenco Second Skin
Spenco
P.O. Box 2501
Waco, TX 76702-2501

Vigilon
Bard Home Health Division
C.R. Bard, Inc.
111 Spring Street
Murray Hill, NJ 07974
(201) 277-8000
(800) 526-4493

HYDROCOLLOID DRESSINGS

Duoderm (Convatec)
E.G. Squibb and Sons
P.O. Box 4000
Princeton, NJ 08450

Intact
Bard Home Health Division
C.R. Bard, Inc.
111 Spring St.
Murray Hill, NJ 07974
(201) 277-8000
(800) 526-4493

J & J Ulcer Dressing
Johnson & Johnson
New Brunswick, NJ 07903

Restore
Hollister Incorporated
2000 Hollister Dr.
Libertyville, IL 60048
(312) 680-1000

HYDROCOLLOID ABSORPTION POWDERS, PASTES, AND GRANULES

Bard Absorption Dressing
Bard Home Health Division
C.R. Bard, Inc.
111 Spring St.
Murray Hill, NJ 07974
(201) 277-8000

Comfeel Ulcus Powder
5610 W. Sligh Ave.
Tampa, FL 33634
(813) 886-5634
(800) 237-4555—outside FL

BIOSYNTHETIC AND BIOLOGIC DRESSINGS

Biobrane
Woodruff Laboratories, Inc.
3100-7 Harvard Street
Santa Ana, CA 92704
(714) 557-7860

FOAM PRD

Biogard Critical Care Floatation Unit
Bio Clinic Corporation
10670 Acacia St.
P.O. Box 1528
Rancho Cucamonga, CA 91730
(714) 989-2535
(800) 854-2369—except CA

Clinisert Pressure Relief System
Support Systems International, Inc.
4349 Corporate Rd.
Charleston, SC 29405
(800) 845–2478
(800) 821-8913—in SC

WATER PRDs

Lotus Pressure Equalizer
Lotus Health Care Products
Naugatuck Industrial Park
31 Sheridan Dr.
Naugatuck, CT 06770
(203) 723-1494
(800) 243-2362

HMT-STEBCO Water Floatation Systems
Health & Medical Techniques, Inc.
1175 Post Rd. E.
P.O. Box 829
Westport, CT 06881
(800) 243-6375
(203) 226-4445

GEL PRDs

Action Pad
Action Products, Inc.
22 N. Mulberry St.
Hagerstown, MD 21740
TELEX: 322619
FAX: (301) 733-2073

Elasto Gel
Southwest Technologies, Inc.
1510 Charlotte
Kansas City, MO 64208
(816) 221-2442
TELEX: 43-4081

STATIC AIR PRDs

Sof·Care
Gaymar Industries, Inc.
10 Centre Drive
Orchard Park, NY 14127

Roho Cushion
Roho Incorporated
P.O. Box 658
Belleville, IL 62222
1-800-851-3449

DYNAMIC AIR PRDs

Grant APP
Grant Airmass Corporation
1011 High Ridge Road
Stamford, CT 06905
1-800-243-5237

Betabed
Huntleigh Technology Inc.
227 Route 33 East
Manalapan, NJ 07726
1-800-223-1218

LOW AIR LOSS PRDs

Flexicare
Support Systems International, Inc.
4349 Corporate Rd.
Charleston, SC 29405
(800) 845-2478
(800) 821-8913—in SC

Kinair
Kinetic Concepts, Inc.
P.O. Box 8588
San Antonio, TX 78208
(800) 531-5346
TELEX: 4620414

Mediscus Mark V-A
Mediscus Products, Inc.
13135 Champions Dr., Suite 120
Houston, TX 77069
(713) 583-9232—in TX
(800) 922-9065
TELEX: 820-736

AIR FLUIDIZED PRDs

Clinitron
Support Systems International, Inc.
4349 Corporate Rd.
Charleston, SC 29405
(800) 845-2478
(800) 821-8913—in SC

SMI Air-Fluidized Support System
Surgi-Med, Inc.
815 Terminal Rd.
Lansing, MI 48906
(800) 221-4736
(517) 321-2202

Fluid-Aire
Kinetic Concepts, Inc.
P.O. Box 8588
San Antonio, TX 78208
(800) 531-5346
TELEX: 4620414

CHAPTER 10

Treatment of Wounds Due to Vascular Problems

Joseph M. McCulloch, Ph.D., P.T.
John Hovde, M.S., P.T.

Wounds caused by vascular problems typically occur in the leg. Vascular wounds of the upper extremity are far less common.[1,2] Chronic leg ulcers are reported to occur in 1 percent of the adult population. Venous disease is associated with the majority of the ulcerations. In a study of 600 patients with 827 leg ulcers, 76 percent of the ulcerated legs had evidence of venous disease and 22 percent had signs of arterial insufficiency.[3] Roughly half of the legs with arterial insufficiency had coexisting signs of venous disease. A wide range of diseases and causative factors are responsible for the remaining small percentage of leg ulcers.

The principal objective of this chapter is to guide clinical decision making in the evaluation and treatment of wounds of vascular system origin. To aid decision making, the chapter is limited to commonly encountered ulcers. Through the discussion, the reader should gain understanding of the pathology, presentation, and treatment of common vascular wounds and the ability to identify those wounds that are atypical. The reader is referred to other sources for discussion of vascular disorders associated with atypical ulcers. Brief reviews of vascular anatomy, physiology, and wound etiology are followed by discussions of evaluation and treatment.

VASCULAR STRUCTURE AND FUNCTION

Blood flow from the aorta through the peripheral vessels occurs because of a pressure gradient. During systole the pressure in the large arteries normally rises to approximately 120 mmHg and decreases to 80 mmHg during diastole. As blood flows into smaller arteries, the average pressure decreases slightly while the flow and pressure remain pulsatile. As blood flows into the arterioles, the pressure drops significantly to approximately 40 mmHg. The pulsatile flow is then converted to a continuous flow. Pressures in the beginning and end of the capillaries are 35 mmHg and 15 mmHg, respectively, while pressures in the venous system range from 15 mmHg in the venules to near zero at the right atrium. The pressure changes noted in the vascular system are related to the structure of the vessels.[4]

Blood vessels are composed of five major elements: endothelial cells, basement membrane, elastic tissue, smooth muscle, and collagen.[5] These structures are integrated to form three layers — the intima, media, and adventitia.[6] The inner layer, the intima, is composed of endothelial cells, basement membrane, and elastic tissue. Endothelial cells cover the luminal surface and regulate the exchange of blood components across the vessel wall. The basement membrane encircles the endothelial cells, providing a supporting structure. Much of the support is provided by a prominent band of elastic tissue that surrounds the basement membrane. The middle layer, the media, consists principally of smooth muscle surrounded by a less prominent band of elastic tissue. The outside layer, the adventitia, is formed mainly by inelastic and tough collagenous connective tissue. The proportions of the five elements vary in different parts of the vascular system from aorta to veins, giving each part a distinct structure and function.

Large elastic arteries, such as the aorta, subclavian artery, and common iliac artery, have characteristically thick walls with large quantities of elastic tissue in the media. These properties allow the large arteries to act as low-resistance conduits and as a pressure reservoir.[7] The larger lumens of the arteries are kept open by the thick vessel walls. The large lumens provide for a relatively low resistance to blood flow. During systole, the walls stretch to accommodate the volume of blood ejected by the heart. The passive recoil of the artery walls during diastole meanwhile maintains high pressure to drive blood through the distal tissue. Branches of the large arteries such as the femoral, popliteal, and tibial possess a medial layer made mostly of smooth muscle. These arteries are able to change in caliber according to the demands of the tissues they perfuse.

Arterioles are small unnamed vessels that branch from small arteries. Arteriolar radii are under precise control of the sympathetic nervous system. The degree of arteriolar smooth muscle constriction within organs and tissue is regulated by the amount of smooth muscle contraction and consequently determines the blood flow distribution.[8]

Capillary walls are made of a very thin layer of endothelial cells that perform the ultimate function of the vascular system, the exchange of nutrients and metabolic end products. The capillary wall has a ring of smooth muscle at the arteriolar end. This smooth muscle ring functions in flow regulation. Venules emerging from capillary beds have less muscle and elastic tissue than corresponding-sized arterioles. The venules unite to form larger veins that combine in turn to form larger vessels.

A major factor distinguishing veins from corresponding arteries is the thickness of their walls. Veins have much thinner walls. The muscle and elastic portion of venous walls are less developed than arterial walls and the venous adventitia is proportionally thicker.[6] Vein walls are much more distensible than artery walls, allowing veins to accommodate variations in blood volume and store blood. More than 60 percent of the body's blood volume is contained in veins and venules.[7] Another principal difference between veins and arteries is the presence of valves that allow veins to regulate the direction of blood flow toward the heart.

In the leg, deep and superficial veins are connected by perforating veins that penetrate the fascia between the two. Valves direct the flow of blood from superficial to deep veins in the legs. In contrast, the valves in the foot direct blood from deep to superficial veins, which is how the saphenous veins are filled without direct contact with the capillary beds.[9] Because of the valves, blood flow in the legs is assisted by contractions of skeletal muscle. Blood flow in the abdomen and chest is assisted by movement of the diaphragm. These are known respectively as the *skeletal muscle pump* and *respiratory pump*.[7]

The lymphatics are thin-walled, permeable vessels that are not part of the blood circulatory system. Lymphatics have blind ends through which interstitial fluid and components such as proteins diffuse. The fluid is carried to where the largest lymph vessels empty into the veins in the lower neck. Thus, lymphatics carry fluid from interstitial spaces back into the blood.[7]

VASCULAR PATHOLOGY

In general, clinical problems from vascular disease result from occlusion of the affected vessel. Arterial obstruction leads to ischemia, whereas venous and lymphatic occlusion produce congestion and edema.[10] Because vascular diseases are customarily classified as arterial, venous, or lymphatic disease, they will be discussed separately. The following section begins with an overview of arterial disease and arterial wounds, followed by discussions of specific arterial diseases that cause wounds more commonly encountered in clinical practice. After a discussion of venous pathology, venous wounds, and lymphatic pathology, the section ends with a discussion of the interaction of vascular disease and causative factors.

Arterial Insufficiency

Arterial disease is often classified anatomically as affecting visceral tissue, cerebral tissue, or the extremities. Anatomic classification stems from the great variation in resulting pathologies such as bowel necrosis, stroke, or leg ulceration, respectively. Occlusion of large, named vessels to the extremities can lead to tissue necrosis, whereas occlusion of small, unnamed arteries, arterioles, and capillaries rarely does so. Arterial disorders can also be classified as either acute (such as thrombosis) or chronic (such as arteriosclerosis obliterans). Both acute and chronic occlusive disease may result in ischemic ulcerations. Alternately, arterial disease can be viewed as either organic or functional. In organic disorders, structural changes in the artery wall or lumen may obstruct blood flow. Functional arterial disorders such as Raynaud's disease are reversible vasomotor disturbances. These diseases, which frequently affect upper extremities, more than likely cause pain and pallor rather than ischemic necrosis. Livedo reticularis is a functional disorder associated with dilated capillaries and venules. Individuals develop a purplish discoloration, which can lead to leg ulceration. Finally, arterial lesions can be classified by morphology into one of four types—obstruction, disruption (from trauma), fistula, or dilatation (aneurysm). The first three are associated with tissue necrosis, while dilatative disorders are not.[2]

Wounds from arterial insufficiency result as follows. When blood flow to a given tissue is impaired, the tissue becomes ischemic. If resulting tissue hypoxia leads to irreversible cell damage, the condition is recognized by pathologists as ischemic coagulative necrosis.[10] When tissue death is clinically visible the condition is termed *dry gangrene*. The term *gangrene* can be applied to a dry, dark, cold, mummified, contracted toe or to a pinhead-sized bit of necrosis on a fingertip. Whether the gangrene affects the toe, foot, leg, or trunk depends on the location and extent of the arterial impairment.[1] When gangrene affects a patch of skin, the necrotic tissue sloughs off and a skin ulcer is produced. Further necrosis enlarges the ulcer.[11] The term *wet gangrene* is applied by some to tissue changes caused by a combination of hypoxia and bacterial infection.[10] Others apply the term to the wet, swollen, necrotic part of a diabetic extremity with or without infection.[10]

The most significant arterial disease in terms of frequency of ulcer production is *arteriosclerosis obliterans. Arteriosclerosis* is a general term for thickening and hardening of the arterial wall.[12] By far, the most common type of arteriosclerosis is *atherosclerosis.* Nonatheromatous forms of arteriosclerosis, such as Mönckeberg's sclerosis or arteriosclerosis, typically do not cause ulceration. The term *arteriosclerosis obliterans* is used to describe atheromatous lesions of the aorta and its branches.[13] Arteriosclerosis obliterans usually affects the arteries to the lower extremities and is responsible for 95 percent of patients with chronic occlusive arterial disease.

The pathology of atherosclerosis is well known.[12] The characteristic lesion is the atheromatous plaque that develops in the intima of the artery wall. The plaque contains lipids, calcium, and fibrous tissue. The lesion progressively gets larger, causing the vessel lumen to narrow. The disease progresses slowly for many years. Blood flow does not become affected until the lumen cross-sectional area is reduced by 75 percent. Collateral circulation develops in an attempt to compensate for the obstruction and maintain viability of the affected extremity. However, the collateral circulation often is inadequate to provide blood to an exercising muscle. This event leads to the symptom of intermittent claudication, pain that occurs on walking but is relieved when the subject rests. Intermittent claudication typically affects calf muscles regardless of which proximal artery is obstructed. This occurrence is due to the great demand for oxygen required by the calf muscles. Complete obstruction of the lumen and collaterals can occur with plaque enlargement, leading to the symptoms of rest pain, ulceration, and gangrene. Thrombosis may occur due to turbulence of blood flow at the site of a plaque. When thrombosis occurs, collateral circulation obviously does not have time to develop. This event necessitates surgical correction to prevent gangrene and limb loss.

The progression of atherosclerosis is related to age. The ideally normal intima exists in the fetus and neonate. With age comes progressive intimal proliferation and thickening. The relationship between normal intimal thickening and atheromatous plaque formation is not clear, but a direct causal relationship is not likely. Symptoms of arteriosclerosis obliterans usually occur in persons older than age 50 but are not uncommon in younger individuals.

Smoking, diabetes mellitus, hyperlipoproteinemia, and hypertension are factors known to increase the risk of arteriosclerosis obliterans.[2] Between 60 and 70 percent of patients with atherosclerosis have two of the four risk factors. Of patients with obstructive arterial disease, 73 to 90 percent are smokers. Smoking induces the entry of cholesterol into arterial endothelium in animals. Smoking also raises blood lipids and affects peripheral blood flow. How these effects specifically influence arteriosclerosis obliterans is unknown.

As with smoking, the exact relationship of diabetes mellitus to arteriosclerosis obliterans is unknown. Of patients with obstructive arterial disease, 7 to 30 percent are diabetics, however. Persons with diabetes have more extensive arterial disease and have the disease at younger ages than nondiabetics. Diabetics also tend to display less involvement of the aorta and iliac arteries and more involvement of the popliteal and tibial arteries.

Hypertension has been reported in 29 to 39 percent of patients with obstructive arterial disease. Excessive, constant pressure and turbulence may lead to intimal damage. Hyperlipoproteinemia has been related to the occurrence of atherosclerosis. Hyperproteinemia is reported to exist in 31 to 57 percent of patients with obstructive arterial disease. As with the risk factors, exact causal relationships are not known.[14]

Thromboangiitis obliterans, known as Buerger's disease, is the second most common chronic occlusive disease, though rare compared with arteriosclerosis obliterans. Both diseases cause tissue ischemia. Thromboangiitis obliterans is distinctive in affecting younger men who are smokers and by the intense inflammatory component that leads to occlusion of both arteries and veins. Small distal vessels and middle-sized arteries are affected with proximal progression ensuing. The symptom of cold sensitivity and signs of ulcers and gangrene occur in upper and lower extremities alike. The marginal collateral circulation in the toes and fingers leads to early tissue necrosis when obstruction does occur.[12,13]

Less common causes of ischemic wounds are grouped under the term *necrotizing vasculitides*. This broad group of disorders is characterized by inflammatory reactions in the blood vessels, leading to necrosis and destruction of the vessel wall. The resulting pathologies vary greatly and are beyond the scope of this chapter. Examples of vasculitis known to cause wound development are Takayasu's arteritis, polyarteritis nodosa, rheumatoid arthritis, and systemic lupus erythematosus.

Acute interruption of blood flow to an extremity is a severe condition warranting emergency treatment. Generally, if circulation is not restored within 6 to 8 hours after paresthesias develop, the chance of limb loss is great. Common causes of acute arterial occlusion include trauma, embolism from the heart, or thrombosis at the site of a pre-existing chronic arterial occlusive disease. The embolus may be fat, air, or aggregates of cholesterol, but the usual material is thrombus that arises from the wall of an atrium and lodges at an arterial bifurcation. The symptoms of acute occlusion include pain, pallor, loss of pulses, paresthesia, and paralysis. The extent of tissue necrosis depends on many factors such as site of the occlusion, suddenness of the occlusion, extent of collateralization, and duration of the ischemia.[15]

Sickle cell anemia is another vascular problem that warrants attention. While often considered an arterial problem, sickle cell disease really affects the arterial and venous systems at the microvascular level. The ulcerations that result tend to be more closely aligned with those of venous insufficiency. Sickle cell anemia is classified as a chronic hemolytic anemia. When red cells containing sickle hemoglobin become deoxygenated at the capillary level, the red cell assumes a rigid sickle shape. This process takes about 3 seconds to occur. By this time, many of the sickled cells have already been transported into the larger vessels of the venous system. Cells that are delayed in passing through the capillaries become trapped in the microcirculation, and infarction results. Infarction, in turn, leads to a venous ulceration.[16,17] Management of ulcerations in these patients is the same as that for patients having venous insufficiency and is discussed later in the chapter.

Venous Insufficiency

The manner in which veins react to injury or disease appears limited in comparison to the previously discussed arterial system. As the title of this section implies, we are dealing with situations that prevent veins from effectively performing their job, that is, returning blood to the cardiopulmonary system. Four major disruptive mechanisms warrant discussion in this area, *thrombosis, obstruction, dilatation,* and *hemorrhage*.

Venous thrombosis, like arterial thrombosis, begins with the adherence of platelets to the endothelial wall. As this aggregation continues, a fibrin mesh is deposited, which in turn encourages further platelet adherence, until finally the vessel lumen is occluded. In the ensuing days to weeks, several events potentially occur.

Within days of occlusion, fibrinolysins begin to act upon the thrombus. At this stage, the individual becomes very susceptible to embolization. Meanwhile, an inflammatory process is occurring in the vessel wall adjacent to the thrombus. In many instances, embolization does not occur; instead, the area becomes recanalized during the process of inflammatory repair. Unfortunately, during this entire sequence of events, valve damage has usually occurred.[18] This then places the patient at risk for future venous problems.

The extent to which venous obstruction leads to significant dysfunction and resultant ulcerations is most dependent on the anatomic location of the involved segment. Obstruction of superficial veins or even their surgical excision seldom causes major consequences due to the number of collateral veins left behind. Should a significant segment of a deep vein become obstructed, however, major peripheral problems could result. Edema is one variable that can serve as an indicator of the degree of obstruction.

The third major problem causing venous insufficiency is *venous dilation* or *varicosity*. While generally accepted in the past as being caused by persistent increases in pressure, varicosity is more recently felt to be due to an inborn defect since the condition can often be noted just after adolescence. Whether the defect lies in the valves, the venous wall, or both is not fully understood.[19] Varicosities are frequently subdivided into primary and secondary, depending upon whether they are hereditary or due to an obstructive phenomenon, respectively.

The final factor contributing to venous insufficiency is *hemorrhage*. Hemorrhage can really be considered a possible concurrent problem with any of the previously identified factors. Any hemorrhage can result in the development of a hematoma or more seriously the loss of significant blood volume.

Venous Ulceration

While it is accepted that venous ulcerations result from the skin and subcutaneous tissue receiving poor nutrition, the exact mechanism by which nutrition becomes compromised remains unclear. Numerous researchers have hypothesized causative factors that are felt to contribute to abnormally high venous pressure at the ankle. These hypotheses range from increased lower extremity pressure present during relaxed standing to excessively high pressure transmitted from deep to superficial veins during calf muscle contraction.[20-23]

Until recently, two major theories existed related to the cause of venous ulcerations. One theory, focusing on the stasis or pooling of venous blood, was advanced by Homans[24] who suggested that tissue anoxia and cell death occurred due to blood lying stagnant within dilated veins. This theory gained support from DeTakats and others,[25] who noted a decreased oxygen content of blood taken from varicose veins. These findings were challenged by Blalock,[26] who suggested that the decreased oxygen concentration was due to the dependent posture of the extremity during sampling. Although support for this theory has been lacking since 1929, the concept is still taught today.[27]

A second theory on the cause of venous ulcerations was provided in 1953 by Puilacks and Vidal Barraquer.[28] They noted that blood appeared to move faster through veins whenever a varicosity or ulceration was present. This event was caused by the presence of an arteriovenous fistula. The shunting of blood which thereby occurred supposedly caused certain areas of the skin to receive improper oxygenation, which, in turn, led to cell death. Direct observations of such fistulas have been lacking. In addition, subsequent studies have failed in supporting this theory.[29]

A NEW THEORY IS PROPOSED

Browse and Burnand,[30] following the work of Landis,[31] noted that patients with chronic venous ulcerations had enlargement of the local capillary bed. Further examination revealed that the large molecule fibrinogen was escaping the vascular system at the capillary level. The capillary defect was directly related to the degree of damage to the calf pump. Additionally, histologic studies revealed a layer of fibrin to be present around the capillaries.

Normally, fibrin is broken down by the fibrinolytic system of the blood. This system has been found to be significantly compromised in patients with postphlebitic extremities, however. Because of this compromise, fibrinogen polymerises to form insoluble fibrin. The fibrin in turn deposits around the capillary, creating a barrier to the passage of oxygen and other nutrients. The result is tissue necrosis.

A dysfunctional fibrinolytic system may be one of the primary causes of damage to the venous system. Figure 10–1 graphically represents one possible model of the process, according to Browse and Burnand.[30]

The changes that occur in the skin before an ulcer develops have been termed *lipodermatosclerosis* or *liposclerosis*.[32] Liposclerosis initially presents as erythema or pigmentation of the skin. Subsequent thickening of the skin occurs accompanied by an increased warmth. At this stage, the condition is often mistaken for cellulitis or superficial thrombophlebitis. All of the classic signs of inflammation occur—redness, heat, pain, and swelling. In addition, the area begins to become indurated due to the organization of tissue fluid. As the situation progresses, actual pigment changes occur in the skin. The brownish discoloration, so classically seen in venous insufficiency, is produced by hemosiderin. Hemosiderin, a by-product of hemoglobin lysis, permanently stains the tissues. As the process worsens, the pigmentation darkens and ultimately skin breakdown occurs. The resulting ulceration is generally characterized by having irregular

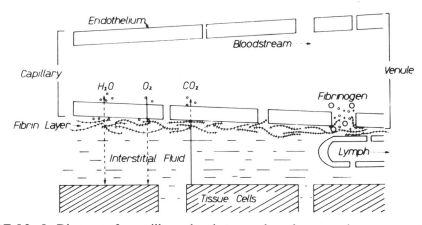

FIGURE 10–1. Diagram of a capillary, showing an enlarged pore at the venous end leaking fibrinogen into the interstitial fluid where it polymerises to form an insoluble layer of fibrin (From Browse, and Burnand,[30] p. 244, with permission).

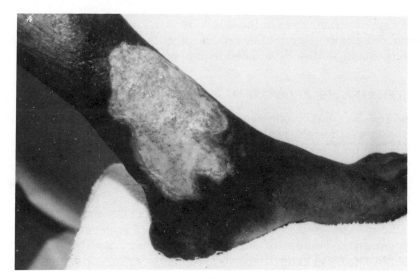

FIGURE 10–2. Ulceration secondary to venous insufficiency.

margins and a significant bed of granulation tissue. The healthy granulation tissue is frequently noted to be growing from an area of fibrosis.[33]

While venous ulcerations can occur anywhere in the lower leg, they are most frequently located just proximal to the medial malleolus (Fig. 10–2). The predilection of this area for ulcer development is felt to be due to high pressures in incompetent perforating veins being directly transmitted to the capillaries in the region in addition to the poor arterial supply to the area.[34]

FACTORS CONTRIBUTING TO WOUND ETIOLOGY

The vascular diseases previously described can individually lead to wound development. More often, related factors such as poor nutritional status, immobility, and trauma contribute to wound development. The role these factors play in causing wounds requires thorough understanding for optimal treatment and prevention.

The importance of nutrition in wound healing is well known. Vitamin C, vitamin A, zinc, and amino acids are directly involved in the metabolic process of healing. Vitamin C is essential for collagen formation. Deficiency of this vitamin causes delayed wound healing and poorly formed scar tissue of low tensile strength.[10] Vitamin A influences the differentiation of healing epithelium.[35] Zinc plays an important role in protein synthesis; its deficiency adversely affects wound healing. Chapter 6 addresses the relationship between nutrition and healing in detail.

Immobility promotes wound development. As stated in the discussion of vascular physiology, muscle contraction assists the return of venous blood to the heart. Immobility leads to the development of thrombophlebitis and edema, especially when the lower limb is in a dependent position, as often occurs when a person's upper body is propped up in bed. Edema is harmful to healing wounds. Edema fluid is an excellent culture medium for infecting bacteria, and its presence may compress low-pressure collateral vessels. Immobility helps cause pressure sores with their all too well-known disastrous consequences.

Trauma to dysvascular limbs plays a more obvious role in causing wounds than does nutrition or immobility. Three types of trauma should be considered: mechanical, thermal, and chemical. In one study of a large group of patients having amputated ischemic limbs, 62 percent of the amputations resulted from mechanical, thermal, or chemical trauma as the initiating event.[36] A common form of mechanical trauma is poorly given nail and callus care. Further information relating trauma to wounds is found in Chapter 11.

Some examples of trauma known to cause severe wounds in dysvascular limbs are a limb struck by a softball, a foot soaked in hot water, and homemade concoctions of topical agents applied to dry skin or small ulcers. In each of the examples cited, the same trauma to a normally vascularized limb would probably have resulted in inconsequential tissue damage, if any. The underlying dysvascular state, whether arterial or venous, made the tissue damage severe. Ischemic limbs are especially susceptible to thermal damage, either heat or cold. Normal peripheral vascular systems are capable of adjusting to local or systemic temperature changes. Skin circulation, which controls body temperature, is under control of the sympathetic nervous system. A local increase in skin temperature causes a segmental vasodilation of the limb vessels to increase blood flow and dissipate the heat. When the blood flow does not increase adequately in a diseased system, the heat concentrates at the source and quickly burns the skin. Likewise, when a limb with arterial insufficiency is cooled, the vessels cannot dilate to keep the skin warm, thus leading to frostbite.

Many of the aforementioned factors commonly coexist with vascular pathology and with other factors not mentioned, such as poor hygiene. Although vascular diseases and factors related to wound etiology are discussed individually, it is probable that few wounds have only one cause. The clinician managing the patient must assess the many factors that may cause wounds and prolong or prevent healing. Consider the example that follows. A patient with a history of alcohol-related malnutrition, diabetes, smoking, and bilateral arteriosclerosis obliterans arrived at an emergency room with three gangrenous toes and a deep ischemic ulcer on the lateral malleolus of the right leg. The opposite limb was ulcer free on admission but developed a deep pressure sore on the heel within 48 hours of admission. The patient ultimately had a right below-knee amputation but, with meticulous limb protection, nutrition correction, and wound care, the left heel ulcer healed. This type of patient presents a special challenge to the clinician.

CLINICAL SIGNS AND SYMPTOMS

Wounds of the lower extremity can usually be categorized into one of three groups: arterial, venous, or neurotrophic, according to the principal underlying pathology. The relatively infrequent wound that does not fit into one of these groups is associated with a wide range of medical problems. Careful clinical inspection is usually enough to classify a wound into one of the three groups. A complete medical examination and history are needed to elucidate all factors related to wound development. Special diagnostic procedures such as angiography or Doppler ultrasound studies are often needed for a precise diagnosis.

Wounds related to arterial insufficiency have distinct characteristics. They are usually located on the toes, interdigital spaces, foot, or lateral malleolus (Fig. 10–3). Ischemic ulcers can be very deep with exposed tendons. Because capillaries are a principal component of granulation tissue, the base of an ischemic ulcer is probably

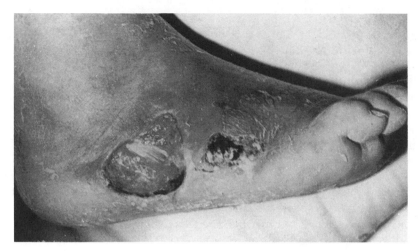

FIGURE 10–3. Ulcerations secondary to arterial insufficiency.

necrotic, lacking granulation tissue. The border of an ischemic ulcer lacks epithelium and often has rough, steep edges. Black, gangrenous skin may surround or be adjacent to the ulcer. Ischemic wounds are usually painful. Gangrene of the toes or foot is easily recognized as dark mummified tissue often with a distinct line of demarcation between viable and necrotic tissue. Ischemic wounds are preceded by symptoms of arterial insufficiency, decreased pulses, intermittent claudication, pallor on elevation, rubor on dependency, slow nail growth, and atrophic skin.[2,11]

Venous ulcers have characteristics related to venous obstruction—namely, pigmentation, liposclerosis, and edema. Pigmentation is produced by hemosiderin deposits when fragile venules are ruptured.[11] Liposclerosis is recognized as the thick, tender, hard skin and subcutaneous tissue. Venous ulcers typically occur on the medial side of the ankle but may extend up, down, or around the entire lower leg. The size of venous ulcers varies greatly. The fascia and deep structures are not usually exposed. The base of the wounds may have a covering of fibrous debris, but the ulcers usually have a firm bed of granulation tissue. The borders of venous ulcers are flat, sloping into a shallow crater. Epithelium can be seen at the borders during the healing process. A large amount of fluid seepage occurs and the skin below an ulcer is often wet and eczemic. Venous ulcers, though often painless, can cause pain that is typically less severe than that experienced with arterial ulcers. Venous ulcers tend to develop slowly and can exist for many years—even decades.

Neurotrophic ulcers typically present as deep punched-out ulcers on the plantar surface of the foot. These ulcers are described in detail in Chapter 11.

TREATMENT

From the previous discussion of wound etiology, one can ascertain that a wound is not a disease but rather the manifestation of a disease process. The disease usually progresses silently until the presentation of symptoms late in the process. For a successful outcome, clinical decisions regarding treatment depend on understanding the disease process, factors related to wound development, and the effects of specific interventions.

Local wound care is important but by no means the essential part of wound management. The decisions about what type of dressing, wound cleansing, or topical agents to use are seldom the key determinant of success or failure in treating a wound. Many wounds heal with no treatment or with simple measures such as bed rest. Because of the tendency for wounds to heal, many claims arise regarding the effectiveness of certain dressings, agents, or procedures. Hovde treated a venous ulcer on a patient who repeatedly stated that dog saliva had healing properties because a previous wound of his had healed after being licked by a dog. The account by the patient no doubt was truthful, but a cause-and-effect relationship between the two events is unlikely. Clinicians must avoid making similar claims about treatments of their choosing. Details of local wound care are presented in Chapter 9.

Care of Limb with Wounds Secondary to Ischemia

Conservative management of ischemic wounds consists of local wound care, bed rest, reduction of risk factors, and limb protection. Bed rest is indicated to avoid excessive muscular activity, which causes a redistribution of blood flow from skin and foot circulation to exercising muscle.[37] Bed rest with the head of the bed elevated 5 to 7 degrees produces an increase in oxygen tension and skin temperature in ischemic toes.[14] Tilting the bed too high or hanging the limb while the patient is in a seated position induces leg edema, which should be avoided. Leg elevation decreases blood flow to the foot and should also be discouraged.

Of the risk factors previously identified, that which is most easily identified and eliminated is smoking. All practitioners involved in the care of a patient should actively reinforce the need for the patient to stop smoking. Diabetes mellitus, hypertension, and hyperlipoproteinemia require appropriate medical and dietary management.

The importance of limb protection is often not stressed enough. An ischemic limb with an open wound should be placed in a protective environment equivalent to a cocoon: all resting surfaces should be softly padded. Cotton or lamb's wool can be placed between toes to prevent pressure or moisture accumulation. The ambient temperature should be kept comfortably warm. Skin lotion should be applied to intact dry skin to prevent cracking. Vigorous active exercise should be avoided to maintain optimal skin circulation. Passive movements of the limbs or resting splints may be indicated to preserve joint mobility and soft-tissue length. Patients on bed rest are particularly apt to develop plantarflexion contractures. Any ambulation necessary should not allow pressure on gangrenous or ischemic tissue. A walker, crutches, or other assistive devices may be needed to allow safe ambulation. When the wound is healed, limited walking should begin only with adequate protective footwear, as described in Chapter 11. Careful limb monitoring is required as activity is increased.

A complete review of medications given to patients with ischemic wounds is beyond the scope of this chapter. Medications prescribed include thrombolytic agents, anticoagulants, and vasodilators. The purpose of thrombolytic agents is to lyse obstructive lesions in order to improve blood flow. Anticoagulants, not commonly prescribed, might prevent thrombosis in diseased vessels. Vasodilators are prescribed to increase blood flow. Many of the drugs in these categories are beneficial to patients with ischemic ulcers. However, the types of drugs mentioned have not been shown to have specific enough therapeutic effects on wound healing to warrant further discussion.[14]

Approval was recently given by the Food and Drug Administration (FDA) for the marketing of a therapeutic device that may show promise in the management of

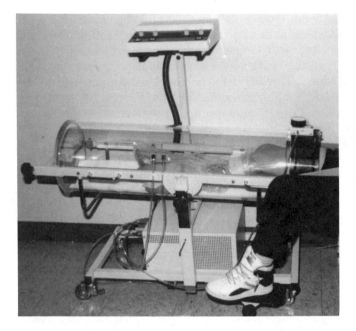

FIGURE 10–4. Patient receiving therapy in the Vasotrain 447 vacuum-compression unit.

wounds in ischemic limbs. This device, the Vasotrain 447* (Fig. 10–4), is designed to provide vacuum-compression therapy (VCT) to the extremities. The VCT consists of a rhythmically applied series of alternating positive- and negative-pressure phases. In the negative-pressure phase, blood vessels are theoretically enlarged and blood is drawn into the extremity. The positive-pressure phase then assists removal of blood from the extremity. The operator may adjust the time and pressure of each phase. Controlled studies with the Vasotrain 447 are currently underway by McCulloch and colleagues at Louisiana State University Medical Center, New Orleans.

Overview of Surgical Procedures

Surgical procedures used on ischemic limbs are generally quite different than those used on limbs with venous disease. In cases of ischemia, the goal of surgery is to improve or restore blood flow past occluded segments of arteries. In cases of venous disease, the goal is usually to restore the effectiveness of the skeletal muscle pump. Debridement and amputation procedures may be performed in cases of either arterial or venous insufficiency. Debridement is discussed in Chapter 9.

Amputation, the surgical removal of a limb or limb segment, is performed when gangrene and infection of necrotic tissue threaten the individual. The goals of amputation are removal of dead tissue to relieve pain and allow primary healing, and construction of a stump suitable for function or fitting of a prosthesis. An amputation can be viewed as a destructive event or failure of therapy. However, a successful amputation is of great benefit to a patient, much more so than prolonging the event with ineffective conservative measures.[38]

---

*Vasotrain 447, Enraf-Nonius, P.O. Box 483, 2600 AL Delft, Holland. Marketed in the United States by Henley International, 10518 Kinghurst, Houston, TX 77099.

Surgical procedures employed in the management of patients with ischemic wounds include arterial reconstruction, endarterectomy, angioplasty, and sympathectomy. Surgical procedures require a detailed diagnosis that usually includes vascular laboratory studies and angiography, in addition to clinical history and physical examination. Doppler studies are described in Chapter 8. Translumbar aortography is a means of visualizing the extent of most lower extremity obstructive lesions. Other special angiographic techniques, involving vasodilators or postischemic reactive hypoxemia, are used when severe obstruction of proximal arteries prevents identification of smaller outflow vessels that may be patent.

Arterial reconstruction is revascularizing a limb by surgically attaching a conduit above and below a diseased portion of an artery, so that blood bypasses the occlusion. The bypass graft material may be knitted Dacron or a vein such as the saphenous or cephalic vein. When veins are used, the valves must be cut or, if left intact, the vein must be removed and the proximal and distal ends reversed to allow blood flow in the correct direction. Vein bypass grafts may be anatomic or extra-anatomic. In the former, the graft conduit parallels the diseased vessel. Two common anatomic procedures are aortofemoral grafts for aorta and iliac disease and femoropopliteal bypass for superficial femoral artery disease.

Endarterectomy is the excision of the occlusive plaque followed by repair of the vessel. Endarterectomy is performed when the diseased segment of the vessel is short. The procedure is usually done on large vessels such as the aorta, iliac artery, and common femoral artery.

Percutaneous transluminal angioplasty is a procedure that is also performed on a short segment of diseased artery. A balloon-tipped catheter is inserted into the artery and pushed to the occluded segment. The balloon is inflated to compress the occlusion and enlarge the lumen of the artery by permanently overstretching the media and adventitia.

Sympathectomy is the excision of lumbar sympathetic ganglia, which results in the loss of vasoconstrictive properties in the artery. Blood flow is increased in the skin and foot but not in muscle with this procedure. Sympathectomy, therefore, is ineffective as a treatment for intermittent claudication. Sympathectomy is reported to enhance healing of small ulcers, minor gangrene, and chronically moist ulcers between the toes, but is ineffective in treating larger gangrenous areas such as the entire toe or foot.[15,38]

Care of Limb Wounds Secondary to Venous Insufficiency

The literature abounds with suggested methods of managing patients with chronic venous ulcerations. As is frequently the case in medicine, the debate centers on the conservative versus the surgical approaches. Because one of the primary purposes of this text is to present contemporary perspectives on conservative management, most of our effort is spent in this area. However, a brief discussion of the other point of view is justified.

Ligation of incompetent calf and ankle perforating veins has been advocated by many as providing good results with patients in controlled studies.[39-41] Others, however, have not found results of such procedures to be as promising[42,43] and have even gone so far as to advise no surgical intervention in such cases.[44] Negus and Friedgood,[45] however, have recently reported improved results following subfascial ligation of all incompetent calf and ankle perforators. In addition, they advocate the ligation and stripping of the saphenous veins when these are shown to be incompetent.

Sclerotherapy has been proposed as another means of treating the venous incompetence that leads to ulceration. This procedure, which involves the injection of a sclerosing agent into the vein, is typically reserved for very small varices that cannot be surgically removed. This procedure was used a great deal in the past and has recently started to regain its popularity as a more cost-efficient means than surgery of dealing with varicose veins.[46]

The conservative management of chronic venous ulceration has historically focused on cleansing of the ulcer in combination with elevation and compression of the extremity. The primary goal of such treatment was to reduce venous hypertension and allow swelling to subside.[34] Various extremity wraps have been designed to control edema. The least effective of such wraps appears to be the standard elastic wraps, which tend to loose elasticity with use and are, in addition, difficult to apply with uniform pressure. Work by Lippmann and Briere[47] revealed that elastic wraps do little if anything to assist the muscle pump mechanism of the calf. Instead, as the muscle contracts the elastic wrap stretches, thus failing to assist the movement of venous blood from the extremity. Rather a pliable, nonstretchable dressing should be used that maintains leg contour during muscle contraction. The effect is to move venous blood out of the extremity. One such wrap, which meets the previously mentioned criteria, is Unna's boot (Fig. 10–5). Marketed under various brand names, such as Medicopaste* and Primer,† the wraps differ only in terms of the additives used in each. There is little in the literature to substantiate the benefits of any of the additives in accelerating wound healing. Instead, the major benefits of these dressings come from their semirigid nature.

Another technique used in controlling edema and breakdown are custom-fitted stockings. "Custom-fitted" is emphasized to draw attention to the fact that commercially produced over-the-counter elastic stockings cannot possibly mold to each individual's leg in such a manner as to give any uniform pressure. One downfall of custom-fitted support stockings, however, is not in the stockings but in the practitioner's tendency

---

*Medicopaste, Graham-Field, Inc., Hauppauge, NY 11788.
†Primer, Glenwood, Inc., Tenafly, NJ 07670.

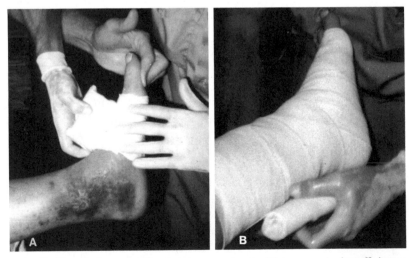

FIGURE 10–5. Unna's boot application to a patient with a avenous insufficiency ulceration. Application begins distally (*A*) and proceeds in a spiral fashion up the lower leg (*B*).

to fit the patient for such garments while the extremity is enlarged. Doing so only ensures that the limb will retain its present size.

Hydrotherapy is another form of intervention used a great deal in the treatment of venous ulcerations. Hydrotherapy in wound care got its start from the use of full body immersion tanks with air turbines as an aid in the debridement of devitalized tissue from burn patients. The beneficial effects of the treatment were logically (and often illogically) applied to the treatment of various other types of wounds. This area has grown so rapidly that the primary use of hydrotherapy equipment is in wound care.

The primary effects of hydrotherapy are tissue hydration, increased circulation, and debridement of devitalized tissues. If one pauses for a moment and examines the findings that exist in most venous ulcerations, one sees that the patient is primarily suffering from a venous hypertension situation. Certainly, increasing blood supply to an area that already cannot handle the blood volume present would not be desirable. Second, placing an extremity into a dependent position with warm water for a standard 20-minute treatment session would very likely increase the dependent edema. In addition, tissue hydration is seldom lacking in venous ulcerations, and the swirling effects of the water have essentially no effect in debriding the dense, firmly adherent fibrotic tissue seen in most chronic venous ulcerations. The question, then, is: Why do practitioners continue to treat patients in this manner? Routine and ritual are difficult to change.

Earlier in this chapter, the theoretic framework of Browse and Burnand[30] was presented. They noted that providing increased external pressure is one means of lowering the venous hypertension and, it is hoped, preventing further liposclerosis. We concur with this approach and advocate external compression as a major component of management in patients with chronic venous ulceration.

The treatment proposed in most cases of chronic venous ulceration begins with a gentle cleansing of the leg and ulceration via spray lavage or a very brief (less than 5-minute) soaking and cleansing in tepid water. This phase is followed by compression pumping of the entire lower extremity with an intermittent compression pump. To prevent soiling of the compression sleeve, the extremity is first placed in a plastic bag and the sleeve is applied. The pump is usually set to a pressure less than diastolic, at a ratio of 90 seconds on to 30 seconds off. Treatment time is variable but usually lasts about 1 hour. Following compression, the extremity is wrapped in a nonelastic dressing such as Unna's boot to keep the limb reduced to the post-treatment size until the next clinic visit. Girth or volume measurements are taken at periodic intervals until the limb size has plateaued. At this point, custom-fitted stockings should be ordered. As previously mentioned, if patients are fitted with stockings before the edema resolves, the limb will, at best, remain the same size. This particular method of treatment was used in a case study performed in 1981. The patient had a large ulceration that measured 14 by 7 cm and had been present for 3 years, despite various forms of therapy. Using compression therapy as the sole treatment modality, the ulcer healed completely in 3 months.[48] Controlled studies on this form of therapy are currently underway.

CLINICAL DECISION MAKING

In this section, several treatment scenarios are given that correlate with the patient examples presented in Chapter 7 on patient examination. Read each of the scenarios, and answer the questions that follow. When finished, check your answers against those provided.

Case A

Mr. Jones was suffering from arterial insufficiency and as a result had developed an ischemic ulceration. Please answer the following questions related to how you would manage this case.

1. Should intermittent compression be used in healing this ulcer?
2. To prevent any further swelling from occurring, should you instruct the patient to elevate his leg while in bed?
3. Should you keep the patient in a warm environment?
4. Would this patient benefit from some form of compression stocking?
5. Should the patient be told to elevate the head of his bed?

Solution

1. As a general rule, intermittent compression would not be indicated in the presence of arterial insufficiency. The poor arterial functioning could become further compromised with any form of external support. At times, these types of patients also have edema in the lower extremities. We have successfully treated such patients with low-pressure intermittent compression (less than 40 mmHg) with the extremity in a dependent position.
2. Swelling is minimal in this case and is probably not of major consequence. Elevating the legs, in the presence of arterial insufficiency, would likely lead to rest pain from claudication.
3. Placing the patient in a generalized warm environment is suggested. Such an environment encourages a reflex vasodilation and can possibly increase arterial flow in the compromised extremity. In the past, infrared bakers were used for this purpose. This practice is discouraged because many of these patients have decreased sensation and a burn could result.
4. As previously addressed, any form of external compression could further compromise circulation and should be discouraged.
5. Some relief from claudication pain is frequently obtained when the lower extremities are placed in the dependent position. This position can be achieved by placing the head of the bed on shock blocks, thus putting the legs below the level of the heart.

Case B

Mr. Conrad has chronic venous insufficiency, and his ulcer is secondary to the venous incompetence. Please answer the following questions concerning how the case should be managed.

1. Should your treatment consist of whirlpool for debridement followed by wet-to-dry saline dressings and intermittent compression?
2. If the patient did receive compression pumping, you could dress him afterward with either an Unna's boot or an elastic wrap. Would these approaches be equally good in controlling edema?
3. Should the patient be discouraged from doing any type of walking exercise until the ulcer has healed?

4. Would this patient benefit from being placed on crutches, non–weight-bearing on the right?

Solution

1. As has been discussed, intermittent compression may be of value in treating ulcers secondary to venous insufficiency. Whirlpool, however, has little to offer this type of patient and may even encourage more swelling. If used for its cleansing effect, the treatment should be brief (less than 5 minutes). Likewise, wet-to-dry dressings are of questionable benefit. There is a great tendency to overuse this type of dressing. Wet-to-dry dressings are primarily used for debridement in cases when there is necrotic tissue that sticks to the dry dressing and is debrided as the dressing is removed. Most venous ulcerations are denser than other wounds and do not debride easily. Experience has shown that the body will take care of healing the wound if the edema is controlled.

2. As discussed, for the muscle pump to effectively move fluid through the incompetent venous system, the calf needs to remain fairly constant in size as the muscles contract. Elastic wraps tend to stretch, in addition to applying uneven pressure. Unna's boots, on the other hand, provide a semirigid support to the leg and prevent further swelling from occurring.

3. Exercise is not contraindicated in patients who have venous insufficiency. If the patient should exercise, two points need to be emphasized. Support garments should be worn while exercising, and whenever possible the lower extremities should be elevated after exercise until the heart rate returns to normal. Both techniques minimize edema.

4. As identified in the response to the previous question, exercise is not contraindicated if properly performed. Placing a patient with venous insufficiency into a non–weight-bearing situation serves only to encourage dependent edema. Such management of the condition is strongly discouraged.

SUMMARY

This chapter has provided a review of the structure and function of the vascular system and has presented a discussion of how disease processes affecting this system result in the development of dermal wounds. The most commonly occurring problems were discussed, with greatest emphasis placed on those conditions most likely to cause the development of ulcerations of the lower extremities. Clinical signs and symptoms that help to differentiate wounds of varying etiologies were given.

Treatment methods outlined in this chapter emphasized the clinical decision-making approach and stressed the importance of addressing the cause of the lesion in any and all therapies that may be instituted. This strategy was carried through in the clinical decision-making examples.

The chronic nature of vascular wounds means that many people may be involved in caring for a given wound. The list of care takers may include physicians, nurses, physical therapists, the patient, attendants, and family members. The possibility of conflicting efforts by different care takers is great. Clear communication between practitioners is essential to create an effective team approach. The key to coordinated wound management is education of the patient or family members when the patient is unable to participate in his or her own care. When wound management is successful, the patient must not be led to think that the disease has been cured. The vascular disease remains and the right combination of causative factors might easily occur and a wound develop again. Appropriate care of the limb must continue.

REFERENCES

1. Fairbairn, JF, II: Clinical manifestations of peripheral vascular disease. In Fairbairn, JF, II, Juergens, JL, and Spittel, JA: Peripheral Vascular Diseases, ed 4. WB Saunders, Philadelphia, 1972, p 20.
2. Barnes, RW: The arterial system. In Sabiston, DC (ed): Essentials of Surgery. WB Saunders, Philadelphia, 1987, p 857.
3. Callan, MJ, et al: Arterial disease in chronic leg ulceration. An underestimated hazard? Br Med J 294:929–931, 1987.
4. Guyton, AC: Textbook of Medical Physiology, ed 7. WB Saunders, Philadelphia, 1986, p 230.
5. Lie, JT and Brown, AL: Normal structure of the vascular system and general reactive changes of the arteries. In Fairbairn, JF, II, Juergens, JL, and Spittel, JA: Peripheral Vascular Diseases, ed 4. WB Saunders, Philadelphia, 1972, pp 45–62.
6. Grollman, S: The Human Body, Its Structure and Physiology, ed 2. Macmillan, New York, 1969, pp 191–196.
7. Vander, AJ, Sherman, JH, and Luciano, DS: Human Physiology, The Mechanism of Body Function. McGraw-Hill, New York, 1975, pp 246–267.
8. Shepherd, JJ: The physiology of blood flow in the limbs. In Fairbairn, JF, II, Juergens, JL, and Spittel, JA: Peripheral Vascular Diseases, ed 4. WB Saunders, Philadelphia, 1972, pp 63–77.
9. Lofgren, EP: Chronic venous insufficiency. In Spittell, JA (ed): Clinical Vascular Disease. FA Davis, Philadelphia, 1983, p 135.
10. Robbins, SL and Angell, M: Basic Pathology. WB Saunders, Philadelphia, 1976, p 265.
11. Menendez, CV: Ulcers of the Leg. Charles C Thomas, Springfield, IL, 1965, p 12.
12. Petersdorf, RG, et al: Harrison's Principles of Internal Medicine. McGraw-Hill, New York, 1983, p 1465.
13. de Wolfe, VG: Chronic occlusive arterial disease. In Spittell, JA (ed): Clinical Vascular Diseases. FA Davis, Philadelphia, 1983, pp 15–35.
14. Coffman, JD: Principles of conservative treatment of occlusive arterial disease. In Spittell, JA (ed): Clinical Vascular Disease. FA Davis, Philadelphia, 1983, pp 2–14.
15. Hollier, LH: Principles and techniques of surgical treatment of occlusive arterial disease of the lower extremities. In Spittell, JA (ed): Clinical Vascular Diseases. FA Davis, Philadelphia, 1983, pp 37–48.
16. Huntsman, RG: Sickle Cell Anemia and Thalassemia. Canadian Sickle Cell Society, St John's, Newfoundland, Canada, 1987.
17. Trainor, F, et al: Venous ulcer in a sickle cell patient. J Am Podiatr Med Assoc 76:12, 692–694, 1986.
18. Ludbrook, J and Jamieson, GG: Disorders of the systemic veins. In Sabiston, DC (ed): Textbook of Surgery. WB Saunders, Philadelphia, 1977, p 1826.
19. Regan, B and Folse, R: Lower limb venous dynamics in normal persons and children with varicose veins. Surg Gynecol Obstet 132:15, 1971.
20. Bauer, G: Insufficiens av vena femoralis-poplitea. Svensk Lakartidning 44:1757–1769, 1947.
21. Linton, RR and Hardy, IB: Postthrombotic syndrome of the lower extremity. Surgery 24:452, 1948.
22. DeTakats, G: Thrombo-embolism J Int Chir 8:903–921, 1948.
23. Arnoldi, CC and Linderholm, H: On the pathogenesis of the venous leg ulcer. Acta Chir Scand 134:427–440, 1968.
24. Homans, J: The aetiology and treatment of varicose ulcers of the leg. Surg Gynecol Obstet 24:300–311, 1917.
25. DeTakats, G, et al: The impairment of the circulation in the varicose extremity. Arch Surg 18:671, 1929.
26. Blalock, A: Oxygen content of blood in patients with varicose veins. Arch Surg 19:898–905, 1929.
27. Schanzer, H and Peirce, EC: A rational approach to surgery of the chronic venous stasis syndrome. Ann Surg 195:25–29, 1982.
28. Piulacks, P and Vidal Barraquer, F: Pathogenic study of varicose veins. Angiology 4:59–100, 1953.
29. Lindemayr, W, et al: Arteriovenous shunts in primary varicoses: A critical essay. Surgery 6:9–14, 1972.
30. Browse, NL and Burnand, KG: The cause of venous ulceration. Lancet 2:243–245, 1982.
31. Landis, EM: Microinjection studies of capillary blood pressure in human skin. Heart 15:404–453, 1930.
32. Browse, NL and Burnand, KG: The postphlebitic syndrome: A new look. In Bergan, JJ and Yao, JST (eds): Venous Problems. Year Book Medical Publishers, Chicago, 1978, pp 395–404.
33. Browse, NL: Venous ulceration. Br Med J 286:1920–1922, 1983.
34. Skillman, JJ: Venous leg ulcers. In Menaker, L (ed): Biologic Basis of Wound Healing. Harper and Row, Hagerstown, MD, 1975, pp 113–120.
35. Klein, P: Vitamin A acid and wound healing. Acta Dermatol (Suppl)74:171–173, 1975.
36. Weiss, AV and Fairbairn, JF, II: Trauma, ischemic limbs and amputation. Postgrad Med 43:111–115, 1968.

37. Abramson, DI: Physiological basis for the use of physical agents in peripheral vascular disease. Arch Phys Med Rehabil 46:216–244, 1965.
38. Way, LW: Current Surgical Diagnosis and Treatment. Lange Medical Publications, Los Altos, CA, 1985, pp 680–703.
39. Bertelsen, S and Gammelgaard, A: Surgical treatment of post-thrombotic leg ulcers. J Cardiovasc Surg 6:452, 1965.
40. Hansson, LD: Venous ulcers of the lower limb. Acta Chir Scand 128:269–277, 1964.
41. Field, P and VanBoxall, P: The role of the Linton flap procedure in the management of stasis dermatitis and ulceration in the lower limb. Surgery 70:920–926, 1971.
42. Recek, E: A critical appraisal of the role of ankle perforators for the genesis of venous ulcers in the lower leg. J Cardiovasc Surg 12:45, 1971.
43. Burnand, KG, et al: Relation between postphlebitic changes in the deep veins and results of surgical treatment of venous ulcers. Lancet 1:936–938, 1976.
44. Kiely, PE: Diagnosis of deep vein incompetence and the avoidance of surgical interference in these patients. Personal communication as reported in Negus, D and Friedgood, A: The effective management of venous ulceration. Br J Surg 70:623–627, 1983.
45. Negus, D and Friedgood, A: The effective management of venous ulceration. Br J Surg 70:623–627, 1983.
46. Lofgren, EP: Chronic venous insufficiency. In Spittell, JA (ed): Clinical Vascular Disease. FA Davis, Philadelphia, 1983, p 141.
47. Lippman, HI and Briere, JP: Physical basis of external supports in chronic venous insufficiency. Arch Phys Med 52:555–559, 1971.
48. McCulloch, JM: Intermittent compression for the treatment of a chronic stasis ulceration. Phys Ther 61:10, 1452–1453, 1981.

CHAPTER 11

Treatment of Wounds Caused by Pressure and Insensitivity

George Hampton, M.P.H., P.T.
James Birke, M.S., P.T.

Early descriptions suggested vascular deficiency as the primary etiologic factor in plantar ulceration in patients with Hansen's disease, diabetes mellitus, and other neuropathies.[1] Recent laboratory and clinical studies, however, have identified mechanical forces as the primary cause of tissue necrosis in these patients.[2-4]

Clinical observation confirms that patients with diminished or absent sensation are at an increased risk of pressure-induced wounds. Patients with sensory neuropathy may be grouped into two general categories: (1) those with central nervous system injury or disease who are either nonambulatory or limited in ambulation and (2) those with normal or moderately limited motor function who are ambulatory. The first group includes patients with spinal cord injury, tumors, and cerebrovascular accidents. Prevention and treatment of pressure sores in these patients is based on frequent pressure relief and materials or devices that minimize pressure and irritation at the interface between skin and the supporting surface. In spite of the understanding of etiology and treatment of pressure sores in spinal cord injury patients, pressure sores still remain one of the most common complications in patients treated in the United States Regional Spinal Cord Injury Centers.[5,6] The second group includes patients with diabetes mellitus;[7] spina bifida; syringomyelia; sensory neuropathy of traumatic, toxic, or familial origin; and Hansen's disease.

This chapter addresses the management of soft-tissue wounds in ambulatory patients with sensory neuropathy. However, the rationale and methods described here have some direct application to more disabled patients who are confined to a wheelchair or bed. Many of the techniques developed for treatment and prevention of hand and foot ulcers of Hansen's disease patients are also applicable in the management of other neuropathies.[3,8,9] A clear understanding of the effects of mechanical forces on insensitive tissues; evaluation and education of the patient at risk for mechanical or thermal injury; evaluation and treatment of pressure ulcers; and prevention of recurrent ulceration are emphasized.

MECHANICAL FORCES

The three primary factors in mechanical force injury are pressure, time, and direction of forces. Pressure is determined by dividing force by the area over which the force is applied. Thus, a relatively low force applied to a small area may result in high pressure. The amount of time that pressure is applied to tissues is equally important. In 1959, Kosiak[10] demonstrated in an animal experiment that relatively high pressure (500 mmHg) applied for 2 hours would cause tissue ulceration. In contrast, a pressure of 150 mmHg took 9 hours to produce ulceration. Figure 11–1 shows the time-pressure relationship documented by Kosiak. The direction of applied force determines whether the resulting tissue stress will be in the form of compression, tension, or shear.[11,12] *Normal* forces are identified as compression or tension forces applied perpendicular to the tissue surface, and *shear* is described as a force applied parallel or oblique to the surface[11,12] (Fig. 11–2).

A combination of normal compressive forces and shear forces occurs frequently and is responsible for much of the soft-tissue injury in patients with sensory neuropathy. Two examples will illustrate this point. First, the quadriplegic patient seated in a wheelchair for 2 hours gradually slides forward in the wheelchair seat and experiences skin breakdown over the sacrum. In the second example, a patient with lower extremity sensory deficit wears a new pair of shoes for 30 minutes and develops blisters on both heels due to friction where the top of the shoes rubbed his heels with each step.

Brand[9] states that there are five types of injury to which sensory neuropathy patients are susceptible:

1. "Continuous pressure causing necrosis from lack of blood supply;
2. Concentrated high pressure, causing cutting or crushing by mechanical violence;
3. Heat or cold, causing burning or frostbite;
4. Repetitive mechanical stress of moderate degree causing inflammation and autolysis; and
5. Pressure on infected tissues resulting in the spread of infection."

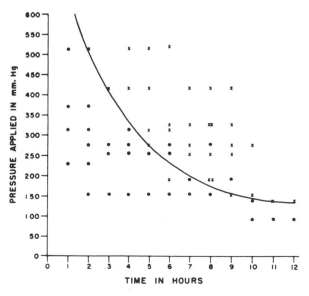

FIGURE 11–1. Pressure–time relationship noted in 62 separate experiments on 16 dogs: x = ulceration; · = no ulceration (From Kosiak,[10] p. 66, with permission).

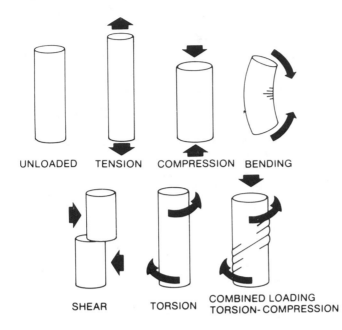

UNLOADED   TENSION   COMPRESSION   BENDING

SHEAR   TORSION   COMBINED LOADING TORSION-COMPRESSION

FIGURE 11–2. Normal verses shear stress (From Soderberg,[11] p. 68, with permission).

Repetitive stress of moderate degree is the most subtle form of injury to insensitive tissues. The person with normal sensation will experience discomfort or pain after a period of exposure to low-level repetitive stress and will either stop the activity or shift the stress to another area. The uninformed patient with sensory deficit will continue the activity in exactly the same way until the number of repetitions exceeds tissue tolerance and skin breakdown occurs. This clinical observation has prompted research on denervated animals to determine tolerance levels to repetitive stress and to identify methods of detecting early signs of tissue damage.[13,14]

From data on the study of rat footpad responses to controlled repetitive stress, Beach and Thompson,[13] report:

1. Denervated tissue may tolerate the same level of stress as normal tissue, but tissue damage occurs with fewer repetitions.
2. Inflammatory changes persist for periods as long as 1 week after repetitive stress sessions when early autolysis of tissues occurs.
3. If repetitive stress is resumed while tissues are still inflamed, necrosis will occur.
4. Callus formation occurs in response to repetitive stimuli and protects the foot if the callus is not excessively thick.

FORCE-RELATED RISK FACTORS

Ambulatory patients with sensory neuropathy experience varying degrees of risk relative to the extent of sensory loss, vascular deficiency, loss of skin resiliency, decreased thickness of weight-bearing soft tissues, scar formation over weight-bearing tissues, skeletal deformity, and decreased area of weight-bearing surface.[1,2,7–9] With the presence of one or more of these factors, tissue tolerance is decreased and the pressure or shear stress is usually increased.

Studies have shown that loss of sensation and abnormal pressure are the primary cause of plantar ulcerations in patients with diabetes mellitus, leprosy, and other diseases.[15-17] The level of sensory loss necessary to predispose a patient to foot injury has been referred to as loss of protective sensation. A precise method for determining loss of sensation is not possible. Nylon sensory filaments, however, have been shown to be acceptable tools for clinically identifying patients at risk of plantar ulceration.[8] Static and dynamic forces acting on the sole of the foot during ambulation have been analyzed with pressure transducers attached to weight-bearing surfaces[18] and with the subject walking barefoot across a force plate.[15,19-21] These studies reveal a high correlation between the site of plantar ulceration in diabetic patients and the sites of maximal force load on the sole of the foot. The most common sites of plantar ulceration in patients with diabetes mellitus and Hansen's disease are the first metatarsal head and great toe.[8] A study of 21 ambulatory patients with diagnoses of spina bifida, spinal cord tumor, and incomplete paraplegia revealed a different pattern, with the heel being the most common site of ulceration.[17] In this study, the most common foot deformities were prominent calcaneus, calcaneocavus, calcaneovalgus, and heel valgus.

The concentration of forces on the insensitive foot with normal alignment and surface area is essentially the same as that observed for normal subjects. Risk of ulceration is related to ischemia from continuous unrelieved pressure or prolonged repetitive stress that exceeds tissue tolerance. When foot deformity occurs, the distribution of forces changes and the sites likely to ulcerate will change accordingly. For example, in equinovarus the most likely site for ulceration is the fifth metatarsal head. In hallux valgus, the dynamic force on the big toe at push-off is reduced and peak load on the first metatarsal head is increased, with an increased risk of ulceration at that site.

FOOT SCREENING EXAMINATION

Timely foot screening and risk classification are the most important components of a prevention program. The foot screening examination should not be excessively time consuming, yet it should provide sufficient data to evaluate the presence of or history of ulceration, loss of sensation, areas of high pressure, and predisposing factors to injury such as foot deformities and improper footwear.[22] A risk classification scheme identifies those patients who are most likely to develop plantar ulceration and who, therefore, are most likely to benefit from protective footwear and patient education. Screening and identification of risk can provide an overall savings to the patient population.

A foot screening form (Fig. 11-3) provides a basis for easy recording of clinical findings and is readily adaptable to a computer data system. The areas selected for testing in the foot screen provide information directly related to assessing the patient's risk of ulceration.

Subjective Examination

Patients are asked if they have ever had an open sore on the bottom of their feet. Nonplantar lesions are not typical of neuropathic ulceration. If a positive history is found, the specific sites of ulceration will direct the clinician to the areas of the foot at highest risk of injury and in most need of protection. Patients are also asked if they have felt a recent loss of strength or sensation in the foot. This finding may alert the clinician to patients with unstable disease and in need of more frequent follow-up.

DATE _____

COMPLAINTS _____

Sensation and strength since last seen: Worse _____   Same_____   Improved _____
History of ulcer on the bottom of the feet: Yes _____ No_____ If yes, location__

STRENGTH

RIGHT		LEFT
	Anterior Tibialis	
	Extensor Hallucis Longus	
	Flexor Hallucis Longus	
	Posterior Tibialis	
	Peroneus Longus	
	Gastroc/Soleus	

	Intrinsics (S/W/A)	

SKIN/PLANTAR SENSATION

SENSORY LEVEL
1 = 01 g(4.17, Mean + SD for normals)
2 = 10 g(5.07, Protective sensation)
3 = 75 g(6.10, Loss of protective sensation)
4 = No perception of 75 g

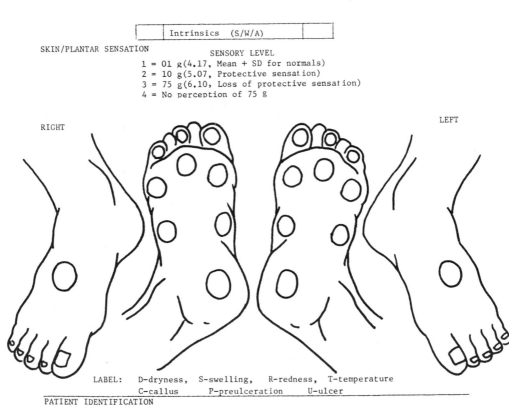

RIGHT   LEFT

LABEL: D-dryness,   S-swelling,   R-redness,   T-temperature
         C-callus   P-preulceration   U-ulcer

PATIENT IDENTIFICATION

FIGURE 11–3. Foot screening form.

Strength

The strength of the foot's intrinsic and extrinsic muscles is assessed. Weakness within the foot results in deformities secondary to motor imbalance. These deformities result in an uneven pressure distribution on the foot. Intrinsic weakness predisposes the foot to cavus and claw toe deformities. Peroneal nerve extrinsic weakness may result in equino-adducto-varus deformities. Tibial nerve extrinsic weakness may result in calcaneo-abducto-valgus deformities.

DEFORMITIES

RIGHT	LEFT	
____	____	Hammer/Claw Toes _____.
____	____	Bony Prominence _____.
____	____	Drop Foot _____.
____	____	Charcot Foot _____.
____	____	Hallux Limitus _____.
____	____	Rear or Forefoot Varus_____.
____	____	Plantar Flexed First Ray_____.
____	____	Equinus _____.
____	____	Partial Foot Amputation/Absorption_____.

ISCHEMIC INDEX

____	____	Ankle/Arm
____	____	Foot/Arm

FOOTWEAR

Type: Standard____Special____Describe_____.

Adequate____Inadequate____Describe_____.

ASSESSMENT

____ 0 No protective Sensory Loss

____ 1 Loss of Protective Sensation(no deformity or plantar ulcer history).

____ 2 Loss of Protective Sensation and Deformity (no plantar ulcer history).

____ 3 History of Plantar Ulcer.

PLAN

____ Patient Education

____ Footwear_____.

____ Therapeutic Exercises_____.

____ Nerve Conduction Studies

____ Referral (Medical, surgical, orthotic, x-ray.)

____ Follow-Up _____.

Comments _____

_____

_____.

_____

Signature

7/88

FIGURE 11–3. *Continued*

Sensation

The bioesthesiometer and Semmes-Weinstein filaments have been shown to be sensitive and objective methods in measuring sensory deficit in the foot.[20,23] Of the two methods, the Semmes-Weinstein nylon filaments are easier to administer and result in fewer false-negative results.[24] Sensation is evaluated using nylon monofilaments cali-

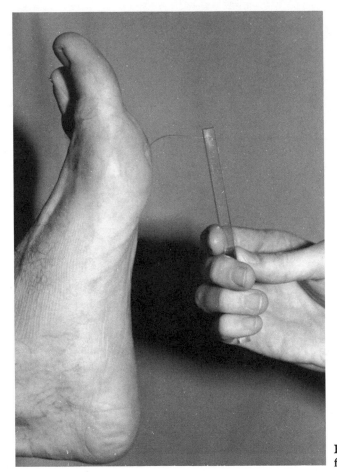

FIGURE 11–4. Nylon sensory filament.

brated at 1-gram, 10-gram, and 75-gram bending forces as described by Birke and Sims.[8] The 1-gram filament is the threshold for normal sensation, and the 10-gram filament is the threshold level for protective sensation. Loss of protective sensation exists when a patient is unable to feel the 10-gram filament. Selected sites of the foot are tested (as illustrated on the screening form) to obtain a general sensory profile. The filaments are applied perpendicular to the skin until the filament bends (Fig. 11–4). The patient, with eyes closed, reports "yes" when touch is perceived. Repeated applications are made in a random pattern.[25] If the patient repeatedly responds inappropriately, an area localization procedure should be followed.[26]

Skin Inspection

The skin is inspected for areas of high pressure. Such areas may be identified as callus, preulceration, or ulceration. Callus must be trimmed before an underlying ulceration can be ruled out. A *preulceration* is an injured area of tissue that has not yet formed an open ulceration. Preulcerations are characterized by ecchymosis or hematoma.[27] Other skin problems to be noted include dryness, discoloration, warmth, and swelling.

Dryness predisposes the foot to cracking and fissuring. In the neuropathic foot, dryness results from a loss of function of the autonomic nervous system. Redness, warmth, or swelling are signs of tissue inflammation. Inflammation may be due to soft-tissue stress, infection, or underlying neuropathic fracture.[28] A neuropathic fracture can be confirmed only by radiologic examination, since patients with neuropathic fractures do not usually complain of pain. Neuropathic fractures are serious complications that can rapidly progress to serious unstable foot deformities. Localized inflammation that persists for 30 to 60 minutes indicates that the skin and subcutaneous tissues are being subjected to potentially damaging stresses.[29,30] The examiner's hands can usually detect a temperature difference of 2°C or greater, but for more accurate or prospective assessment, a skin thermistor, infrared radiometer, or infrared thermography should be used.[31]

Deformities

There are several foot deformities that directly result in a maldistribution of pressures on the foot. Claw toes have been shown to increase the stress on the metatarsal heads, as well as the dorsal aspect of the proximal interphalangeal joint. Hammer and mallet toes may result in greater pressures on the distal end of the toes. Bony exostoses or prominences are associated with high stress. Commonly the metatarsal head may be a bony prominence as a result of a plantarflexed ray. In the midfoot, bony prominence is often secondary to deformity associated with a neuropathic fracture. Hallux limitus, or limitation of first metatarsophalangeal joint extension, is believed to cause great toe ulceration in the neuropathic foot by increasing the pressure on the plantar surface of the toe during the propulsive phase of gait.[32] Forty-five degrees of extension are considered necessary for normal gait.[33,34] Equinus, or limitation of ankle dorsiflexion, similarly increases the risk of ulceration on the insensitive foot as a result of early and increased stress on the forefoot during walking.[35] Normal gait requires about 10 degrees of ankle dorsiflexion.[34,36] Footdrop associated with peroneal nerve paralysis results in the foot slapping the ground in a position of equino-adducto-varus. This position develops increased stress and potential ulceration on the lateral border of the foot. Forefoot and rearfoot varus results in abnormal forefoot pressures.[35,37] The area of localization of stress on the forefoot is relative to the degree of compensatory motion of the subtalar and midfoot joints. For example, a compensated rearfoot and forefoot varus results in a pronated foot with increased medial forefoot pressures; an uncompensated varus may result in a supinated foot with increased lateral forefoot pressures. Plantarflexed first ray results in increased pressures on the first metatarsal head. Charcot's foot (neuropathic fractures) may result in a variety of deformities, but the most classic is the rocker-bottom foot.[22] This deformity is the result of midfoot collapse and predisposes the midfoot to high pressures (Fig. 11–5). Absorption or partial amputation of the foot creates a greater pressure load on the remaining foot. Amputation of the first toe especially results in shift of pressure to the remaining first ray, referred to as a transfer lesion.[22]

Foot/Brachial Ischemic Index

An ischemic index may be used as one means of evaluating the vascular status of the foot. A Doppler ultrasound device is used to determine the ratio between systolic blood pressure (SBP) in the foot compared with that in the arm (Fig. 11–6). An ischemic

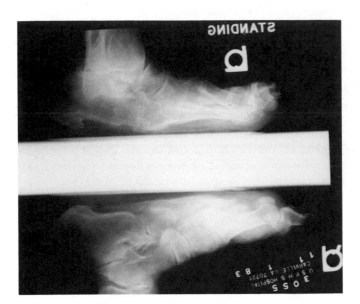

FIGURE 11–5. Neuropathic fracture involving the talus on the left (top).

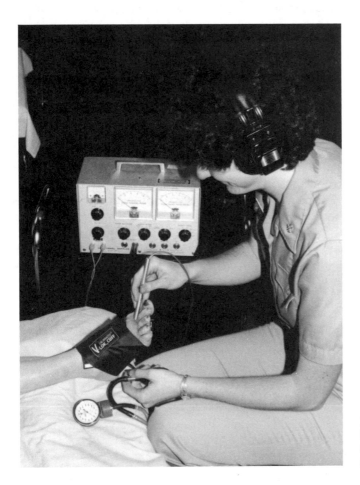

FIGURE 11–6. Systolic blood pressure determination in the foot using a Doppler instrument.

index greater than 0.44 (Foot SBP/Arm SBP) has been shown to be useful in determining the potential for healing the ulcerated diabetic foot.[38,39] For more information on the Doppler examination, the reader is referred to Chapter 8.

Footwear

The footwear of the patient should be assessed for evidence of abnormal wear and inadequate fit. Proper shoe fit should be checked with the patient sitting and standing.[40] For footwear to fit properly, (1) shoe length should exceed foot length by approximately $\frac{1}{2}$ inch, (2) the toebox must be deep enough to avoid pressure on the dorsum of the toes and wide enough to avoid medial and lateral pressure on metatarsal heads; (3) the heel counter should fit snugly and be stiff enough to prevent excessive calcaneal movement during weight bearing, and (4) heel height greater than 2 inches should be avoided as it shifts body weight forward and increases pressure on the metatarsal heads and toes.[40] Leather is considered to be the best material for the upper parts of the shoe because it has some resiliency and adapts to the shape of the foot. Rubber or crepe soles are preferred over leather soles because they afford better accommodation to walking stresses. Heels and soles should be glued or stitched (rather than nailed) to the shoe to eliminate the risk of injury from a protruding nail.

MANAGEMENT OF PLANTAR ULCERS

Prevention of Plantar Ulcers

A management plan may be based on the risk classification scheme (Table 11–1). The plan should include patient education, special footwear, and appropriate medical, surgical, and radiologic referrals.

PATIENT EDUCATION

Patients with loss of protective sensation (Categories 1, 2, and 3) should be taught techniques for foot care,[41] foot inspection,[42] and appropriate footwear.[43]

Foot Care. To effectively hydrate the skin, the feet should be soaked daily for 10 to 20 minutes in lukewarm water.[44] The feet are then partially dried (skin should remain moist to the touch) and petroleum jelly, mineral oil, or oil-based lotion is applied to trap moisture in the skin. Nails should be trimmed straight across. A soft toothbrush or similar device can be used to clean beneath toenails. Calluses should be kept level with the surrounding skin by using an emery board or callus file.[45] The patient should realize that callus protects the underlying tissues from shear stress unless the callus becomes hard and elevated above the adjacent uncallused skin. Hypertrophic nails or heavy calluses should be referred to a podiatrist or other experienced clinician.

TABLE 11–1. Classification for Risk of Plantar Ulceration

Category 0 — No loss of protective sensation
Category 1 — Loss of protective sensation (no deformity or history of plantar ulcer)
Category 2 — Loss of protective sensation and deformity (no history of plantar ulcer)
Category 3 — History of plantar ulceration

Foot Inspection and Injury Prevention. Foot inspection must become part of the patient's daily routine whenever the shoes are removed. The feet must be examined for inflammation, swelling, redness, blisters, hematomas, or wounds. Before donning shoes, socks should be inspected for wrinkles, bunching at the toes, or holes. Shoe inspection includes examining the inside for foreign objects; checking the insole for wrinkling or tears; and looking at the outer sole and heel for sharp objects that may have penetrated the shoe. For injury prevention, patients must be constantly aware of their level of activity. Walking 2 miles a day may be safe for a particular patient, but 3 or 4 miles a day may precipitate tissue injury. (The author is reminded of a young Hansen's disease patient who had been maintained ulcer free in shoes with custom insoles for 2 years. At a neighborhood party, he played in a pick-up basketball game for 20 minutes. The shear stresses from sudden stops and jumping avulsed scar tissue over the metatarsal heads of both feet and necessitated 3 weeks in a cast to provide sufficient healing for him to resume limited ambulation.)

Walking barefoot should be avoided. Brand[9] recommends changing shoes at least twice during the day. New shoes initially should not be worn for more than 1 hour at a time. They should be broken in gradually and the feet should be carefully inspected for injury each time new shoes are removed.

Patients should also understand the potential thermal injury from contact with objects that are hot or cold. Normal sensitive skin or a thermometer should be used to test the temperature of an object such as bath water to avoid tissue injury.

Footwear Selection. An experienced clinician should check the fit of new shoes and not rely completely on size number. The patient needs to understand that size may vary greatly between shoe brand and style. An oxford-type shoe or a jogging shoe is preferred and should provide a snug heel fit, secure fit across the midfoot, adequate room in the toebox, and $\frac{1}{2}$ inch of space beyond the longest toe. Laces are preferred over buckles or elastic straps because laces provide a more even distribution of pressure and prevent excessive shoe movement. Leather or fabric uppers will stretch as the shoe is broken in, and crepe, vibram, or rubber soles are recommended. Style often conflicts with protection (especially in dress shoes with high heels and pointed toes), and special occasions may require a compromise. Injury from these shoes can usually be prevented if lengthy periods of standing or walking are avoided. Patients with loss of protective sensation often benefit from soft-molded insoles that spread stress over a large area and reduce energy absorption demands on weight-bearing tissue.[46] The toebox should allow adequate depth for insoles to avoid increased stress on the toes or sides of the foot. Extra-depth shoes and jogging shoes usually provide adequate space for insoles.

Treatment of Plantar Ulcers

Successful treatment of plantar ulcers caused by pressure and insensitivity is best achieved by a well-organized interdisciplinary team approach. The team may include physician, nurse, physical therapist, podiatrist, surgeon, and prosthetist/orthotist. The specialists' interests and experiences in the neuropathic foot are more important than their respective disciplines. The physical therapist may be a major contributing member of the team providing expertise in foot screening, wound management, patient education, orthotics, and footwear modification.

In the United States, the majority of plantar ulcers are secondary complications of diabetes mellitus. Though most diabetic plantar foot ulcers are the result of neuropathy, vascular disease may also cause tissue damage or compromise wound healing. Primary

TABLE 11–2. Ulcer Classification

0 — Intact skin
1 — Superficial ulcer
2 — Deep ulcer
3 — Infected ulcer
4 — Partial foot gangrene
5 — Full foot gangrene

vascular disease should be ruled out before an ulcer management plan is considered. The ischemic index has been previously discussed. With appropriate management, most diabetic plantar ulcers heal at a rate comparable to ulcers seen in other diseases.

Wagner[39] presented a foot ulcer classification system that may be used to select lesions that are appropriate for conservative (nonsurgical) wound healing techniques (Table 11–2). A Grade 0 cannot be determined until heavy callus is removed over a potentially ulcerated area. The presence of an ulcer underlying a large plantar callus is not unusual. The scheme shown in Figure 11–7 has been successfully used for treatment of diabetic and nondiabetic plantar ulcers. The scheme is appropriate for Grade 1 and 2 plantar ulcers or Grade 3 plantar ulcers following the medical treatment of infection with bed rest and antibiotics. These approaches are not recommended for gangrenous lesions of the foot.

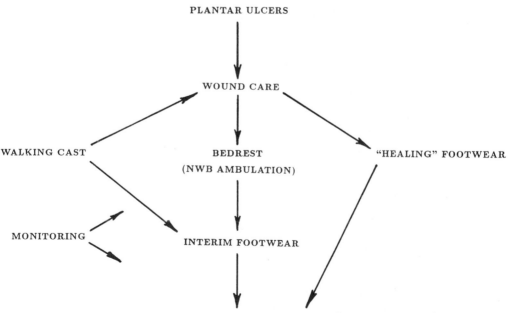

FIGURE 11–7. Management scheme for plantar ulceration of the foot (From Birke, JA and Sims, DS: The insensitive foot. In Hunt, GC (ed): Physical Therapy of the Foot and Ankle. Churchill Livingstone, New York, 1988, p. 152, with permission).

WOUND CARE

Differentiation of a Grade 1 from a Grade 2 ulcer is based on the assessment of wound depth. The wound should be gently probed with a sterile instrument to determine if it tracks to bone, tendon, or joint.[22] If synovial joint tissue is probed, a clear, bubbly fluid may be seen. Lytic enzymes present in synovial fluid are believed to interfere with wound healing. The presence of necrotic bone or tendon in the wound may also inhibit healing. Grade 2 ulcers should be evaluated by the surgical member of the treatment team.[4,47]

The size of the ulcer can be easily traced on sterilized exposed x-ray film placed over the wound (Fig. 11–8). This record is convenient for reassessment of the wound and viewing by the patient and staff. Patients are better motivated to comply with treatment plans when they can see the benefits of treatment. Specific methods of debriding and dressing wounds are covered in Chapter 9. In general, the wound should be debrided of necrotic tissue, cleaned, and covered with sterile dressings. Heavy callus typically forms around the border of the ulcer and should be trimmed to promote epithelial growth.[48–50] A topical antiseptic effective for the flora found on the wound is also recommended. No specific topical agent has been found to have any major contribution in the healing rate of neuropathic ulcers.

REDUCING FORCES

Bed Rest. Critical to the healing process of a plantar ulcer is the reduction of the weight-bearing stresses on the foot. Bed rest, though easiest to recommend, is usually not practical for long periods of time and requires complete compliance by the patient to

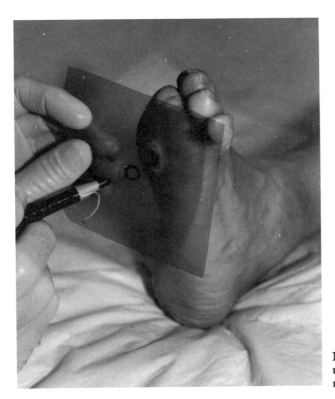

FIGURE 11–8. Ulcer tracing using sterilized x-ray film and a marking pen.

be effective. Often the patient will take short walks in his or her room or to the bathroom with the foot relatively unprotected. Bed rest is effective only if the patient remains completely non–weight bearing when out of bed. A long period of bed rest is especially deleterious to the general health of the diabetic patient.

Walking Casts. For many decades, walking casts have been used in the treatment of plantar ulcers in leprosy patients. Only in recent years have walking casts become a popular method for treating plantar ulcers in this country. Walking casts have been shown to be effective in healing plantar ulcers by reducing pressures during walking, reducing edema, and protecting the wound from traumatic re-injury.[51-53] Relative contraindications for the use of walking casts on the insensitive foot include infection, edema, and fragile hypotrophic skin. Once swelling and/or infection is controlled, a cast may be safely applied.

Total contact casts are considered the most effective casting method (Fig. 11–9).[54,55] Padding is selectively located over bony prominences (tibial crest, malleoli, navicular tuberosity, posterior heel, and toes) rather than over the entire leg as in standard casting methods. The inner layers of plaster are applied without tension and carefully molded to obtain an optimal total contact fit. The combination of minimal padding and careful

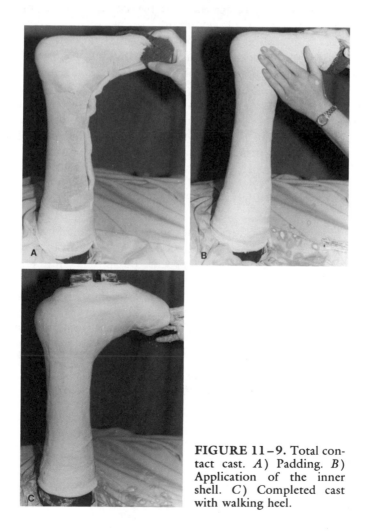

FIGURE 11–9. Total contact cast. *A*) Padding. *B*) Application of the inner shell. *C*) Completed cast with walking heel.

TABLE 11–3. Summary of Wound Healing Rates Using Casting

Author	No. Ulcers	Rate (days)	% Healed	Diagnosis
Pring, 1982	24	42	75	Leprosy
Pollard, 1983	8	21–56	100	Diabetic
Joseph, 1983	26	~28	65	Leprosy
	(24)		(12)	(controls)
Lang-Stevenson, 1985	26	70	100	Spina bifida or spinal injury
Diamond, 1987	1	39	100	Diabetic
Sinacore, 1987	33	44	82	Diabetic
	3	129	100	Nondiabetic
Walker, 1987	30	31	—	Diabetic forefoot
	25	42	—	Diabetic rearfoot
Birke, 1988	39	39	93	Diabetic
	69	43	93	Nondiabetic
Kaplan, 1988	24	41	—	Leprosy

molding of the inner shell provides a snug fit and better distribution of pressures. The toes are enclosed by plaster to protect the foot from direct trauma or from objects entering the cast. A ¼-inch piece of plywood and a rubber walking heel are applied to the bottom of the cast at a location 60 percent of the distance from the heel to the toe. This location creates a smooth rocker motion during walking.[43,53] The effectiveness of walking casts in healing diabetic and nondiabetic foot ulcers has been demonstrated in several studies[17,56–63] (Table 11–3).

Healing Footwear. Not every patient will accept, or is a candidate for, a walking cast. In these cases, alternatives to casting should be devised. Walking splints have been developed (Fig. 11–10); they are popular with patients and staff and have been very effective. The walking splint is functionally a half cast that is secured to the leg by an elastic wrap or Velcro closures. The shell is made of plaster reinforced by fiberglass taping (3M Orthopedic Products, Atlanta, GA), and relief for the posterior heel and plantar lesion is provided with adhesive backed padding (Contemporary Products, Corona, CA).

The cut-out sandal is another device that can be used as an alternative to casting.[22] The footbed of a molded Plastazote sandal is cut out or relieved from beneath to reduce pressure under the plantar lesion (Fig. 11–11). Care must be taken to ensure that edge pressures are not produced by the modification.[12]

Felted foam padding is useful for small Grade 1 ulcers or lesions that are almost healed.[64] An ulcer relief is cut out of a piece of ¼-inch felted foam (Stein Foot Specialty, Union, NJ). The relief must be trimmed closely to the posterior margin of the lesion but extend well distal to the lesion to provide a dynamic pressure reduction during walking (Fig. 11–12). The pad is then attached to the foot with rubber cement and secured with Kling (Johnson and Johnson Products, New Brunswick, NJ) or Fabco bandage (Fabco, Springfield, MA). The foot is fit into a castboot or plastazote sandal.

INTERIM FOOTWEAR

When proper techniques are followed, insensitive foot lesions heal without difficulty. The challenge is to prevent reulceration. The major mistakes in management of the neuropathic ulcer occur during the initial period after the ulcer is closed. The first mistake is not providing the patient with temporary protective footwear at the time of

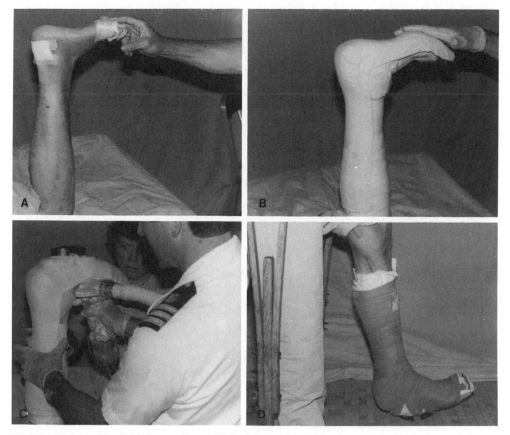

FIGURE 11–10. Walking splint. *A*) Padding. *B*) Inner layer of plaster in the form of a posterior splint. *C*) Fiberglass casting tape is used to reinforce the plaster and secure the heel; the layers of fiberglass covering the dorsum of the foot are removed with a cast saw. *D*) An elastic wrap is used to secure the walking splint to the foot.

healing but permitting the patient to return to the activities that originally created the ulcer. The patient must begin wearing protective footwear immediately after healing devices are removed. A molded Plastazote sandal[40] such as the one seen in Figure 11–13 is a good choice for interim footwear. This sandal can be easily fabricated to the patient's foot within several hours.

The second mistake that often results in reulceration of the foot is failure to instruct the patient to resume walking activities slowly. Partial weight-bearing ambulation with crutches is advised for the first 4 to 6 weeks after the ulcer is closed. The newly closed ulcer will not be fully healed for several months. New epithelium is thin and fragile at this time and may be adhered to deeper structures by scar tissue. Resilience to shear stresses is limited.[7] Another important consideration at this time is the osteoporotic changes in the bones of the foot due to immobilization. Patients who do not gradually resume activity are at a high risk of neuropathic fracture (Charcot's foot).[65]

The best way to monitor the progress of the patient's activities after healing is by measuring the temperature difference between the involved and uninvolved foot areas. Normal feet should have a difference in temperature less than 1°C. The foot undergoing a healing inflammatory process will often have a several-degree Celsius difference

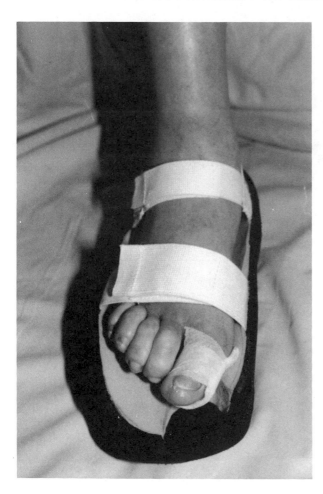

FIGURE 11–11. Cut-out sandal.

between feet, but this difference should slowly decrease during the weeks following closure of the wound. If the patient is too active, this difference will increase due to stress-induced inflammation. The patient must be cautioned that the first evidence of injury to the bones of the foot (Charcot's foot) is swelling and warmth.

DEFINITIVE FOOTWEAR

For the purpose of discussion, plantar ulcers will be grouped into three areas of the foot: forefoot, midfoot, and heel. Most plantar ulcerations of the foot occur at forefoot (toes, metatarsal heads).[8] This results from high stresses acting on the forefoot during the propulsive phase of gait. The midfoot is a common site of ulceration in the partially amputated foot or in the foot with rocker-bottom or pronatory deformities secondary to neuropathic fracture. Heel ulcers may result from direct trauma, like stepping on a nail, or may be the result of abnormal pressure from ankle calcaneus deformity. Ankle calcaneus often results from weakness of the tibial (S 1) innervated musculature of the leg, commonly seen in neuropathy secondary to spina bifida.[17]

A successful initial molded orthotic device is one made of soft thermoplastic materials such as a combination of ¼-inch Plastazote 1 and 2 (BXL Plastics Limited, ERP

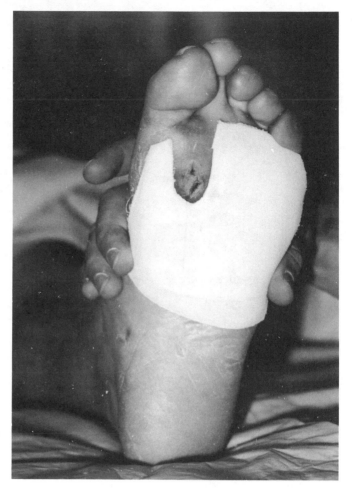

FIGURE 11–12. Felted foam (From Birke, JA and Sims, DS: The insensitive foot. In Hunt, GC (ed): Physical Therapy of the Foot and Ankle. Churchill Livingstone, New York, 1988, p. 158, with permission).

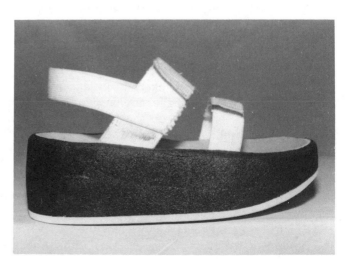

FIGURE   11–13.   Molded Plastazote sandal.

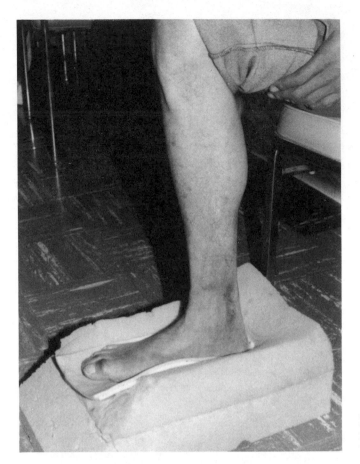

FIGURE 11–14. Technique for molding low temperature, thermoplastic materials.

Division, Croydon Surrey, CR9 3AL, England) (Fig. 11–14). The material properties of Plastazote provide optimal accommodation of the stresses on the foot; however, the insole is not durable. Plastazote material is not suitable for definitive orthotics because it quickly "bottoms out" under areas of high stress. After the ulcer is fully healed, firmer orthotic materials should be used so that insole failure will not be the cause of reulceration.

The patient with a forefoot ulcer should be fit with a molded orthotic designed to spread the plantar forces over a greater surface area.[66] A relief may be necessary on the underside of the orthosis to further reduce forces at a site of high pressure. Reliefs made under the orthosis are less likely to produce edge pressures.[14] There is evidence to support the use of a rocker sole modification for forefoot ulcers.[67,68] The rocker has been shown to reduce pressures on the forefoot during propulsion. Rocker modifications have not been well accepted by patients because of their appearance. Lower profile rockers of a clog type have been recommended as the optimal shape to use on the neuropathic foot.[69]

Midfoot ulcers associated with the shortened foot should also be fit with molded insoles and shoes with a rocker sole (Fig. 11–15). Probably the most effective shoe for the shortened foot is a short custom-molded boot. The short boot minimizes ground reaction forces on the foot by shortening the toe lever, thus reducing the forces acting on the bottom of the foot[22,40] (Fig. 11–16). Others have recommended standard length

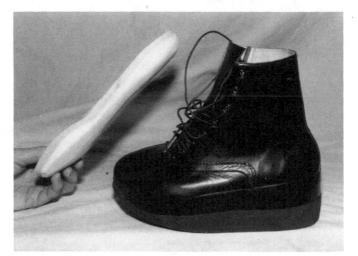

FIGURE 11–15. Custom molded boot with a molded insert.

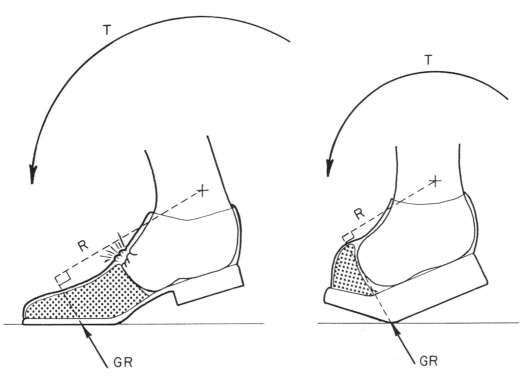

FIGURE 11–16. Comparison of the torque [torque (T) = ground reaction force (GR) times the perpendicular distance from the axis of rotation (R)] acting on a short foot walking in a long shoe verses short rocker shoe (From Birke, JA and Sims, DS: The insensitive foot. In Hunt, GC (ed): Physical Therapy of the Foot and Ankle, Churchill Livingstone, New York, 1988, p. 164, with permission).

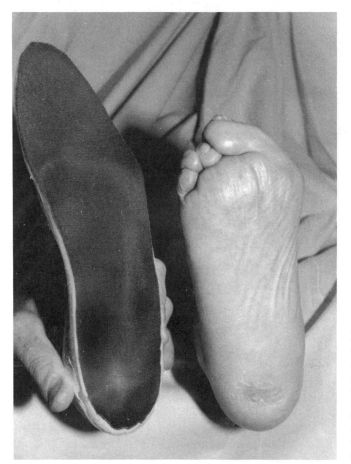

FIGURE 11-17. Foot orthosis with a molded and relieved heel cup made of suborthalene* and covered with ⅛ inch poron† used after a heel ulceration.
*JMS Berkshire Resource, Inc., Garfield, NJ 07011.
†AliMed Inc., Dedham, MA 02026.

footwear with a metatarsal bar carefully placed behind the distal end-bearing surface of the foot.[46] Midfoot ulcers secondary to Charcot's deformities usually require a custom-molded, deeply molded, low-quarter boot to accommodate the large midfoot bony prominence.

Heel ulcers may be managed with rigid, heel-cupped orthoses and shoes with a modified heel (Fig. 11-17). The heel cup is formed from a positive model of the foot and is relieved at the site of previous ulceration. The shoe heel is trimmed or cushioned to shorten the heel lever and thus reduce stresses on the heel at heel strike.

EVALUATION OF FOOTWEAR

Footwear and orthotics fabricated for the patient with an insensitive foot must be carefully evaluated to ensure a proper fit. Pressure testing is an effective way of assessing the fit of footwear. Pressure transducers and electronic force plates have been used in clinical studies but are not widely available for clinical use. Harris' mat[14,27] and microcapsule slipper socks[46,70] are practical methods of assessing the location and magnitude of static and dynamic forces on the foot. Details of fabrication and use of Harris' mat and microcapsule slipper socks have been previously described.[27,40,70]

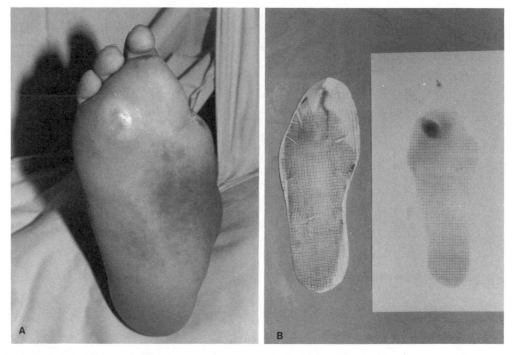

FIGURE 11–18. Harris Mat foot pressure test of a diabetic patient with a bony prominence of the fourth metatarsal head. *A*) Footprints. *B*) demonstrate area of high pressure walking barefoot (right) and reduction in pressure walking in a modified shoe (left).

The Harris' mat footprint test includes:

1. The patient stands on the mat on a hard floor. Dark areas identify high pressure on the sole of the foot (Fig. 11–18A).
2. The patient walks across the mat placed on a hard floor to determine pressure distribution during stance phase of gait.
3. A thin (1-mm) Harris' mat that is trimmed to fit inside the shoe shows pressure distribution with the shoe in place. The examiner must be careful to avoid smearing the ink on the paper or wrinkling the paper as the shoe is placed on the foot.

To use the microcapsule slipper socks, special socks containing pressure-sensitive dye capsules are placed on the feet. The shoes are carefully donned with laces fully loosened. The patient is instructed to walk 30 paces at his or her normal cadence, or at a cadence determined by the examiner. Shoes are then carefully removed to avoid friction and the slipper socks are turned inside out. Dark-blue stains indicate high pressure or shear stress, and light-blue stains indicate areas of moderate stress.

If either Harris' mat or the microcapsule tests reveal small areas of high stress, insole or footwear modifications are indicated to reduce the stress. The test should then be repeated after the modifications are initiated (Fig. 11–18B).

CLINICAL DECISION MAKING

The treatment of ulcers in the sensory neuropathy patient should be based on the evaluations described in this chapter and the general medical status of the patient. The long-term goal should be to prevent recurrence of the ulcer, and short-term goals are to unload the area of ulceration and protect the site from injury or infection while wound healing takes place. The choice of treatment(s) may, according to the severity of the condition, range from bed rest with medications to simple alteration of shoe or sandal for reduction of stress at the site of injury.

Case A

A 50-year-old male diabetic patient is seen in physical therapy for foot evaluation and determination of need for therapeutic footwear. A hard 3-mm thick callus under the right first metatarsal head is trimmed level with the adjacent skin surface. Skin underlying the callus is intact but a "Grade 0" preulcer measuring 1.5 cm in diameter is present. Sensory testing with Semmes-Weinstein nylon filaments reveals loss of "protective sensation" in both feet. Foot alignment is normal and skin is intact on the plantar surface of both feet. The skin is dry to touch and superficial cracking is noted around the lateral border of both heels.

GOALS

1. Promote healing of Grade 0 preulcer
2. Protect skin from excessive dryness and cracks
3. Protect feet from mechanical force injury

TREATMENT CHOICES

1. Walking cast
2. Custom-made soft sandal
3. Soft insoles for both shoes with pressure relief under right first metatarsal head
4. Patient education regarding skin hydration, foot inspection, activity level, and safe footwear

DECISION

Soft insoles in well-fitting shoes with adequate toebox depth would be appropriate for this patient. Limitation of activity, instruction in foot care, daily inspection of feet, and weekly follow-up visits to document healing of preulcer would be indicated for this patient.

SUMMARY

Wound prevention and healing in sensory neuropathy patients require a good understanding of the mechanisms of soft-tissue injury and the techniques and materials available for effective treatment. Relatively low levels of repetitive stress during a period of hours or days is thought to be the most common cause of pressure ulcers in ambulatory patients. The physical therapist, other clinicians, and the patient must employ frequent visual inspection, assessment of inflammatory changes, and protective footwear as a substitute for the patient's loss of protective sensation.

Mechanical forces in soft-tissue injury, types of injury, foot screening examination, classification of risk of injury, management and prevention of plantar ulcers, patient education, and evaluation of footwear have been presented in this chapter.

REFERENCES

1. Hall, OC and Brand, PW: Etiology of the neuropathic plantar ulcer. J Am Podiatric Assoc 69:173, 1979.
2. Price, EW: Studies on plantar ulceration in leprosy. Leprosy Review 31:159, 1960.
3. Brand, PW: The Effects of Pressure in Human Tissues. Rehabilitation Services Administration, United States Department of Health and Human Services, Washington, DC, 1977.
4. Brand, PW: The insensitive foot (including leprosy). In Jahss, MH (eds): Disorders of the Foot. Vol 2. WB Saunders, Philadelphia, 1982, p 1266.
5. Young, JS, et al: Spinal Cord Injury Statistics: Experience of the Regional Spinal Cord Injury Systems. Good Samaritan Medical Center, Phoenix, 1982, p 85.
6. Fine, PR, et al: The state of the National Spinal Cord Injury Database. National Spinal Cord Injury Statistical Center, University of Alabama, Spain Rehabilitation Center, Birmingham, 1985.
7. Brand, PW: The diabetic foot. In Ellenberg, M and Rifkin, H (eds): Diabetes Mellitus: Theory and Practice, ed 3. Medical Examination Publishing, New York, 1983, pp 829–849.
8. Birke, JA and Sims, DS: Plantar sensory threshold in the insensitive foot. Leprosy Review 57:261, 1986.
9. Brand, PW: Management of the insensitive limb. Phys Ther 59:8, 1979.
10. Kosiak, M: Etiology and pathology of ischemic ulcers. Arch Phys Med Rehabil 40:62, 1959.
11. Soderberg, GL: Kinesiology: Application to Pathological Motion. Williams and Wilkins, Baltimore, 1986, p 67.
12. Thompson, DE: The effects of mechanical stress on soft tissue. In Levin, ME and O'Neal, LW (ed): The Diabetic Foot, ed 4. CV Mosby, St Louis, 1988, p 91.
13. Beach, RB and Thompson, DE: Selected soft tissue research: An overview from Carville. Phys Ther 59:30, 1979.
14. Brand, PW: Repetitive stress in the development of diabetic foot ulcers. In Levin, ME and O'Neal, LW (eds): The Diabetic Foot, ed 4. CV Mosby, St Louis, 1988, p 83.
15. Ctereteko, GC, et al: Vertical forces acting on the feet of diabetic patents with neuropathic ulceration. Br J Surg 68:608, 1981.
16. Sabato, S, et al: Plantar trophic ulcers in patients with leprosy. Int Orthop 6:203, 1982.
17. Lang-Stevenson, AL, et al: Neuropathic ulcers of the foot. J Bone Joint Surg 67B:438, 1985.
18. Bauman, JH and Brand, PW: Measurement of pressure between foot and shoe. Lancet 1:629, 1963.
19. Stott, JR, Hutton, WC, and Stokes, LA: Forces under the foot. J Bone Joint Surg 55B:335, 1973.
20. Boulton, AJ, et al: Dynamic foot pressure and other studies as diagnostic and management aids in diabetic neuropathy. Diabetes Care 6:26, 1983.
21. Duckworth, T, et al: Plantar pressure measurements and the prevention of ulceration in the diabetic foot. J Bone Joint Surg 67B:79, 1985.
22. Birke, JA and Sims, DS: The insensitive foot. In Hunt, GC (ed): Physical Therapy of the Foot and Ankle. Churchill-Livingstone, New York, 1988, pp 133–168.
23. Chockinov, RT, Ullyot, GL, and Moorhouse, JA: Sensory perception thresholds in juvenile diabetes and their close relatives. N Engl J Med 286:1233, 1972.
24. Graham, S, Theriot, S, and Birke, JA: Comparison of sensory testing methods in the neuropathic foot. Unpublished study. GW Long Hansen's Disease Center, Carville, LA, 1987.
25. Birke, JA, Sims, DS, and Theriot, SM: Foot Screening Examination. Instructional videotape, produced by the Training Branch, GW Long Hansen's Disease Center, Carville, LA, 1985.
26. Von Prince, K and Butler, B: Measuring sensory function of the hand in peripheral nerve injuries. Am J Occup Ther 21:385, 1967.
27. Shipley, DE: Clinical evaluation and care of the insensitive foot. Phys Ther 59:13, 1979.
28. Harry, JR and Brand, PW: Patterns of disintegration of the tarsus in the anesthetic foot. J Bone Joint Surg 48B:4, 1966.
29. Bergtholdt, HT and Brand, PW: Temperature assessment and plantar inflammation. Leprosy Review 47:212, 1976.
30. Bergtholdt, HT: Temperature assessment of the insensitive foot. Phys Ther 59:18, 1979.
31. Bergtholdt, HT and Brand, PW: Thermography: An aid in the management of insensitive feet and stumps. Arch Phys Med Rehabil 56:205, 1975.
32. Barrett, JP and Mooney, V: Neuropathic and diabetic pressure lesions. Orthop Clin North Am 4(1):43, 1973.
33. Mann, RA and Hagy, JJ: Running, jogging, and walking: A comparative electromyographic and biomechanical study. In Bateman, JE and Trott, AW (eds): The Foot and Ankle. Brian C. Decker, Thieme-Stratton, New York, 1980, pp 167–175.
34. Fromherz W: Examination. In Hunt, GC (ed): Physical Therapy of the Foot and Ankle. Churchill-Livingstone, New York, 1988, pp 59–90.
35. Hunt, GC and Brocato, RS: Gait and foot pathomechanics. In Hunt, GC (ed): Physical Therapy of the Foot and Ankle. Churchill-Livingstone, New York, 1988, pp 39–57.
36. McPoil, TG and Brocato, RS: The foot and the ankle: Biomechanical evaluation and treatment. In Gould, JA, III, and Davis, GJ (eds): Orthopedic and Sports. Vol 2. CV Mosby, St Louis, 1985.
37. Root, ML, Orien, WP, and Weed, JH: Normal and Abnormal Function of the Foot; Clinical Biomechanics, ed 1. Vol II. Clinical Biomechanics, Los Angeles, 1977.

38. Raines, JK, Darling, RC, and Buth, V: Vascular laboratory criteria for the management of peripheral vascular disease of the lower extremities. Surgery 79:21, 1975.
39. Wagner, W: A classification and treatment program for diabetic, neuropathic, and dysvascular foot problems. American Academy of Orthopedic Surgeons Instructional Course Lecture, Vol 28, 1979.
40. Coleman, WC: Footwear in a management program of injury prevention. In Levin, ME and O'Neal, LW (eds): The Diabetic Foot, ed 4. CV Mosby, St Louis, 1988, p 293.
41. Birke, JA, Sims, DS, and Theriot, SM: Your Feet, Skin Care: A Guide for Patients with Insensitive Feet. Produced by the Training Branch, Gillis W. Long Hansen's Disease Center, Carville, LA, 1983.
42. Birke, JA, Sims, DS, and Theriot, SM: Your Feet, Self-Inspection. Produced by the Training Branch, Gillis W. Long Hansen's Disease Center, Carville, LA, 1983.
43. Birke, JA, Sims, DS, and Theriot, SM: Your Feet, Footwear Selection. Produced by the Training Branch, Gillis W. Long Hansen's Disease Center, Training Branch, Carville, LA, 1983.
44. Boeker, MJ and Leu, MM: A study of the effects of hydration and emollients on the feet of the aged. J Am Podiatr Med Assoc 68:402, 1978.
45. NIAMDD Fact Sheet: Foot Care for the Diabetic Patient. United States Department of Health and Human Services, United States Government Printing Office, Washington, DC, 1980.
46. Hampton, GH: Therapeutic footwear for the insensitive foot. Phys Ther 59:27, 1979.
47. Fritschi, EP: Surgical reconstruction and rehabilitation in leprosy. The Directory for Southern Asia Leprosy Mission, New Delhi, India, 1986.
48. Jones, RO: Ulceration in the neuropathic foot of Hansen's disease. J Am Podiatr Med Assoc 72:299, 1982.
49. Peacock, EE and Van Winkle, W: Wound Repair, ed 2. WB Saunders, Philadelphia, 1976, pp 119–127.
50. Srinivasan, H and Mukherjee, SM: Trophic ulcers in leprosy III. Leprosy Review 36:186, 1964.
51. Mooney, V and Wagner, FW: Neurocirculatory disorders of the foot. Clin Orthop Rel Res 122:53, 1977.
52. Pollard, JP, Le Quesne, LP, and Tappin, JW: Forces under the foot. J Biomed Eng 5:37, 1983.
53. Birke, JA, Sims, DS, and Buford, WL: Walking casts: Effect on plantar foot pressures. J Rehabil Res Devel 22:18, 1985.
54. Coleman, WC, Brand, PW, and Birke, JA: The total contact cast. J Am Podiatry Med Assoc 74:548, 1984.
55. Helm, PA, Walker, SC, and Pullium, G: Total contact casting in diabetic patients with neuropathic foot ulcerations. Arch Phys Med Rehabil 65:691, 1984.
56. Pring, DJ and Casiebanca, N: Simple plantar ulcers treated by below-knee plaster and moulded double-rocker plaster shoe: A comparative study. Leprosy Review 53:261, 1982.
57. Pollard, JP and LeQuesne, LP: Method of healing diabetic forefoot ulcers. Br Med J 286:436, 1983.
58. Joseph, B, Joshua, S, and Fritschi, EP: The moulded double-rocker plaster shoe in the field treatment of plantar ulcer. Leprosy Review 54:39, 1983.
59. Diamond, JE, Sinacore, DR, and Mueller, MJ: Moulded double-rocker plaster shoe for healing a diabetic plantar ulcer: A case report. Phys Ther 67:1550, 1987.
60. Sinacore, DR, et al: Diabetic plantar ulcers treated by total contact casting. Phys Ther 67:1543, 1987.
61. Walker, SC, Helm, PA, and Pullium, G: Total contact casting and chronic diabetic neuropathic foot ulcerations: Healing rates by wound location. Arch Phys Med Rehabil 68:217, 1987.
62. Birke, JA, Koziatek, E, and Coleman, WC: Healing rates in diabetic and non-diabetic plantar ulcers. Unpublished study, Gillis W. Long Hansen's Disease Center, Carville, LA, 1988.
63. Kaplan, M and Gelber, RH: Care of plantar ulcerations: Comparing applications, materials, and non-casting. Leprosy Review 59:59, 1988.
64. Frykberg, RG: Podiatric problems in diabetes. In Kosak, GP, et al (eds): Management of Diabetic Foot Problems. WB Saunders, Philadelphia, 1984, pp 45–67.
65. Warren, G: Tarsal bone disintegration in leprosy. J Bone Joint Surg 53B:688, 1971.
66. Reed, JK: Footwear for the diabetic. In Levin, ME and O'Neal, LW (eds): The Diabetic Foot. CV Mosby, St Louis, 1983, pp 360–377.
67. Bauman, JH, Garling, JP, and Brand, PW: Plantar pressures and trophic ulceration. J Bone Joint Surg 45B:652, 1963.
68. Coleman, WC: The relief of forefoot pressures using outer shoe sole modications. Proceedings of the International Conference on Biomechanics and Kinesiology of Hand and Foot, Madras, India, December, 1985.
69. Nawoczenski, D, Birke, JA, and Coleman, WC: The effect of rocker sole design on plantar forefoot pressures. J Am Podiatr Med Assoc 78:455–460, 1988.
70. Brand, PW and Ebner, JD: Pressure sensitive devices for denervated hands and feet. J Bone Joint Surg 51:109, 1969.

CHAPTER 12

Electrical Stimulation in Tissue Repair

Luther C. Kloth, M.S., P.T.
Jeffrey A. Feedar, P.T.

Information presented in previous chapters has described some of the complex events related to the unique processes of self-repair of wound tissues. Unfortunately, in chronic wounds, any one or a combination of the "normal" healing processes including progressive blood clotting events, inflammation, cellular proliferation, and scar remodeling may be hampered by factors such as compromised blood flow and oxygen supply to the tissues, infection, desiccation, and disease, to mention a few.

Despite the fact that for centuries, electrical charge from various sources has been applied to facilitate healing of injured tissue,[1-3] only during the past 20 years have controlled research studies on humans and animals provided rather convincing documented evidence that electrically augmented bone healing is best facilitated by invasive cathodal (rather than anodal) stimulation with between 5 and 20 microamperes (μA) of direct current[4-9] (less than 1.0 mA constitutes μA current). In contrast, during the same time period most of the research related to electrically augmented healing of human chronic dermal ulcers has indicated that healing is promoted by injection of μA currents via the anode to the wound tissue[10-14] and that the negatively biased electrode suppresses both healing and infection.[10,15] Interestingly, other studies, in which μA currents were applied to severed tendons in animals, have reported that both the anode and cathode effectively enhance healing and increase the breaking strength at the site of severance.[16,17] These findings suggest that injured bone, tendon, and dermal/subdermal tissues composed of different cellular constituents and having dissimilar biochemical and biomechanical properties, respond differently to positive and negative microamperage currents.

The purpose of this chapter is to discuss the use of biostimulating electric currents to augment healing of chronic dermal wounds. This will be accomplished by (1) reviewing pertinent clinical literature; (2) discussing relevant animal, cellular, and cutaneous oxygen studies; (3) identifying and describing the types and characteristics of therapeutic currents that are appropriate for wound healing applications; (4) discussing theories postulated to explain why external electrical stimulation enhances soft-tissue healing by stimulating endogenous bioelectric circuits; (5) identifying contraindications to using electrical stimulation to promote wound healing; and (6) selecting treatment protocols to augment wound healing based on clinical decision-making processes.

LITERATURE REVIEW

Charged Gold Leaf

Perhaps the earliest recorded documentation related to the use of electrical charge to enhance tissue healing appeared in "Choice and Experimental Receipts in Physik and Chirurgery," originally published in 1688 by Sir Kenelm Digby with republication of portions of these folk treatments completed in 1925 by Robertson.[1] Among the remedies discussed in Digby's "Receipts" was the application of charged gold leaf to smallpox lesions that were observed to heal without scarring. In the 1960s, interest in using gold leaf to heal resistant dermal wounds was revived when Kanof[18] reported that charged gold leaf accelerated the healing of pressure sores but produced excessive granulation tissue formation when used in treating burn wounds. In the same year, Gallagher and Geschickter[19] reported that electrostatically charged gold leaf applied to surgical wounds caused hemostasis of injured arteries and veins and could be used in surgery to stop capillary bleeding. In a 1966 pilot study, Wolf and associates,[20] perhaps motivated by the previous reports of the effects of gold leaf, used the metal foil to treat 25 ischemic ulcers of various etiologies on 13 patients. Twenty were pressure sores that had existed from 1 week to 4 years. One wound resulted from diabetic small-vessel disease, one from chronic lower extremity venous insufficiency, and three coexisting decubiti served as controls. Results indicated that the surface area of 20 of the ulcers treated with gold leaf, which was reapplied every 48 hours, decreased an average of 62 percent during a time period ranging from 7 days to 9 weeks. During the same time period, the three control ulcers increased in size an average of 96 percent. Although the number of wounds treated and controlled was too limited to be of statistical significance, nevertheless the outcomes reported suggest that μA currents generated by electrostatic charge from gold leaf may have enhanced wound healing.

Smith and coworkers[21] compared the effects of gold leaf, aluminum foil, flexible collodion, and polyethylene film in treatments administered to 44 patients with 64 dermal ulcers that were first subjected to surgical debridement. They measured the surface area of each ulcer before and after treatment, and progress was reported as the percentage re-epithelialized per day. The metal foils placed on the wounds were covered with an eye pad that was secured with a bandage, and the entire dressing was changed every 5 to 7 days (unlike Wolf and associates,[20] who changed the gold foil every 48 hours). In contrast to the findings of Wolf and colleagues, the healing rate with gold leaf was found to be only as effective as the control wounds, which were treated with a simple dressing. Ulcers occluded with aluminum foil or polyethylene film failed to produce re-epithelialization, and the wounds treated with flexible collodion showed an indication of healing only after the formation of desiccated crust.

Although others have reported positive outcomes following the use of gold leaf to treat dermal ulcers, their findings are reported from studies that either did not involve a control group[22] or represented a single case study.[23] In addition, histologic findings from experimental wounds treated with gold leaf are inconclusive and have not been replicated.[24]

Thus, today gold leaf is seldom used to treat wounds. Perhaps the lack of establishing gold leaf as an efficacious treatment can be attributed to certain clinical conditions that have not been consistently satisfied in the studies that have been published. For example, Kanof[18] and Wolf and colleagues[20] found optimal healing effectiveness of gold leaf to be dependent on establishing a firm electrostatic bond between the gold leaf foil and the tissue being treated. This bonding was accomplished by creating a dielectric interface with ethyl alcohol that was used to cleanse the area before applying gold foil to the wound. With only one or two layers of gold foil tightly adhering to the irregular wound surface, tiny breaks occurred in the fragile sheets. To create an unbroken gold foil surface over the wound that would provide a uniform charge distribution to the wound tissues, four to eight layers of gold leaf were required and were usually left in place for about 48 hours after which the crumbling gold foil was removed with the aid of normal saline irrigation. When repeated, this procedure was found by Wolf and associates[20] to be most effective in enhancing wound healing when the blood hemoglobin level was 12 g per 100 cc or higher. In fact, they observed that when the hemoglobin level fell below this value, the healing process augmented by gold leaf was halted and resumed again only when the value was restored.

Although the exact mechanisms by which charged gold leaf promotes healing are unclear, perhaps its effectiveness results from an electrochemical influence that causes a mild foreign body reaction that stimulates healing.[19] Maybe, through the low-level electrostatic negative charge produced, gold leaf promotes migration of epithelial cells across the wound surface;[21] or perhaps the charge present in gold leaf has no effect at all on tissues or cells, but instead, healing is promoted by the superimposed layers of gold leaf which create the effect of an occlusive dressing and an accompanying moist wound healing environment with low oxygen tension.

Clearly, additional controlled clinical research is needed to provide objective information related to mechanisms and effectiveness of gold leaf in healing wounds. Additionally, the quantity of charge generated by gold leaf at the interface between the gold foil and wound tissue should be determined. Perhaps this charge quantity, through perturbation of certain cells (e.g., angioblasts, fibroblasts, or epidermal cells), can be shown to be responsible for their proliferation, migration, or more appropriate orientation for tissue repair processes. If the mechanism is identified, then a variety of charge dosages may be selected from other μA sources and applied to chronic wounds to determine the most appropriate type and dosage of current needed to accelerate tissue repair.

Low Voltage, Constant Microamperage, Direct Current

Apparently motivated by the earlier clinical findings of Kanof,[18] and their own clinical results related to the effectiveness of charged gold leaf in promoting repair of chronic dermal ulcers,[20] Wolcott and colleagues[10] developed a battery-powered device capable of delivering 200 to 1000 μA of constant current to wound tissue via an anode or cathode. They used this constant, microamperage direct current (CMDC) device in an 18-month clinical trial study to test the hypothesis that electric charge injected into tissues of ischemic dermal ulcers from the anode would accelerate the rate of healing in comparison to control wounds. All wounds were initially treated with the cathode for 3 days or until infected wounds were aseptic. When anodal treatment resulted in a healing plateau, polarity was reversed until healing recommenced, after which anodal stimulation was reapplied. They reported that out of 75 ulcers treated with direct current, 45 percent healed completely in an average of 9.6 weeks at a rate of 18.4 percent a week. In contrast, 55 percent of the ulcers healed incompletely to an average volume decrease of 64.7 percent in 7.2 weeks at a rate of 9.3 percent a week. The average healing rate for all wounds was 13.4 percent per week. In addition, eight other patients, six of whom were paraplegics, who had bilateral ischemic ulcers of comparable size and location served as the control group. The eight control ulcers were managed the same way as the eight treated, contralateral ulcers, except they did not receive electrical stimulation. The mean healing rate for the control ulcers was 5 percent per week compared with 27 percent per week for their treated counterparts. Interestingly, 71 percent of all the patients in this study were paraplegics whose rate of tissue repair was about 40 percent slower than for patients with other primary diagnoses. Despite the overall slower rate of wound healing for the spinal-cord–injured patients, the treatment protocol, which called for 2 hours of anodal μA stimulation, followed by a 4-hour nonstimulation interval three times in a 24-hour period for an average of 7.7 weeks, was successful in producing an 81.8 percent wound volume decrease at a healing rate of 13.4 percent per week for the 75 treated ulcers.

Using the same protocol, similar results were reported by Gault and Gatens,[12] who treated 100 ischemic skin ulcers with the same CMDC device and protocol used by Wolcott and associates.[10] In addition, six patients with bilateral symmetrical ulcers served as the control group. The six control ulcers healed at a rate of 14.7 percent per week compared with 30 percent per week for the six treated ulcers. Three of the six treated ulcers healed completely while two of the untreated control wounds increased in size during the 4-week treatment period. The 100 ulcers treated with μA stimulation healed at a similar rate of 28.4 percent per week, which resulted in complete healing of 48 percent of these ulcers in 4.7 weeks.

In both of these studies, a paucity of control wounds is clearly evident. Possibly recognizing this common deficiency, Carley and Wainapel[13] designed a clinical study around a modified protocol of Wolcott and coworkers,[10] in which 30 hospital inpatients with chronic dermal ulcers ranging in duration from 2.3 to 12.3 months were paired according to age, diagnosis, and wound etiology, location, and size. One member of each pair was randomly assigned to an experimental group and received wound treatment consisting of CMDC stimulation, while the other member was assigned to a control group and was treated with either wet-to-dry dressings or hydrotherapy. The 15 patients in the treatment group received 300 to 500 μA of direct current if their wound tissues were normally innervated or 500 to 700 μA if their wound tissues were denervated. The electrical stimulation was applied to the wound via the anode following cathodal stimulation for the first 3 days. Polarity was reversed for 3 days if a plateau in healing was observed. The treatment regimen based on the protocol of Wolcott and associates[10] was modified such that the treatment schedule allowed for 2 hours of stimulation twice daily, 5 days a week, rather than 2 hours of stimulation three times daily, 7 days a week.

Overall, wounds of patients in the μA-current treatment group showed a 1.5 to 2.5 times faster healing rate than wounds of patients assigned to the control group. A nonparametric statistical analysis of data collected for the two groups revealed a statistically significant and progressively increased difference between them after 3, 4, and 5 weeks of treatment.

The three studies just discussed share some commonalities that may be unique to the chronic wound treatment protocol that uses CMDC. The commonalities are either consistent with or modified from the protocol of Wolcott and associates[10] and, as reported, do produce favorable clinical outcomes. They include (1) initial application of the cathode to the wound for 3 or more days for bactericidal effects, followed by (2) anodal wound stimulation for 2 hours, two or three times daily 5 to 7 days per week; (3) reversal of polarity daily or every 3 days after a plateau in healing is observed; and (4) constant current stimulation at an amplitude of 200 to 1000 μA. Notice that these microamperage values are substantially higher than the 5 to 20 μA range mentioned earlier, for which constant direct current applied invasively has been documented to augment healing of bone in cases of delayed and/or non-union fracture. Perhaps in future clinical studies it will be shown that constant direct current applied at less than 300 μA as effective in stimulating repair of dermal ulcers as current greater than 300 μA. Indeed, in a controlled study, Alvarez and colleagues[25] have demonstrated a significant increase in dermal collagen synthetic capacity and re-epithelialization in induced wounds in pigs treated with 50 to 300 μA of CMDC from the anode. Their results suggested to them that electric charge can favorably influence the proliferative and migratory capacity of epithelial and connective tissue cells involved in tissue regeneration and repair.

In contrast to the favorable outcomes reported in previous clinical studies following anodal wound stimulation, eight venous-insufficiency leg ulcers in existence from 8 months to 5 years were treated with 50 to 100 μA of CMDC produced from a 0.2 to 0.8 voltage source.[26] All ulcers healed in an average of 30 days and none recurred during a follow-up period of more than 3 years. Unlike previous clinical studies cited[10,12,13] not only was the current amplitude considerably lower but also it was applied to the wound tissues via the cathode. The results reported are surprising in view of the well-known fact that sclerotic effects are produced by an acidic pH at the anode of constant current and sclerolytic effects are produced by an alkaline pH at the cathode. Nevertheless, on histologic examination of biopsy scar tissue from the area of the pre-existing ulcer of one patient 1 year after the ulcer was healed, Assimacopoulos[26] observed dense connective tissue rich in hyalinized collagen fibers that were oriented parallel to the surface. Typical of scar tissue, elastic fibers were also present but no sebaceous glands, sweat glands, or hair follicles were present. These observations were considered to be "histologic proof" that "very strong scar" tissue was produced by the influence of negative CMDC.[24] In another report by the same author, similar results were observed in a controlled animal study using the same μA and voltage amplitudes applied via the cathode to treat induced wounds in rabbits.[27] Wounds treated with CMDC healed in 17 to 18 days whereas control wounds required 25 to 26 days to heal. Histologically, wounds of control animals were covered with a small scar and consisted of epidermis and fibrous connective tissue with collagen fibers arranged perpendicular to the surface. Scars treated with negative μA current were larger and stronger and consisted of epidermis and dense connective tissue with hyalinized collagen fibers oriented parallel to the surface.

Although the reported histologic findings from induced animal wounds treated with cathodal direct current are similar to findings observed in human wounds treated with negative direct current, the animal findings only support and do not totally confirm the human study findings. Clearly, existing published clinical research provides more support for anodal wound stimulation with CMDC than for cathodal stimulation. Additional double-blind, controlled research is needed to more rigorously evaluate the efficacy of anodal and cathodal μA currents in healing chronic dermal ulcers.

IONTOPHORESIS

Constant direct current applied at mA levels has also been used to promote wound healing by repelling either zinc or histamine iontophoretically into wound tissue at the anode. The use of zinc to promote healing dates back to ancient Egyptians, who used the metal in the form of calamine, a mixture of ferric and zinc oxides still in use today.[28] On one patient, Cornwall[29] reported using iontophoresis to repel zinc oxide in a 0.1 M solution into bilateral dermal ulcers present on the tibial crests of a 71-year-old man. Initially, the ulcers measured 15.6 cm² on the left leg and 7.74 cm² on the right leg. Before each iontophoresis treatment, the patient's ulcers were treated with a whirlpool bath to which povidone-iodine was added. After treating each ulcer iontophoretically with 4 to 5 mA daily, 6 days a week, for a total of 20 days, the ulcers decreased in size to 0.2 cm² and 0.04 cm², respectively. Calculations to determine reduction in wound area revealed a 98.7 percent closure on the left and a 99.5 percent closure on the right. Because no control wounds were available, the assumption can be made that healing may have occurred as a result of the daily whirlpool treatments.

Abramson and coworkers[30] used histamine immersion iontophoresis to treat limb ulcers on 15 patients with a variety of conditions. Ulcers on hands, feet, or lower leg were immersed in a 1:10,000 histamine diphosphate solution. The anode was attached to the inner surface of the container and the cathode was applied to the patient's back. Treatments, administered with direct current at 3 to 12 mA were given two or three times a week for 5 to 20 minutes. The iontophoresis treatment was preceded by 15 minutes of hydrotherapy followed by debridement of necrotic tissue. Although 10 of the 15 ulcers reportedly healed in periods of a few weeks to several months, healing may possibly have been promoted by whirlpool and/or debridement procedures. In a concurrent study, the authors demonstrated that histamine by ion transfer did not raise oxygen uptake but did markedly increase blood flow; therefore histamine iontophoresis for wound healing may be beneficial even in the presence of impaired arterial circulation. From the paucity of clinical studies, the efficacy of iontophoresis for wound healing is apparently not established, and additional controlled clinical studies are needed to support or refute its use.

Low Voltage, Pulsed Microamperage Current

Although μA current from CMDC was used in studies previously cited, its generation is not limited to devices that generate CMDC. Because μA currents have an amplitude of less than 1.0 mA, they may also be produced by devices that deliver biphasic and monophasic currents. Barron and associates[31] used μA current generated via a modified biphasic square wave at an amplitude of 600 μA and a frequency of 0.5 pps to treat decubitus ulcers in six geriatric patients. There was no mention of control or placebo wounds, but within 1 month, five of the six wounds that had been treated three times a week, by placing a pair of metal probe electrodes 2 cm from the wound edge, had essentially healed. Additional controlled clinical research using low voltage, monophasic or biphasic pulsed μA current delivered from metal probe electrodes to the wound perimeter is needed to provide support or to refute the efficacy of these devices for wound healing.

High Voltage, Monophasic, Pulsed Current

The use of high voltage, monophasic pulsed current (HVPC) to enhance tissue healing dates back to 1966, when a veterinarian applied this form of current to the hind limb of four dogs whose hind limb circulation had been compromised for 12 hours by proximal tourniquet application. Twenty-four hours after removal of the tourniquet, each dog was treated with HVPC for 5 minutes daily for 14 days at 150 volts, a frequency of 12 to 14 pulses per second and a pulse duration of 4 microseconds. A control group of four dogs did not receive HVPC after tourniquet removal. Dogs in the control group developed pronounced hind limb edema and superficial necrosis. At the end of the study, dogs in the treatment group walked without limping and had no observable differences between the normal and traumatized hind limb. All dogs in the control group developed severe gangrene.[32]

Two case reports[33,34] and two clinical studies[14,35] have provided some preliminary evidence that HVPC augments healing of chronic dermal ulcers. Thurman and Christian[33] attributed to HVPC treatment the healing of a purulent septic abscess on the foot of a 43-year-old female patient with juvenile-onset diabetes mellitus. They placed electrodes adjacent to the patient's abscess and elicited muscular contractions at a nontetanizing frequency in an attempt to improve blood flow. Blood flow was observed to improve and the abscess responded favorably after 2 weeks of HVPC treatment provided twice daily on weekdays and once daily on weekends. Impending amputation of the patient's limb was unnecessary, and the wound healed completely after 6 months of HVPC treatment.

In two patients who were treated with HVPC following podiatric surgery, Ross and Segal[34] implied that HVPC was used to enhance tissue healing. However, the only reported benefits were pain and edema reduction, with no mention of the effects on tissue healing.

Akers and Gabrielson[35] compared the rate of healing of decubitus ulcers in human subjects using three different treatment procedures. Fourteen patients with pressure sores were assigned to one of three treatment groups: (1) whirlpool bath once a day, (2) a combination of whirlpool bath and HVPC twice a day, and (3) HVPC twice a day. There was no control group, no mention of the numbers of patients in the three treatment groups, the number or duration of treatments, or the stimulus characteristics. Based on microcomputer wound area analysis, the authors reported that patients who received only HVPC treatment (who were either spinal cord denervated or had the involved limb partially denervated) experienced the greatest rate of change in wound size followed by patients who received both whirlpool and HVPC treatments. Patients who received whirlpool treatment alone experienced the least change. Statistically there was no difference between the three groups.

In a controlled clinical study, Kloth and Feedar[14] randomly assigned 16 patients with Stage IV dermal ulcers to either a treatment or a control group. They applied HVPC to the wound at 105 pps and set the current amplitude to just below that which produced a visible muscle contraction. Nine patients in the treatment group received 45 minutes of anodal stimulation to the ulcer 5 days a week. Seven patients in the control group received 45 minutes of placebo stimulation to the ulcer 5 days a week. Wounds of patients in the treatment group healed at a rate of 45 percent a week and healed completely in 7.3 weeks. The wound area of patients in the control group increased a mean of 29 percent during a mean period of 7.4 weeks. The wounds of three patients assigned to a control subgroup increased in area by 1.2 percent during 8.7 weeks. However, when these three patients were reassigned to a treatment subgroup their wounds healed at a rate of 38 percent a week and were completely healed in 8.3 weeks.

One other report has published findings from a pilot study in which HVPC was used to treat wounds of 15 patients with diabetic foot ulcers. Although there was no control group, the wounds of 12 of the 15 patients healed completely in a mean period of 2.6 months with anodal stimulation applied for 1 hour, 3 days a week.[36]

These findings, when compared with those of other clinical studies[10,12,13] suggest that HVPC is as effective as CMDC in augmenting wound healing. In addition, based on information currently available, HVPC treatment appears to be more cost effective than CMDC because complete healing of wounds treated with HVPC has been achieved with between 3 and 4 hours of electrical stimulation per week for 7 to 9 weeks[14,36] compared with complete healing with CMDC (excluding iontophoresis), which reportedly requires 20 to 42 hours a week for 5 to 10 weeks.[10,12,13] Additional controlled clinical studies with both types of current are needed to clearly establish optimal healing dosages and duration of treatments needed to most effectively provide the optimal healing rates. A summary of select controlled and noncontrolled clinical studies is presented in Table 12–1.

Low Voltage, Pulsed Milliamperage Current

All of the previous clinical studies reviewed used direct or pulsed current with the anode or cathode placed directly on or immediately adjacent to the wound during treatment. With the exception of studies in which iontophoresis was used, all of the studies used μA levels of bioelectric current. In contrast to these studies, Kaada[37] successfully treated 10 patients with 19 leg ulcers of various etiologies with burst mode from a traditional TENS device. He applied 15 to 30 mA for 30 to 45 minutes, three times daily via two bursts per second of cathodal stimulation to the webspace between the first and second metacarpals of the ipsilateral hand. The anode was positioned at the ulnar border of the same wrist. All of the ulcers, which had resisted treatment for several months to 4 years, healed completely in response to the remote pulsing stimulation of muscles underlying the electrodes on the hand and wrist. Kaada[37] proposed that the remote electrical stimulation of hand muscles resulted in improved microcirculation in tissues of the ipsilateral lower extremity as evidenced by increased temperature of the toes and healing of the leg ulcers. He further proposed three mechanisms that may explain how remote electrical stimulation of hand muscles causes vasodilation of small vessels in the ipsilateral lower extremity. The mechanisms include (1) activation of a central serotonergic link that inhibits sympathetic vasoconstriction; (2) activation and release of vasoactive intestinal polypeptide (VIP) into the plasma; and (3) activation of a segmental axon-reflex leading to vasodilation.[37] In support of the first mechanism is the finding that serotonin inhibitors were found to block the vasodilation response, but the response was not affected by the opiate antagonist naloxone or by antagonists of humoral vasodilators.[38–42]

Other investigators have also reported vasodilation responses of hand and digital vessels to remote transcutaneous stimulation of the skin over the spinal cord[43] or ulnar nerve[44] at mA levels of current flow. As usual, not all studies using mA levels of electrical stimulation are in agreement with these findings. In fact, one study reported a drop in digital temperature, suggesting vasoconstriction of digital vessels following sensory and motor excitation elicited by noninvasive stimulation of acupuncture points.[45] Ernst and Lee[46] applied mA levels of stimulation to the dorsal webspace of the hand with a monophasic pulse having a duration of 800 μsec, delivered below the pain threshold, and reported an increase in sympathetic tone with subsequent vasodilation after 50 minutes. In a controlled study, no change in sympathetic tone was noted following sensory stimulation in patients with chronic pain.[47]

Despite the equivocal research findings related to the use of pulsed mA levels of current and the remote effects produced on circulation in the distal extremities, this approach to treatment of hand, foot, and digital ulcerations may prove to be effective in facilitating wound repair in patients with primary diagnoses of Raynaud's disease, CREST syndrome, and reflex sympathetic dystrophy.

ANIMAL, CELLULAR, AND CUTANEOUS OXYGEN STUDIES

Numerous controlled animal and in vitro studies have provided information that supports using μA current clinically to promote tissue repair and accelerate healing in chronic dermal ulcers. Many of these studies have reported that bioelectric currents produce increased tensile strength of wound scar following application of CMDC.

Assimacopoulos[27] treated induced wounds in rabbits with cathodal CMDC applied continuously at 100 μA until healing was complete. Treated wounds healed 25 percent faster than control wounds, and had larger and stronger scars composed of dense connective tissue and hyalinized degenerated collagen fibers arranged parallel to the surface. Untreated control wounds took longer to heal, were weaker, and had smaller scars with less dense connective tissue and collagen fibers arranged perpendicular to the surface. The breaking load required to fail or rupture the scars healed by bioelectric current was approximately two times greater than the load required to fail control scars. Another study has also reported greater tensile strength of induced wound scars treated with 10 to 20 μA of cathodal CMDC compared with controls.[48] In that same study, wounds treated with anodal CMDC demonstrated decreased tensile strength compared with control wounds. These studies suggest that polarity may be a factor to consider when treating wounds with polarized current. However, other investigators may not support this notion, because reports indicate that tensile strength of wounds treated with CMDC is greater than tensile strength of control wounds, even though polarity was not considered in one study[49] and the anode and cathode straddled treated and control wounds in another study.[50] In two other μA studies, neither current amplitude[51] nor polarity[51,52] affected wound tensile strength to a significant degree.

In two recent studies by Brown and associates,[53,54] HVPC was applied to induced wounds in rabbits to determine the effects of cathodal and anodal polarity on wound closure and tensile strength. In the first study, negative polarity was applied to treatment and control groups of animals for 2 hours twice daily for either 4 or 7 days at 30 to 60 volts, with a pulse duration of 100 μS and a frequency of 80 pps. After 4 days, wound scar tensile strength in treated animals was 36 percent greater than that of control scars; however, this difference was not significant, nor was the percent of wound closure between the two groups. After 7 days, control wounds had closed more than treated wounds and control wound scars had significantly greater tensile strength than treated scars. Because of this latter finding, the authors speculated that perhaps cathodal polarity may have impeded the healing process.[53] In a follow-up study, Brown and colleagues[54] used the same research design, except that the anode was applied to the wounds of animals in the treatment group. After 4 days of positive-polarity HVPC stimulation, wound closure was significantly less for treated than for control wounds, but between 4 and 7 days after injury, wound closure values for treated animals increased from 50 percent to 80 percent, so that at 7 days after injury wound closure was comparable for treatment and control groups. In addition, there was no difference in tensile strength between treatment and control wounds after 4 or 7 days of stimulation, but histologic examination of wounds from both groups revealed that a more rapid rate of epithelialization had occurred in wounds treated with HVPC for 4 and 7 days compared with control wounds examined after the same time periods. Thus, while neither study demonstrated clear-cut differences between treatment and control animals, nevertheless indications from the results suggest that selection of treatment polarity may depend on the polarity of the wound injury potential and that, perhaps, based on the findings of Burr and coworkers,[55] exogenous polarity applied through treatment electrodes should be opposite the polarity of the wound injury potential. This notion

TABLE 12–1. A Summary of Clinical Bioelectric Wound Healing Studies

Author(s)/Journal	No. Patients	Number and Type of Wounds	Current Type and Characteristics	Hours of Treatment/Week	Percent Healing Rate/Week	Percent of Wounds Healed; Mean No. of Weeks for Healing
Wolcott et al[10]	67	75 treatment; 8 control ischemic ulcers	Constant microamperage DC, 200–800 μA; anodal polarity after cathode for 3 or more days	42	Treatment group: 13.4% Control group: 5%	45%; 9.6 wk
Gault and Gatens[12]	76	100 treatment; 6 control ischemic ulcers	Constant microamperage DC, 200–800 μA, anodal polarity after cathode for 3 or more days	42	Treatment group: 29% Control group: 14.7%	48%; 4.7 wk
Carley and Wainapel[13]	30	15 treatment; 15 control indolent ulcers	Constant microamperage DC, 300–700 μA; anodal polarity after cathode for 3 days	20	Treatment group: 18% Control group: 9%	Not reported; 5 wk
Assimacopoulos[26]	3	8 treatment; 0 control venous insufficiency leg ulcers	Constant microamperage DC, 50–100 μA; cathodal polarity	168 (assumed)	Treatment group: not reported	100%; 4.4 wk
Barron et al[31]	6	6 treatment; 0 control decubitus ulcers	Low voltage biphasic microamperage current 600 μA at 0.5 pps; cathode initially for resistant cases	3 (assumed)	Treatment group: not reported	83%; 4 wk

Akers and Gabrielson[35]	14	14 treatment; 0 control decubitus ulcers	High voltage monophasic pulsed current; amplitude frequency and polarity not reported	Not reported	Not reported	Not reported
Kloth and Feedar[14]	16	9 treatment; 7 control, 3 treatment subgroups decubitus ulcers	High voltage monophasic pulsed current 100–160 V (sensory stimulation) 500–800 μA, anodal polarity, 105 pps.	3.7	Treatment group: 46% Control group: 11.6% (increase in wound size); treatment subgroup: 38%	100%; 7.3 wk
Alon et al[36]	15	15 treatment; 0 control decubitus ulcers	High voltage, monophasic pulsed current, below motor response; anodal polarity, 80 pps microamperage currents assumed	3	Not reported	80%; 10.5 wk
Kaada[37]	10	19 treatment; 0 control dermal ulcers	Low voltage, square wave milliamperage current; 15–30 mA, cathodal polarity 2 bursts/sec	Not reported	Not reported	100%; 12 wk

may explain why polarity reversal has been reported to reinitiate wound repair processes following plateaus in healing that has been observed in a number of clinical studies.[10,12-14]

Other animal studies have confirmed that the polar electrochemical effects of CMDC applied at 5 to 20 μA in vivo across canine and rat blood vessels produce blood coagulation and thrombosis within the vessel beneath the anode but not beneath the cathode.[56-60] Additional studies have confirmed that when polarity is reversed the cathode is capable of solubilizing the clot formed beneath the anode.[61-65] These findings provide support for the clinical observation that cathodal CMDC solubilizes necrotic wound tissue especially when it consists of coalesced blood elements. In addition, some clinicians have claimed that cathodal HVPC produces the same effect. However, in theory this claim is not well founded because Newton and Karselis[66] have demonstrated that HVPC does not produce significant acid or base build-up at the anode and cathode, respectively. The empirical assumption then is that the alkaline pH produced at the cathode of CMDC (but not HVPC) is responsible for solubilizing coagulated blood and necrotic tissue through sclerolytic liquefaction. On the other hand, the acid pH produced at the anode of CMDC (but not HVPC) may, through a sclerosing effect, produce hyalinization of collagen leading to formation of a congealed scar. This type of dense scar is often observed following healing of chronic full thickness wounds treated with CMDC. In contrast, wounds treated with HVPC are usually observed to heal with a tissue covering that is less dense but more resilient.

Certainly, in clinical practice HVPC and CMDC devices offer polarity selection. However, because CMDC produces pH and accompanying electrochemical changes in tissues at the anode and cathode but HVPC does not, we may conclude that changes in wound scar tensile strength produced by HVPC do not occur from electrochemical reactions resulting from sclerotic effects at the anode. Clearly, additional research is needed to identify whether sensory levels of HVPC stimulation are capable of producing pH changes in wound tissues. Farther on in this chapter we will show that the total current injected into the tissues from HVPC devices at voltages less than 200 volts is microamperage current of less than 1.0 mA.

Other important responses to the application of electric current to animal tissues and tissue cultures have been reported. These studies have provided important information that has led to the development of theories postulated to explain possible mechanisms by which electrical currents enhance tissue repair. A number of these theories are presented later in this chapter.

Cheng and colleagues[67] analyzed some of the biochemical effects that occur in rat skin tissue during stimulation with electric current. They reported that 10 to 1000 μA of CMDC applied to skin strips 0.5 mm thick for 2 hours in vitro increased the ATP concentration in the skin to five times. Optimal increased production of ATP occurred when the current amplitude was set at 500 μA. At 1000 μA, ATP generation was equal to concentrations measured in control skin. In addition, they also reported that 100 to 500 μA of CMDC increased amino acid uptake by 30 to 40 percent above control levels and that a current amplitude of 50 μA was required to obtain a maximal stimulation effect on protein synthesis.

The ability of electrical currents to increase production of ATP has also been demonstrated following stimulation of the thylakoid membrane in plant chloroplasts[68,69] (despite the absence of light) where photosynthesis occurs and in other animal tissues devoid of any metabolic energy.[70] In plants, energy produced by photosynthesis is stored as a proton gradient across the thylakoid membrane of chloroplasts.[71] In 1968, Mitchell[72,73] was awarded the Nobel Prize in Chemistry for his theory of chemiosmotic bioenergetics, which stated that the source of energy needed to phosphorylate ADP and ATP comes from energy stored as a proton gradient across the thylakoid membrane in chloroplasts of plants and the mitochondrial membrane in animals, rather than from a chemical intermediate containing a high-energy phosphate bond. The chemosmotic theory explains the results of studies that have shown how to maintain life in a plant cell by substituting electrical energy for light.[68,69] This same theory also explains why electrical energy is capable of stimulating repair of tissues compromised by hypoxia, injury, or nutritional deficiency.[74] In this regard, a proton gradient is created across mitochondrial membranes exposed to CMDC. The current produces this gradient when electrons at the cathode react with water to form hydroxyl ions, and acid and protons are formed at the anode. As a result, a proton gradient and a voltage gradient are established across the intervening tissues between the electrodes. The influence of the electric field and the proton concentration difference produce a proton or proticity current that moves from anode to cathode. As the migrating protons cross the mitochondrial membrane-bound H^+-ATPase, ATP is formed.[72,73] The increased ATP production stimulates amino-acid transport and these two factors both contribute to increased protein synthesis,[75,76] a most desirable response in chronic wounds in which protein destruction often exceeds protein generation.

In addition to biochemical changes that occur in animal tissues exposed to μA currents, there are other influences on cells created by currents applied to animal tissues and tissue cultures that may partly explain how biosynthesis of certain cells in vivo is enhanced or perhaps guided by the galvanotaxis influence of exogenously applied direct currents. Erickson and Nuccitelli[77] exposed developing fibroblasts from quail somites, cultured in plasma, to electric fields of between 1 and 10 mV per mm^2 and observed that the fibroblasts migrated toward the cathode. Dunn and associates[78] observed that fibroblast ingrowth and collagen fiber alignment are increased in collagen sponge matrix stimulated with between 20 and 100 μA of cathodal direct current. Bourguignon and Bourguignon[79] stimulated human fibroblasts growing in cell culture with 20 minutes of HVPC applied at various voltages and pulse rates and monitored protein and DNA synthesis using radioactively labeled precursors [^{3}H] proline and [^{3}H] thymidine, respectively. They found that at 2 hours after stimulation the fibroblasts significantly increased their rate of protein synthesis by 160 percent over controls with maximal synthesis occurring at 50 V and 100 pps with the cells positioned close to the cathode. When the fibroblasts were positioned close to the anode, the maximal rate of protein synthesis was only 120 percent of the unstimulated controls and required a stimulus amplitude of 150 V. In addition, these investigators also reported a significant increase in DNA production between 2 and 24 hours after stimulation with maximal synthesis also occurring close to the cathode at 75 V and 100 pps. At these voltages and pulse rate, the time-averaged current flowing through the culture chamber during the 20-minute stimulation period did not exceed 50 μA. This finding suggests that HVPC devices are capable of delivering μA levels of current that are voltage and frequency dependent. The findings reported from this in vitro study further suggest that as a consequence to increasing protein and DNA synthesis by HVPC stimulation, collagen synthesis and fibroblast proliferation also increase. There is also evidence that current levels no greater than 500 picoamperes can stimulate macromolecular synthesis in living cells.[80,81] Unfortunately, various commercial enterprises have extrapolated the information from animal and tissue culture studies to explain how μA currents applied exogenously to injured tissues in vivo restore disturbed endogenous bioelectric activity back to its preinjured state.

Epidermal cell migration may also be influenced by exogenous electric currents.

Cooper and Schliwa[82] have exposed isolated fish epidermal cells to electric currents of 50 mV/mm and higher. They reported that single epidermal cells, cell clusters, and cell sheets migrated toward the cathode. Interestingly, by using a variety of calcium channel antagonists they were able to block the migration of cells that were simultaneously exposed to externally applied electric current field. Alvarez and associates[25] treated induced partial-thickness skin wounds in pigs and, compared with controls, they showed a highly significant increase in the collagen synthetic capacity and rate of epithelialization in wounds treated with 50 to 300 μA of anodal CMDC. Winter[83] has found that epidermal cells undergoing migration during re-epithelialization across wounds in pig skin have their origin in a bordering strip of intact skin less than 0.5 mm wide around the perimeter of the wound. Jaffe and Vanable[84] have shown that a substantial voltage gradient tends to occur in this area and that cellular movement may be enhanced by this endogenous voltage gradient. Of clinical significance is the finding that when the perimeter of superficial wounds is allowed to dry, this lateral voltage gradient is suppressed or eliminated, which probably explains why dry superficial wounds heal more slowly than wounds that are kept moist. As a matter of fact, Winter[83] has demonstrated that moist healing wounds are covered by epidermis twice as quickly as wounds exposed to the air.

Other mechanisms have been proposed to explain the observations that electrical currents accelerate the rate of soft-tissue healing including stimulation of cellular metabolism by elevation of tissue temperature, alteration of the wound microenvironment pH, and release of metallic ions from stainless steel electrodes resulting in cellular biosynthesis. However, neither temperature, ion release, nor pH changes have been demonstrated in previous studies.[66,79]

Effects of Bioelectric Stimulation on Cutaneous Oxygen Supply

Dodgen and associates[85] tested the effects of electrical stimulation on the transcutaneous partial pressure of oxygen (tc-Po$_2$) in 30 diabetic subjects. Ten patients were assigned to one of three groups receiving transcutaneous electrical stimulation either by positive or negative monophasic, paired spiked waveforms or by a symmetric biphasic square waveform. All three groups received submotor stimulation. The tc-Po$_2$ was monitored 30 minutes before stimulation, during the 30 minutes of submotor stimulation, and 30 minutes after stimulation was stopped, and these values were compared with a prestimulation baseline. Compared with prestimulation values, tc-Po$_2$ was found to increase significantly in each of the three groups during stimulation and following stimulation. The authors reported finding no statistically significant differences in tc-Po$_2$ changes among the three different stimulation groups. The mechanism of action of bioelectric stimulation on increasing the tc-Po$_2$ appears to be unrelated to polarity and does not require any net ion flow.[85] These results seem to indicate that electrical stimulation increases cutaneous circulation in diabetic subjects and, therefore, may be useful in augmenting wound healing in diabetics and in other patient populations known to have difficulty in healing skin ulcers—for example, in the elderly and in the spinal cord injured.

Another similarly designed study was carried out in 1988 by Gagnier and co-workers,[86] who tested the effects of electrical stimulation on cutaneous oxygen supply in paraplegics. Ten paraplegic subjects were treated with three different waveforms of electrical stimulation in three separate sessions. Their cutaneous oxygen tension was measured with an oximeter 30 minutes before stimulation, during stimulation, and 30 minutes after stimulation had stopped. The three stimulation waveforms used were monophasic paired spike (MPS) of positive polarity, biphasic pulsed current (BPC), and alternating current (AC). No other stimulus variables were given. The authors found statistically significant increases in cutaneous oxygen tension after 30 minutes of stimulation with MPS and BPC, but not after stimulation with AC. At the end of the poststimulation period (30 minutes after stimulation had stopped), all three waveforms produced significant increases in tc-Po$_2$. Therefore, the authors concluded that any of these three waveforms may be used to enhance wound healing by increasing the cutaneous oxygen tension. Preliminary studies that have used different variations of pulsed and alternating currents to increase the tc-Po$_2$ look promising. However, additional clinical studies are required to further delineate optimal stimulus variables for increasing tc-Po$_2$. The role of tc-Po$_2$ in dermal wound healing also needs additional clarification before clinicians use this treatment approach to facilitate the healing of skin ulcers.

Thus far, we have reviewed pertinent literature to identify how wound tissues in humans and animals, and how cells in tissue cultures and in vivo, are influenced by the application of electrical currents having different characteristics and variables. We have also reviewed how bioelectric stimulation affects cutaneous oxygen tension. Next, we shall discuss the bactericidal effects of electrical stimulation.

Bactericidal Effects of Electrical Stimulation

Wound healing is retarded when infection is present. The use of electrical stimulation to retard or destroy infecting pathogens in in vivo and in vitro models has been documented. Rowley[87] produced bactericidal effects in vitro on Escherichia coli B growth rates using cathodal constant microamperage direct current (CDMC). Rowley and colleagues[88] demonstrated a similar effect using 1.0 mA of CMDC on rabbit-skin wounds infected with Pseudomonas aeruginosa. In another report by Barranco and coworkers,[89] the use of cathodal DC produced a decrease in Staphylococcus aureus growth rates in infected rat and rabbit femurs after stimulation lasting 1 hour.

Wheeler and associates[11] used cathodal direct current to suppress proliferation of pathogens in clinically noninfected human decubitus ulcers during the first 3 days of treatment and also began and continued cathodal treatment of infected ulcers until resolution of infection was determined by pathogen-free cultures. The authors proposed two mechanisms by which cathodal DC stimulation decreased pathogens. First, they postulated that continuous cathodal DC bombarded organisms with electrons, which continually excited cell membranes. They proposed that this stimulation depletes the bacterial substrate and results in death of the organism. The second mechanism they proposed suggested that suppression of diffusion-regulating mechanisms occurred within the protective cell membrane.

Galvanotaxis, or the attraction of cells to the anode or cathode, has been reported in a number of studies. Macrophages migrate toward the cathode,[90] while neutrophils migrate toward both the anode and the cathode.[91,92] However, Dineur[93] and Monguio[91] have reported that leukocytes migrate toward the cathode in regions where infection or inflammation are present. Perhaps the documented bactericidal effect of cathodal CMDC[10,15,94] is the result of attracting phagocytic macrophages and leukocytes to infected tissues rather than from detrimental effects on pathogens caused by electrolysis or raising the tissue pH. Perhaps the galvanotaxis of macrophages to the infected wound tissues exposed to cathodal stimulation occurs secondary to creation of a hypoxic, alkaline environment for which macrophages may have an affinity.

Interestingly, Eberhardt and coworkers[95] have reported an alteration in cell composition of human skin exudate following transcutaneous electrical stimulation. They applied rectangular pulses having a duration of 1 mS and a frequency of 100 pps at 3 to 35 mA for 30 minutes to the skin, 5 cm above and below a 0.5 cm² scarified patch of skin on the flexor surface of the forearm. Between 6 and 9 hours after sensory level stimulation, they found that neutrophilic granulocytes accounted for 63.5 percent of 500 sampled exudate granulocyte and mononuclear cells, compared with 44.7 percent for controls. They also indicated that mononuclear cells such as macrophages and lymphocytes were not observed in the exudate of electrically stimulated forearms until between 9 and 12 hours after stimulation. The authors speculated that because the electrodes straddled the skin injury site, the increased percentage of neutrophils may have been due to an increase in blood flow and that galvanotaxis was not responsible for altering the exudative cell composition.

ELECTRICAL CURRENTS AVAILABLE FOR WOUND HEALING APPLICATIONS

Low Voltage, Constant Microamperage Direct Current (CMDC)

CMDC is the continuous unidirectional flow of charged particles in which the direction of movement of the charged particles does not reverse or cease during the treatment period.[96] This type of current, shown in Figure 12–1A, is delivered to the wound tissues with an electrode that either has a positive (anode) or negative (cathode) charge. Ideally, the amplitude of the current should remain constant, which means that as tissue impedance changes, the voltage also changes to maintain the current at a constant amplitude. Traditionally, this µA current is applied to the wound tissues at between 0.2 and 1.0 mA (200 to 1000 µA). Electrochemical reactions with ions in the tissues may raise the pH to alkalinity forming at the cathode or lower it to acidity forming at the anode. The alkalinity (NaOH) reaction produced at the cathode may be used clinically for its bactericidal effect or as an adjunct to debridement because of its sclerolytic ability to solubilize thrombi[57] and necrotic tissue. The acidity (HCl) reaction produced at the anode has the opposite effect of sclerosing tissue and coagulating blood leaking from small vessels. The latter effect may also augment closure of the wound by producing a congealed scar. Electrotherapeutic devices that deliver CMDC and are specifically intended for wound healing may be commercially available in the near future pending approval by the United States Food and Drug Administration (FDA). However, a low voltage electrotherapeutic device that provides less than 150 V of CMDC with a calibrated digital LED or analog meter readout in the 0 to 1000 µA range would be appropriate if available. A detailed protocol for the use of CMDC is presented later in this chapter. Low voltage, constant direct current devices that provide current output in the mA range may be used to iontophoretically repel select ions into wound tissue to promote healing; however, this technique is not documented by controlled clinical studies.

Low Voltage, Pulsed Microamperage Current

Figure 12–1B shows variations of a waveform that may be generated by low voltage devices that deliver µA current as either constant polarity monophasic pulses or as reversing polarity "biphasic" pulses through paired probe or carbonized rubber

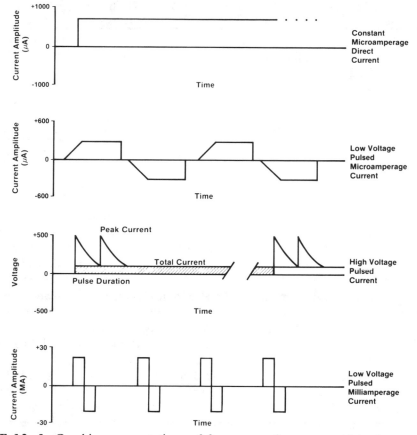

FIGURE 12–1. Graphic representations of four types of current used in the treatment of chronic wounds as described in the literature. *A*) Constant microamperage direct current; polarity may be reversed. *B*) Low-voltage pulsed microamperage current; polarity may be constant or alternately reversed. *C*) High-voltage pulsed current; polarity may be reversed. *D*) Low-voltage pulsed milliamperage current.

electrodes. As mentioned previously, the use of this form of current for treating wounds is poorly documented primarily by testimonial and commercial claims.

High Voltage, Monophasic Pulsed Current

High voltage, monophasic pulsed current is delivered to treatment electrodes as twin-peaked pulses that may be of either positive or negative polarity, with respect to a nontreatment electrode. The duration of the pulse is fixed but varies from one commercial device to another within a range of 45 to 100 μsec. The twin-peaked waveform as shown in Figure 12–1C may be delivered to the tissue at pulse rates between 1 and 125 pps. The voltage required to drive the short-duration, high-peak current pulses into the tissue is necessarily high as explained by the classic inverse relationship between the amplitude of a pulse and its duration. This relationship requires that for very short pulse durations (45 to 100 μsec), the peak currents must be very high (2000 to 2500 mA) and, therefore, the driving voltage must also be high (up to 500 V). However, at this voltage level, the maximal total current reaching the tissues is only 2.5 mA when delivered

TABLE 12–2. Peak and Total Current Generated by a High Voltage Pulsed Current Device at Five Voltage Output Settings

Volts	Peak Current (amperes)	Total Current	
		mA	*μA*
500	2500	2.5	2500
400	2000	2.0	2000
300	1500	1.5	1500
200*	1000	1.0	1000
100	500	0.5	500

*At 200 V, the current delivered to treatment electrodes is approximately 1000 μA. For wound healing applications, the driving voltage is usually closer to 100 V.

through electrodes of standard size. Clinically for wound healing applications, the driving force behind the current need not exceed 200 V, which means that the total current delivered to the tissues per second at sensory perception is in the μA range since it does not exceed 1.0 mA (1000 μA). Table 12–2 shows the relationship between various voltage levels and the total current delivered from an HVPC device. Since, in treating wounds with HVPC, a sensory level of stimulation from the anode has been shown to accelerate tissue repair[14] this means that the voltage level should always be less than 200 V—and usually less than 100 V. Thus, as shown in Table 12–2, the current delivered to wound tissues from HVPC devices at voltages less than 200 V is in the μA current range.

As previously mentioned, HVPC devices deliver monophasic pulses and, therefore, the polarity of the treatment electrodes can be biased with either a positive or a negative charge. However, unlike CMDC, HVPC applied at therapeutically tolerated voltages does not alter skin pH at either the anode or the cathode.[66] This means that the quantity of charge delivered to wound tissues with HVPC devices is insufficient to cause electrochemical reactions. Therefore, HVPC is not direct current and should not be expected to solubilize thrombi and necrotic tissue or to be bactericidal at the cathode; nor should the anode be expected to coagulate blood leaking from small vessels or to form scar tissue through a sclerosing effect. Additional controlled clinical studies are needed to confirm HVPC as an efficacious alternative for treating chronic wounds.

Low Voltage, Pulsed Milliamperage Current

This type of current is characteristic of traditional transcutaneous electrical nerve stimulation (TENS) devices, which often produce symmetric biphasic pulses as shown in Figure 12–1D. Because the quantity of charge contained in the two symmetric phases of each pulse is equal, the accumulation of charge residual in the tissues is zero. When there is zero net charge accumulation in the tissue, there is no polarity and no electrochemical reactions to produce tissue irritation despite the fact that the total current delivered to the tissues may be as high as 30 mA. In some traditional TENS devices, the charge quantity contained in the two phases of each pulse may not be exactly equal. When this phase asymmetry occurs, a small negative or positive charge residual accumulates in the tissues creating slight irritation secondary to minimal electrochemical polarity reactions. In this case when both electrodes are applied to the skin rather than to wound tissue, as they are with traditional TENS devices, the irritation may be observed as a transient skin erythema following treatment.

As previously mentioned, pulsed currents of this type have been applied transcutaneously to the webspace of the hand and through some unknown mechanism, resulted in healing of dermal ulcers in the ipsilateral lower extremity.[37] Traditional TENS devices usually allow the user to select a wide range of pulse rates from 1 to 125 pps and to vary the pulse duration from 20 to 250 μsec. The successful stimulus variables described by Kaada[37,38] include eliciting a motor response with 15 to 30 mA for 30 to 45 minutes, three times daily at two to five bursts per second. Obviously, these studies need to be replicated with patients using a controlled research design.

THEORETIC BASIS FOR USING ELECTRICAL STIMULATION TO STIMULATE ENDOGENOUS BIOCIRCUITS

The generally accepted physiologic wound repair processes were presented in Part I of this text. This section outlines observed endogenous electrical phenomena present in living organisms and presents theories that support the use of electrical stimulation for tissue repair (ESTR) and for stimulating endogenous bioelectric circuits. Investigators have documented the effects of electrical energy on growth and control processes in living organisms for many years. In 1925, Lund[97] demonstrated the presence of potential gradients in the marine organism obelia, a member of the phylum Coelenterata. He found a potential gradient between different parts of the organism's living cells. When an opposing potential difference was introduced across the surface of the organism, the growth of the cells was inhibited. When the potential difference was added, Lund[96] was able to orient the direction of growth toward the positive potential.

Sinyukhin[98] found that by applying extra current (2 to 3 mA) for 5 days to tomato plants whose branches were cut, the branches would grow back up to three times faster than control plants. He also found that the polarity had to match the polarity normally found in the tomato plant in order for these results to occur. In addition, he observed that when the opposite polarity was used, regrowth of the branches was slowed by 2 or 3 weeks. These studies and others[99-102] have demonstrated that endogenous electrical currents do exist in living organisms and that the growth and control of living organisms may be modulated and controlled by exogenously applied currents.

By understanding the relationship between endogenous electrical currents and the effect they may have on the growth and control of living organisms, the clinician may gain additional insight into the treatment of dermal ulcers with electrotherapeutic currents. As these theories are refined and optimal therapeutic currents are identified, wound healing and tissue regeneration, as we know it today, may be revolutionized in the not too distant future.

SKIN BATTERY VOLTAGES

The skin possesses electrical properties that may influence wound healing. In 1860, DuBois-Reymond[103] detected current flowing through wounded mammalian skin. Herlitzka[104] confirmed current flow quantitatively at about 1 μA of current for each millimeter of wounded tissue in human epidermal finger wounds that were immersed in saline. Illingworth and Barker[105] measured currents present in the vicinity of regenerating fingertips immersed in saline, in children who had undergone accidental amputation. These measurements were made at 1- to 7-day intervals following amputation until two successive readings of zero current were obtained. They found that the

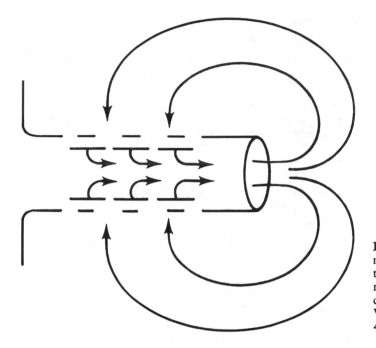

FIGURE 12–2. Endogenous current flow driven by the skin battery in an experimentally amputated salamander limb (From Borgens, Vanable, and Jaffe,[106] p. 4532, with permission).

measurements rose to a peak average current of 22 μA/cm^2 after an average of 8 days. Interestingly, Borgens and associates[106] described a similar peak average current of 60 μA/cm^2 found in injured salamanders after an average of 4 days. In both of these studies, the measured currents flowed out of the injured stump and through a conducting medium forming an electrical shunt between the inside and outside of the skin (Fig. 12–2).

This skin battery potential was also observed in 1945 by Cunliff-Barnes,[107] who detected a positive potential on the inside surface of the intact skin adjacent to wounded tissue. After the wound healed, the positive potential ceased. In 1982, Barker, Jaffe, and Vanable[108] measured skin battery potentials across cavy (guinea pig) skin and found that the interior of the cavy body was always electropositive with respect to the outside of the cavy, and that the negative potentials on the surface ranged from −4 mV, in regions where hair was abundant, to almost −80 mV in areas where hair was sparse (e.g., ear, footpad). Foulds and Barker[109] also found similar patterns when determining skin battery voltages on humans (Fig. 12–3). The surface of human skin was also found to be negative with respect to the inside deeper skin layers. Relatively hairless regions of the feet and hands displayed higher negative potentials than hairy regions such as the scalp. When Jaffe and Vanable[84] made slits into the cavy's skin, they measured a current flow that they described as a positive charge, apparently driven by the cavy's skin battery. They hypothesized that this battery is located in the epidermis or "living layer." When deeper slits were made through the stratum corneum, the current amplitude progressively increased until the depth of the slits approached the dermis (Fig. 12–4). At that depth, the current began decreasing as subsequent slits were made deeper and deeper into the dermis. The potential difference measured across intact skin in relation to wounds that extend through the epidermis is zero, suggesting that the source of the skin battery is the epidermis.

Furthermore, the authors contend that this skin battery is driven by a sodium ion pump. When amiloride (a compound that blocks sodium ion channels of the outer

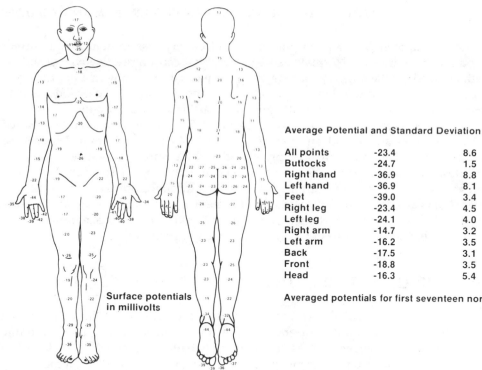

Average Potential and Standard Deviation		
All points	-23.4	8.6
Buttocks	-24.7	1.5
Right hand	-36.9	8.8
Left hand	-36.9	8.1
Feet	-39.0	3.4
Right leg	-23.4	4.5
Left leg	-24.1	4.0
Right arm	-14.7	3.2
Left arm	-16.2	3.5
Back	-17.5	3.1
Front	-18.8	3.5
Head	-16.3	5.4

Surface potentials in millivolts

Averaged potentials for first seventeen normals

FIGURE 12–3. Average human skin battery potential measured on a typical subject aged 29. The exterior of the skin was found to be electro-negative with respect to the inside of the body. Measured in millivolts (from Foulds and Barker,[109] p. 517, with permission).

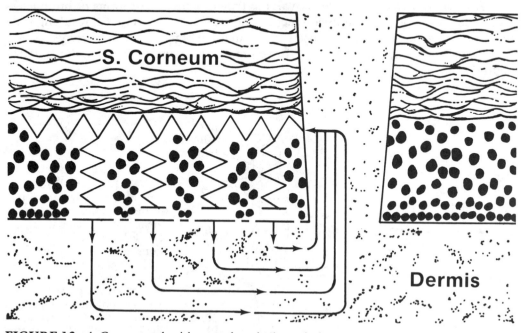

FIGURE 12–4. Current path with wound made through the stratum corneum in the guinea pig skin. The skin battery drives positive charges inward that escape through the wound and returns to the region between the stratum corneum and dermis. Only current on the left side is depicted (from Jaffe and Vanable,[84] p. 36, with permission).

epidermal membrane) was applied, the epidermal battery was inhibited and current flow could not be detected. Normally, sodium ions that carry a positive charge diffuse through channels in the outer membrane of epidermal cells, resulting in a net transport of positive charge across the skin from inside to outside. Therefore, the region closer to the wound is more strongly positive than regions farther from the wound. This closer region is referred to as the lateral voltage gradient (LVG). Jaffe and Vanable[84] measured the LVG six times and found an average value of 140 ± 20 mV/mm. When they applied an external current source to the wound and measured the voltage gradients, current flowed as long as the wound was moistened with Ringer's solution. When the wound was allowed to dry, the current flow stopped. Evidence previously presented in Chapter 9 suggests that a moist wound environment is necessary for optimal wound healing, and these findings further suggest that wound hydration is required if the endogenous electrical properties of skin are to function properly.

CURRENT OF INJURY (INJURY POTENTIALS)

The skin battery potentials previously described following newt limb amputation are characterized by sodium ion currents that flow out of the injured stump[106] and into the proximal stump. Current values found in skin battery potentials just described immediately after injury to the integument are lower than those found when measuring injury potentials that are present following amputation. Skin battery voltages rise to a maximal value some days after injury.[105] Injury potentials, on the other hand, have maximal values immediately after tissue injury, like amputation, and have been explained by Becker and associates[110] to be carried within the body by a DC semiconductor network.

This DC is a constant or slowly varying type of current. All forms of life possess measurable DC potentials on their intact exterior surfaces. The potential resulting from this DC can be measured and has been shown to be an organized field patterned closely to the gross anatomic arrangement of the central nervous system (CNS) as illustrated in Figure 12–5.

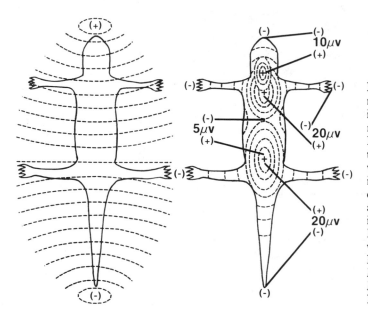

FIGURE 12–5. Direct current field arrangement found in the amphibian by measurement. The potential of the DC field as well as the relationship to the central nervous system is shown. Arrows indicate the location of standard electrode placement and average potentials measured in millivolts (Adapted from Becker,[110] p. 1170. Reprinted with permission from the New York State Journal of Medicine, copyright by the Medical Society of the State of New York).

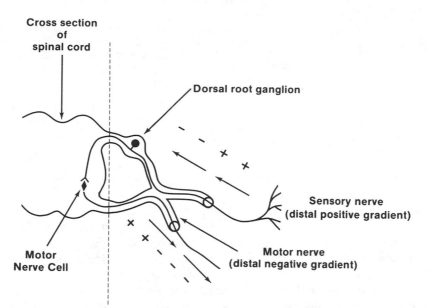

FIGURE 12–6. Cross section of spinal cord and peripheral nerves demonstrating direct current flow and polarity of the motor (output) peripheral nerves and sensory (input) peripheral nerves in the salamander (Adapted from Becker,[110] p. 1173. Reprinted with permission from the New York State Journal of Medicine, copyright by the Medical Society of the State of New York).

This complex electrical field configuration was mapped out on the salamander by Becker and associates[111] who identified areas of relative positive potential over the cranial, brachial, and lumbar cellular aggregates of the neuraxis. These potentials became increasingly negative along the peripheral nerve outflows extending into the extremities (Fig. 12–6). These measured DC potentials have been shown to be completely unrelated to action potentials, which result from membrane depolarization and ion flow. Evidence suggests that there is a continuous flow of moving charges present in this DC system, similar to the size and flow of electrons in a wire connected to a battery.[112] However, conduction similar to that which occurs in a metallic wire can be eliminated from consideration because current flow in tissues does not occur by movement of electrons. Becker[111,113,114] suggests that the DC system operates within the nerve fiber similar to the way a semiconductor works.

Semiconduction occurs, for example, in the germanium crystal when it is "doped" with an impurity. Germanium atoms are normally surrounded by four outer electrons in an orderly lattice-like structure (Fig. 12–7). When an impurity such as an arsenic atom (which has five outer electrons) is added to the germanium atom, there is an extra electron that does not fit into the crystal lattice and is free to move about (Fig. 12–8).

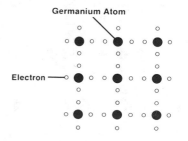

FIGURE 12–7. Schematic of a germanium crystal where each germanium atom is surrounded by four outer electrons in an orderly lattice-like fashion (Adapted from Giancoli, DC: Physics, Prentice-Hall, Inc, Englewood Cliffs, NJ, 1980, p. 502).

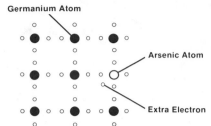

FIGURE 12–8. Schematic of a germanium crystal doped with an arsenic atom. Since arsenic atoms normally have five outer electrons, the fifth or "extra" electron is now free to move about in the crystal lattice. Because the electron is negatively charged and can carry an electric current, this structure is referred to as an n-type semiconductor (Adapted from Giancoli, DC: Physics. Prentice-Hall, Inc, Englewood Cliffs, NJ, 1980, p. 502).

This type of semiconduction is referred to as n-type, because the electrons (negative charge) can carry an electric current.

When an impurity (eg., a gallium atom), which consists of three outer electrons, is added to germanium, a "hole" in the lattice network, like that seen in Figure 12–9, occurs to allow electrons to "jump" into this hole and fill it (Fig. 12–10). The result is that a new hole opens in the lattice next to or adjacent to the original hole, leaving a net positive charge at the new hole. As an electron fills this new hole, another hole opens up and the process repeats itself. This is referred to as p-type semiconduction, because the positive holes carry the electric current. Although semiconductors can carry only small currents, they do allow for mobile electrons to flow as a current over long distance without losing energy.

When a stimulus (trauma, amputation, anesthesia, electricity, and so on) is applied to living organisms, its measured DC surface potentials change. Becker and associates[110] measured these surface DC changes after fracturing one of the long bones in the hind limb of a salamander. They noted DC potential changes, which progressed up the neuraxis to the cranium after a delay of only 2 seconds. This activity suggested that the DC semiconductor system transmits data regarding the injury and that the change in surface potential is a record of the injury data transmitted. After further work, Becker[115] provided evidence that suggests that the postulated DC semiconductor system is composed of Schwann cell sheaths in the periphery, satellite cells in the dorsal root ganglion, and glial cells in the CNS. These structures were previously thought to be only mechanically supportive and nutritive to the CNS. However, when the DC system is stimulated by trauma, Becker[115] has proposed that it produces a "current of injury."

As mentioned earlier, DC surface potentials demonstrate polarity differences. These polarity differences can be measured directly over peripheral nerves with a positive gradient found over sensory nerves and a negative gradient located over motor nerves[110] (Fig. 12–5). This observation provides a theoretic mechanism whereby charges in the DC system can return to their source and complete the electrical circuit. The DC system

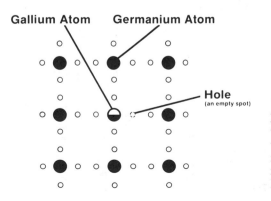

FIGURE 12–9. Schematic of germanium crystal doped with a gallium atom that has only three outer electrons. This configuration results in a "hole" in the lattice structure (Adapted from Giancoli, DC: Physics. Prentice-Hall, Inc, Englewood Cliffs, NJ, 1980, p. 502).

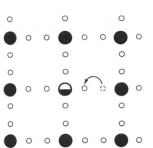

FIGURE 12–10. Schematic of a germanium crystal doped with a gallium atom as in Figure 12–8. An electron "jumps" from the germanium atom to a hole in the gallium atom's outer shell and fills it. This results in "movement" of the hole to the right. This activity is referred to as p-type semi conduction because it leaves a net positive charge at the new hole and these positive holes carry the electric current (Adapted from Giancoli, DC: Physics. Prentice-Hall, Inc, Englewood Cliffs, NJ, 1980, p. 502).

is also thought to operate as a part of the total growth and control system in living organisms. Contributions from local damaged cells and other systems may also stimulate the repair of cells. This notion is depicted in Figure 12–11.

Current of Injury in Regenerating Versus Nonregenerating Species

The current of injury was measured by Becker[116] in 14 salamanders (capable of regenerating amputated body parts) and 14 frogs (not capable of regenerating amputated body parts) after amputation of the right forelimbs between elbow and wrists. The polarity at the stump in the injured frogs and salamanders reversed from about −10 mV to +20 mV at the end of the first day. Voltages in the salamanders then began dropping, and by the third day, the salamanders showed no current at all, while the frog's currents remained about the same. Between days 6 and 10, the salamander's potentials began reversing again from positive to negative. Between days 10 and 20, these currents reached a peak of more than −30 mV just as blastemas began emerging from the salamander stumps. Meanwhile, the frogs exhibited slowly declining positive voltages as their stumps healed over with scar tissue and skin. The injury potentials of both groups of animals returned to the original baseline of −10 mV between days 20 and 25, as seen in Figure 12–12.

Based on these findings, Becker[116] has attempted to complete regrowth in a normally nonregenerating animal by applying negative "injury current" voltages to the amputated forelegs of frogs. After the experiment failed to stimulate full regrowth of amputated frog limbs, he applied 2 μA of positive DC for 5 to 10 minutes to the

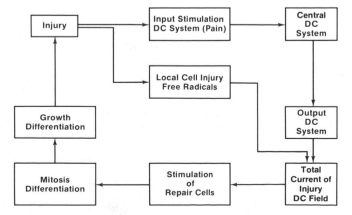

FIGURE 12–11. The theoretic direct current control system involved with local responses to injury (Adapted from Becker,[115] p. 5 Reprinted with permission from the New York State Journal of Medicine, copyright by the Medical Society of the State of New York).

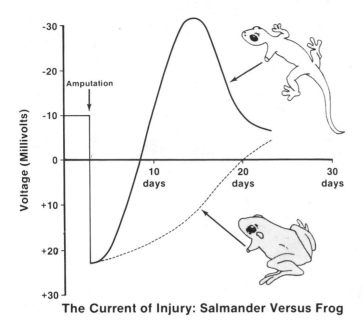

The Current of Injury: Salmander Versus Frog

FIGURE 12–12. Injury potentials measured in regenerating (salamanders) and non-regenerating (frogs) animals. Positive voltages (millivolts) were recorded by the end of the first day in both animals. The salamanders demonstrated a polarity reversal during regeneration while the frogs demonstrated slowly declining positive voltages as they scarred over (Adapted from Becker,[116] p. 73).

amputated limb stumps of salamanders during the 5 days following amputation. His intention was to reinforce the normal positive peak that occurred in the current of injury previously described. To a second group of salamanders, he applied 3 μA of negative current to amputated limbs on the fifth to ninth days, thereby approximating the injury currents that were normally generating negative peaks. Anodal stimulation made the blastemas larger but slowed down limb regeneration. Cathodal stimulation increased the rate of limb regrowth for a week but did not change the time required to regenerate a complete limb.

These failures eventually led Becker to revise and expand his theories to include the electrical properties of the epidermis as well. In 1979, Becker's associate, James Cullen,[117] discovered that when the sciatic nerve in a non-regenerating animal (rat) was sutured to the epidermis after experimental hind limb amputation, electrical potentials could be measured that followed the same injury potential curve characteristics found in the salamander. The only major difference was that the magnitude of the voltage was much greater (Fig. 12–13). Furthermore, as seen in Figure 12–14, they found that in

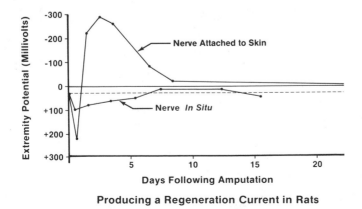

Producing a Regeneration Current in Rats

FIGURE 12–13. Injury potentials measured in rats when an artificial neuroepidermal junction was formed. This injury potential curve exhibits the same potential curves found in the regenerating salamander. The only major difference in potential curves is the amplitude of the voltage (Adapted from Becker,[117] p, 159).

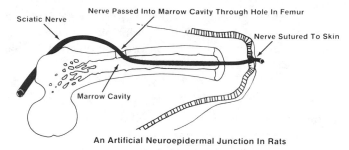

FIGURE 12–14. Artificial neuroepidermal junction in rats (Adapted from Becker,[117] p. 158).

those animals where an artificial neuroepidermal junction was formed (nerve sutured to skin), not only did surrounding tissues regenerate, but partial regeneration of their thigh bones occurred as well. Neuroepidermal junctions consist of nerve fibers joining epidermal cells, and this junction can be likened to a plug fitting into a socket (Fig. 12–15). This "plug-and-socket" arrangement can be viewed as a completion of the DC circuit, allowing for a return of charges to their source. The fact that a neuroepidermal junction was required for experimental bone regeneration to occur in a normally nonregenerating animal is astonishing.

VASCULAR-INTERSTITIAL CLOSED CIRCUIT (VICC)

A third theory suggesting that the body possesses bioelectric circuits and currents contained within the vasculature has been proposed by Nordenstrom.[118] His proposal that a vascular-interstitial closed circuit (VICC) exists in the human body, is based on more than 20 years of research and medical practice and was published in 1983 in his

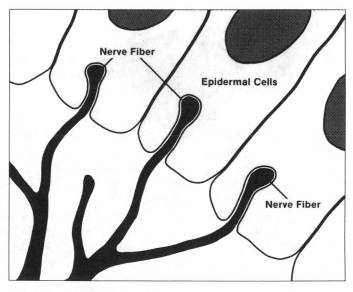

FIGURE 12–15. Schematic of a neuroepidermal junction. The nerve fiber fits into epidermal cells much like a plug fits into a socket (Adapted from Becker,[117] p. 58).

The Neuroepidermal Junction

book.[118] Although most of Nordenstrom's work was performed on cancer patients, an extrapolation of his work and principles applied to soft-tissue healing may prove beneficial once the effects of electrical stimulation on blood flow and angiogenesis are better understood.

Nordenstrom[118] has proposed that bioelectricity is conducted through five main components that may be found in any vascularized part of the body within:

1. Insulating walls of blood vessels
2. Conducting intravascular plasma
3. Insulating tissue matrix (possibly including lymph vessels)
4. Conducting interstitial fluid
5. Electrical junctions for redox reactions (transcapillary junctions)

Nordenstrom reportedly has measured a relatively higher electrical resistance present in the walls of large blood vessels and a relative lower electrical resistance in plasma and interstitial fluids,[118] giving rise to a potential voltage gradient. The vessel walls in this bioelectric circuit act as electrically conducting, insulating cables that carry plasma (the conducting media) and separate it from its surroundings with the other branch of the conducting media (the interstitial fluid) except at its transcapillary junctions (the naturally occurring electrodes in this biocircuit).

The capillary cell membranes act as naturally charged electrodes, which allows ions to move through the cells via gates and vesicles. Additional ions flow between the cells through pores. This local ion flow stops when excess electrons cross enzyme bridges in the capillary walls, closing the pores and gates and thereby closing the local circuit. This occurrence creates a long distance bioelectric circuit in which the ions flow. These capillary cell membranes therefore appear to be the key component in switching the local ion flow across the capillary membranes to long-distance ion flow down the capillary walls.

An accumulation of charge (excessive electrons) can occur as a result of soft-tissue injury or even after normal muscle use. This accumulation of charge can constrict arterial capillaries, switching the current on as previously mentioned. However, venous capillaries do not constrict in an electrical field; therefore, ions and charged cells such as white blood cells can migrate through the pores of a leaky venous capillary near the injury. Because the electric potential from an injury has been found to oscillate, an ebb and flow of charged cells and ions necessary for healing may occur as changes take place in the electrical insulation properties of the capillary membranes. It is unclear how this and other bioelectric circuits function together after exogenous electrical currents are applied to the wound. Because all three theories just described are compatible with one another, healing of wounds with published electrotherapeutic protocols due to one or a combination of these mechanisms.

The therapeutic application of electrical currents for healing is in its infancy. A better understanding of the correlations between inner-injury currents and outer-skin battery voltages will certainly have significant ramifications in selecting and applying electrotherapeutic currents to augment soft-tissue repair. Clearly, electrically mediated repair processes are present in living organisms, and the future may show that exogenous electrical currents will indeed favorably and predictably augment soft-tissue repair, limb regeneration, and growth and control processes. It is hoped that future research will be directly aimed at unlocking and using the regenerative secrets that appear to be inherent to "lower forms" of life. This knowledge may also prove beneficial in fighting various diseases and advancing repairative processes in humans in ways that are inconceivable at present.

CONTRAINDICATIONS TO USING ELECTRICAL STIMULATION TO PROMOTE WOUND HEALING

Before considering electrical stimulation as a treatment intervention for chronic wounds, one should eliminate the diagnosis of osteomyelitis, which is often manifested by deep pain and systemic signs of infection. Osteomyelitis may occur secondary to wound infection and arise at the end of the shaft of a long bone such as the distal tibial metaphysis. Electrical stimulation should not be used to promote wound healing in the presence of osteomyelitis because covering the infected bone with healed soft tissue does nothing to halt the active bone infection that ultimately may form an abscess and recurring breakdown of the healed soft tissue.

Electrical currents should not be applied to wound tissues that contain neoplastic cells. Although there is insufficient evidence, electric currents may enhance proliferation and/or migration of neoplastic cells or may promote cellular dedifferentiation leading to enhancement of cancerous growth.

When topical substances containing metal ions, such as povidone-iodine and mercurochrome, are used in wounds for their bacteriostatic effect, all residues of the ions should be flushed from the wound before treating it with electrical current. This flushing is especially important when CMDC is being used because ions having the same polarity as the DC will be driven iontophoretically into the wound tissue, which may promote development of wound tissue toxicity or irritation. Some individuals may develop allergic reactions to electrical current of any type. This reaction may be manifested by development of dermatitis under an electrode applied to the skin or as an erythematous wheal reaction under the electrode.

Individuals with demand-type cardiac pacemakers should not be treated with electrical stimulation because the electrical current may interfere with the pacemaker rhythm, leading to cardiac arrhythmia. Electrodes from electrical stimulation should not be placed over the thorax tangential to the heart, over the carotid sinus, or over the laryngeal musculature.

CLINICAL DECISION MAKING

The following patient case studies will serve as models for selecting appropriate electrotherapeutic currents and waveforms to stimulate tissue repair, improve microcirculation, and decrease bacterial colonization.

Case A

PATIENT HISTORY

A 65-year-old woman with diabetes mellitus and an infected Stage IV decubitus ulcer on her left greater trochanter is referred for treatment. The ulcer has existed for 6 months.

OBJECTIVE FINDINGS

The ulcer measures 4.6 cm wide × 4.3 cm long × 2.2 cm deep. In addition, tunneling is present that is 0.4 cm wide and extends 2.7 cm inferiorly and parallel to the shaft of the femur. The ulcer is infected with Staphylococcus aureus and has a moderate amount of necrotic tissue over 50 percent of the wound. The patient has an air fluidized pressure-relieving device.

TREATMENT PLAN AND RATIONALE

Cathodal CMDC applied to the wound is recommended at an amplitude of 200 to 1000 μA for 2 to 4 hours, 5 to 7 days per week, until wound asepsis occurs. The anode should be placed closer to the spinal cord or cephalically in relation to the cathode whenever possible (Fig. 12–16A). Cathodal stimulation is used initially for its bactericidal effect, which may occur as a result of the galvanotaxis of macrophages, neutrophils, and leukocytes. Bacteriostatic effects of CMDC may also be occurring because of alkaline tissue pH and/or destruction of bacterial cell membranes. Additionally, cathodal stimulation can solubilize necrotic tissue as a result of its sclerolytic ability.

The tunnelized area must be loosely filled with saline moistened gauze to conduct the current. If the tunneling does not fill in with vitalized granulation tissue or an abscess occurs, then surgical debridement may be necessary. After the infection clears, anodal wound stimulation should begin. The clinician may choose to continue with CMDC or switch to high voltage, monophasic pulsed current (HVPC). Studies previously cited report effective wound healing with HVPC with less daily treatment time, that is, 45 minutes compared with 2 to 4 hours with CMDC. In selecting either type of current for treating the aseptic wound, the cathode should be placed 15 cm caudal or farther away from the spinal cord than the anode whenever possible (Fig. 12–16B). This electrode relationship is used to theoretically amplify the "current of injury" and accelerate tissue repair.

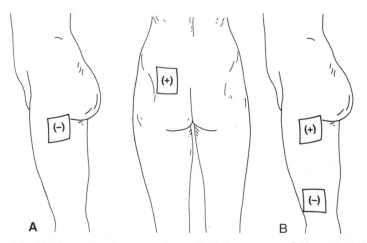

FIGURE 12–16. *A*) Electrode placement for cathodal constant microamperage direct current (CMDC) for bactericidal and sclerolytic effects (Patient case history 1, (−) = cathode, (+) = anode). *B*) Electrode placement for anodal stimulation to amplify "current of injury" and accelerate tissue repair (Patient case history 1, after wound asepsis has occurred).

Case B

PATIENT HISTORY

A 47-year-old woman complains of pain, numbness, and coldness in all digits of both feet and ulcerations of two of her toes. The complaints have been intermittent for 3 years and the ulcerations have existed for 9 months. She was diagnosed with Raynaud's phenomenon 2 years ago.

OBJECTIVE FINDINGS

Physical examination reveals pencil eraser–size Stage III ulcers on the fourth toe of her left foot and on the second toe of her right foot. Both ulcers are clean. The patient complains of pain that increases when her feet are exposed to moisture and drafts, but the pain does not prevent her from performing her normal activities of daily living. Her feet are cold to the touch.

TREATMENT PLAN AND RATIONALE

Cathodal stimulation to the dorsal webspace of both hands for 30 to 45 minutes, three times daily, is recommended (Fig. 12–17). A traditional TENS device may be used with stimulus variables set at 15 to 20 mA, two bursts per second, and a pulse duration of about 100 μsec. This treatment has been shown to cause vasodilation of the small vessels in the ipsilateral lower extremity and presumably assists in the healing of ulcers by improving blood flow to the wound tissues.

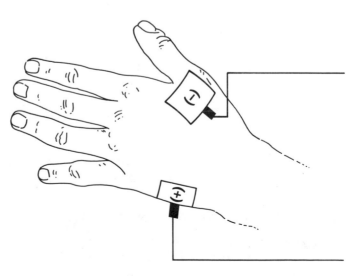

FIGURE 12–17. Electrode placement for treatment of ipsilateral lower extremity wound secondary to Raynaud's phenomena (Patient case history 2).

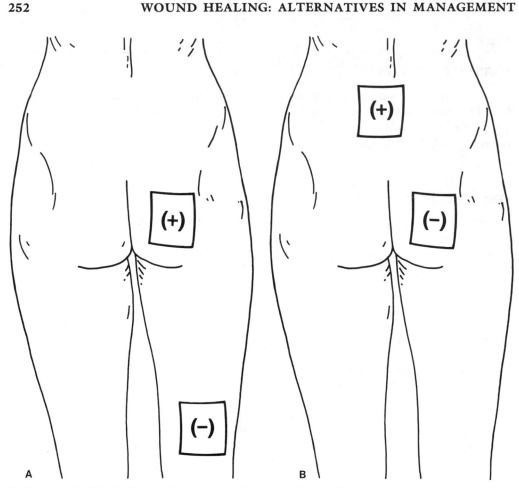

FIGURE 12–18. *A*) Electrode placement for anodal high voltage monophasic microamperage current (HVMMC). Indicated for clean wounds that continue producing granulation tissue formation. *B*) Electrode placement for cathodal HVMMC. Positive—proximal, negative—distal principal used to restimulate "injury current" when/if a plateau in healing occurs.

Case C

PATIENT HISTORY

A 24-year-old man with a history of paraplegia secondary to a motor vehicle accident presents with an ulcer on his right ischial tuberosity. He is wheelchair bound and has had the ulcer for 3 months.

OBJECTIVE FINDINGS

A clean, beefy-red Stage III ulcer, 3.3 cm long × 2.5 cm wide × 1.4 cm deep is present on the patient's right ischial tuberosity. There are no clinical signs of infection.

TREATMENT PLAN AND RATIONALE

HVPC, anodal stimulation to accelerate wound healing, is recommended. There is no need to treat the wound for infection or necrotic tissue; therefore, HVPC is selected and applied with the anode placed over gauze packing the wound. Voltage is set between 75 and 200 V to provide a tingling paresthesia at a pulse frequency of 100 pps (Fig. 12–18A). If a plateau in healing occurs, the polarity should be altered on a daily basis (Fig. 12–18B).

SUMMARY

Electrical currents having various waveform characteristics have been used for decades to augment healing of chronic dermal and subdermal ulcers. This chapter has exhaustively reviewed the history and literature related to the clinical applications of four variations of electrical current and the methods employed to deliver them to wound tissues. Also reviewed were pertinent animal and cellular studies, which provided further scientific information on how wounded tissues and cells respond to exogenously applied electrical stimulation and its clinical relevance to wound healing. Additionally, the theoretic mechanisms by which bioelectric circuits function normally, during trauma, and in response to various clinically applied circuits, were described. Additional controlled clinical research studies are needed to further delineate stimulus variables for using electrical stimulation to augment soft-tissue repair.

REFERENCES

1. Robertson, WS: Digby's Receipts. Ann Med Hist 7(3):216, 1925.
2. Birch, J: Essay on Electricity by George Adams, ed 4. R Hindmarsh, London, 1772, p 519.
3. Lente, FD: Cases of united fractures treated by electricity. NY State J Med 5:5117, 1850.
4. Brighton, CT, et al: Multicenter study of treatment of non-union with constant direct current. J Bone Joint Surg [Am] 63:2, 1981.
5. Brighton, CT, Friedenberg, ZB, and Black, J: Evaluation of use of constant direct current in treatment of non-union. In Brighton, CT, Black, J, and Pollack, SR (eds): Electrical Properties of Bone and Cartilage: Experimental Effects and Clinical Applications. Grune and Stratton, New York, 1979, pp 519–545.
6. Friedenberg, ZB, et al: Stimulation of fracture healing by direct current in rabbit fibula. J Bone Joint Surg [Am] 53:1400, 1971.
7. Heppenstall, RB: Constant direct current treatment for established nonunion of tibia. Clin Orthop 178:179, 1983.
8. Fukada, E and Yasuda, I: On the piezo electric effect in bone. J Physiol Soc Jpn 12:1158, 1957.
9. Peacock, E: Wound Repair. WB Saunders, Philadelphia, 1984, p 420.
10. Wolcott, LE, et al: Accelerated healing of skin ulcers by electrotherapy: Preliminary clinical results. South Med J 62:795, 1969.
11. Wheeler, PC, Wolcott, LE, and Morris, JL: Neural considerations in the healing of ulcerated tissues by clinical electric therapeutic application of weak direct current: Findings and theory. In Reynolds, DV and Sjoberg, AE (eds): Neuroelectric Research. Charles C Thomas, Springfield, IL, 1971, p 83.
12. Gault, WR and Gatens, PF, Jr: Use of low intensity direct current in management of ischemic skin ulcers. Phys Ther 56:275, 1976.
13. Carley, PJ and Wainapel, SF: Electrotherapy for acceleration of wound healing: Low intensity direct current. Arch Phys Med Rehabil 66:443, 1985.
14. Kloth, LC and Feedar, JA: Acceleration of wound healing with high voltage, monophasic, pulsed current. Phys Ther 68:503, 1988.
15. Rowley, B, et al: The influence of electrical current on an infecting microorganism in wounds. Ann NY Acad Sci 238:543, 1974.
16. Stanish, WD, et al: The use of electricity in ligament and tendon repair. Physician Sportsmed 13:109, 1985.
17. Owoeye, I, Spielholz, NI, and Nelson, AJ: Low-intensity pulsed galvanic current and the healing of tenotomized rat achilles tendons: Preliminary report using load-to-breaking measurements. Arch Phys Med Rehabil 68:415, 1987.
18. Kanof, N: Gold leaf in the treatment of cutaneous ulcers. J Invest Dermatol 43:441, 1964.
19. Gallagher, J and Geschickter, C: The use of charged gold leaf in surgery. JAMA 196:105, 1966.
20. Wolf M, Wheeler, PC, and Wolcott, LE: Gold-leaf treatment of ischemic skin ulcers. JAMA 196:105, 1966.

21. Smith, KW, Oden, PW, and Blaulock, WK: A comparison of gold leaf and other occlusive therapy. Arch Dermatol 96:703, 1967.
22. Chick, N: Treatment of ischemic and stasis ulcers with gold leaf and polyethylene film: A preliminary report. J Am Geriatr Soc 17:605, 1969.
23. Risbrook, AT, Goodfriend, SS, and Reiter, JM: Gold leaf in the treatment of leg ulcers. J Am Geriatr Soc 21:325, 1973.
24. Harris, DR and Keefe, RL: A histologic study of gold leaf treated experimental wounds. J Invest Dermatol 52:487, 1969.
25. Alvarez, OM, et al: The healing of superficial skin wounds is stimulated by external electrical current. J Invest Dermatol 81:144, 1983.
26. Assimacopoulos, D: Low intensity negative electric current in the treatment of ulcers of the leg due to chronic venous insufficiency. Am J Surg 115:683, 1968.
27. Assimacopoulos, D: Wound healing promotion by the use of negative electric current. Am Surg 34(6):423, 1968.
28. Bennett, RG: Fundamentals of Cutaneous Surgery. CV Mosby, St Louis, 1988, p 78.
29. Cornwall, MW: Zinc iontophoresis to treat ischemic skin ulcers. Phys Ther 61:359, 1981.
30. Abramson, DI, et al: Physiologic and clinical basis for histamine by ion transfer. Arch Phys Med Rehabil 48:583, 1967.
31. Barron, JJ, Jacobson, WE, and Tidd, G: Treatment of decubitus ulcers: A new approach. Minn Med 68:103, 1985.
32. Young, GH: Electric impulse therapy aids wound healing. Mod Vet Pract 47(14):60, 1966.
33. Thurman, BF and Christian, EL: Response of a serious circulatory lesion to electrical stimulation: A case report. Phys Ther 51:1107, 1971.
34. Ross, CR and Segal D: High voltage galvanic stimulation: An aid to postoperative healing. Curr Podiatry 30(5):19, 1981.
35. Akers, T and Gabrielson, A: The effect of high voltage galvanic stimulation on the rate of healing of decubitus ulcers. Biomed Sci Instrum 20:99, 1984.
36. Alon, G, Azaria, M, and Stein, H: Diabetic ulcer healing using high voltage TENS (abstr). Phys Ther 66:775, 1986.
37. Kaada, B: Promoted healing of chronic ulceration by transcutaneous nerve stimulation (TNS). VASA 12:262, 1983.
38. Kaada, B: Vasodilation induced by transcutaneous nerve stimulation in peripheral ischemia (Raynaud's phenomenon and diabetic polyneuropathy). Eur Heart J 3:303, 1982.
39. Kaada, B and Eielson, O: In search of the mediators of skin vasodilation induced by transcutaneous nerve stimulation. I. Failure to block the response by antagonists of endogenous vasodilators. Gen Pharmacol 14(6):623, 1983.
40. Kaada, B and Eielson, O: In search of the mediators of skin vasodilation induced by transcutaneous nerve stimulation. II. Serotonin implicated. Gen Pharmacol 14(6):635, 1983.
41. Kaada, B and Helle, KB: In search of the mediators of skin vasodilation induced by transcutaneous nerve stimulation: IV. In vitro bioassay of the vasoinhibitory activity of sera from patients suffering from peripheral ischemia. Gen Pharmacol 15(2):115, 1984.
42. Kaada, B, et al: Failure to influence the VIP level in the cerebrospinal fluid by transcutaneous nerve stimulation in humans. Gen Pharmacol 15(6):563, 1984.
43. Dooley, DM and Kasprak, M: Modification of blood flow to the extremities by electrical stimulation of the nervous system. South Med J 69(10):1309, 1976.
44. Owens, S, Atkinson, ER, and Lees, DE: Thermographic evidence of reduced sympathetic tone with transcutaneous nerve stimulation. Anesthesiology 50:62, 1979.
45. Wong, RA and Jette, PV: Changes in sympathetic tone associated with different forms of transcutaneous electrical nerve stimulation in healthy subject. Phys Ther 64(4):478, 1984.
46. Ernst, M and Lee, MHW: Sympathetic vasomotor changes induced by manual and electrical acupuncture of the hoku point visualized by thermography. Pain 21:25, 1985.
47. Ebersold, MI, Laws, ER, and Albers, JW: Measurements of autonomic function before, during, and after transcutaneous stimulation in patients with chronic pain and in control subjects. Mayo Clin Proc 52:228, 1977.
48. Bigelow, JB, et al: Effect of electrical stimulation of canine skin, and percutaneous device — skin interface healing. In Brighton, CT, Black, J, and Pollack, SR (eds): Skin Interface Healing and Electrical Properties of Bone and Cartilage. Grune and Stratton, New York, 1979, p 289.
49. Konioff, JJ: Electrical promotion of soft tissue repair. Ann Biomed Eng 4:1, 1976.
50. Smith, J, et al: The effect of electrical stimulation on wound healing in diabetic mice. J Am Podiatr Assoc 74:71, 1984.
51. Wu, KT, et al: Effects of electric currents and interfacial potentials on wound healing. J Surg Res 7(3):122, 1967.
52. Carey, LC and Lepley, D: Effect of continuous direct electric current on healing wounds. Surg Forum 13:33, 1962.
53. Brown, M and Gogia, PP: Effects of high voltage stimulation on cutaneous wound healing in rabbits. Phys Ther 67:662, 1987.
54. Brown, M, McDonnell, MK, and Menton, DN: Electrical stimulation effects on cutaneous wound healing in rabbits. Phys Ther 68:955, 1988.

55. Burr, HS, Harrey, SC, and Taffel, M: Bio-electric correlates of wound healing. Yale J Biol Med 2:103, 1940.
56. Sawyer, PN and Pate, JW: Bioelectric phenomena as an etiologic factor in intravascular thrombosis. Am J Physiol 175:113, 1953.
57. Sawyer, PN, Suckling, EE, and Wesolowksi, SA: Effects of small electric currents on intravascular thrombosis in the visualized rat mesentery. Am J Physiol 198:1006, 1960.
58. Sawyer, PN, Wesolowski, SA, and Suckling, EE: Experiments in direct current electrocoagulation. Surg Forum 10:435, 1960.
59. Sawyer, PN and Wesolowski, SA: Studies on direct current coagulation. Surgery 49:486, 1961.
60. Sawyer, PN, Dennis, C, and Wesolowski, SA: Electrical hemostasis in uncontrollable bleeding states. Am Surg 154:556, 1961.
61. Sawyer, PN: Bioelectric phenomena and intravascular thrombosis: The first 12 years. Surgery 56:1020, 1964.
62. Sawyer, PN and Deutch, B: Use of electrical currents to delay intravascular thrombosis in experimental animals. Am J Physiol 187:473, 1956.
63. Sawyer, PN and Deutch, B: The experimental use of oriented electric fields to delay and prevent intravascular thrombosis. Surg Forum 5:173, 1955.
64. Sawyer, PN and Pate, JW: Bioelectric phenomena as etiologic factors in intravascular thrombosis. Surgery 34:791, 1953.
65. Wesolowski, SA and Dennis, C (eds): Fundamentals of Vascular Grafting. McGraw-Hill, New York, 1963.
66. Newton, RA and Karselis, TC: Skin pH following high voltage pulsed galvanic stimulation. Phys Ther 63:1593, 1983.
67. Cheng, N, et al: The effects of electric currents on ATP generation, protein synthesis, and membrane transport in rat skin. Clin Orthop 171:264, 1982.
68. Witt, HT, Schloder, E, and Graber, P: Membrane-bound ATP synthesis generated by an external electrical field. FEBS Lett 69(1):272, 1976.
69. Vinkler, C, Korenstein, R, and Farkas, DL: External electric field driven ADP phosphorylation (EFP) in thylakoid membranes. In Oplatka, A and Balaban, M (eds): Biological Structures and Coupled Flows. Academic Press, New York, 1983, pp 113–121.
70. Know, BE and Tsong, TY: Voltage driven ATP synthesis by beef heart mitochondrial Fo Fi-ATPase. J Biol Chem 259(8):4747, 1984.
71. Hinkle, PC and McCarty, RE: How cells make ATP. Sci Am 238(3):104, 1978.
72. Mitchell, P: Vectorial chemistry and the molecular mechanics of chemosmotic coupling: Power transmission by proticity. Biochem Soc Trans 4:399, 1976.
73. Mitchell, P: Keilin's respiratory chain concept and its chemosmotic consequences. Science 206:1148, 1979.
74. Tsong, TY and Astumian, RD: Absorption and conversion of electric field energy by membrane bound ATPases. Bioelectrochemistry and Bioenergetics 15:457, 1986.
75. Kaziro, Y: The role of guanosine-5'-triphosphate in polypeptide chain elongation. Biochim Biophys Acta 505:95, 1978.
76. Keller, FB and Zamecnik PD: The effects of guanosine diphosphate and triphosphate on the incorporation of labeled amino acids into proteins. J Biol Chem 221:45, 1956.
77. Erickson, CA and Nuccitelli, R: Embryonic fibroblast motility and orientation can be influenced by physiological electric fields. J Cell Biol 98:296, 1984.
78. Dunn, MG, et al: Wound healing using a collagen matrix: Effect of DC electrical stimulation. J Biomed Mater Res 22(A2):191, 1988.
79. Bourguignon, GJ and Bourguignon, LYW: Electric stimulation of protein and DNA synthesis in human fibroblasts. Federation of American Societies for Experimental Biology Journal 1:398, 1987.
80. Harrington, DB: Macromolecular synthesis in the differentiated erythrocyte of Rana pipiens following small amounts of electrical current. J Cell Biol 43:50A, 1969.
81. Harrington, DB and Becker, RO: Electrical stimulation of RNA and protein synthesis in the frog erythrocyte. Exper Cell Res 76:95, 1973.
82. Cooper, MS and Schliwa, M: Electrical and ionic control of tissue cell locomotion in DC electric field. J Neurosci Res 13:223, 1985.
83. Winter, GD: Movement of epidermal cells over the wound surface. In Montagna, W and Billingham, RE (eds): Advances in Biology of the Skin. Vol 5. Pergamon Press, New York, 1964, p 113.
84. Jaffe, LF and Vanable, JW: Electric fields and wound healing. Clin Dermatol 2(3):34–44, 1984.
85. Dodgen, PW, et al: The effects of electrical stimulation on cutaneous oxygen supply in diabetic older adults (abstr). Phys Ther 67(5):793, 1987.
86. Gagnier, KA, et al: The effects of electrical stimulation on cutaneous oxygen supply in paraplegics. Phys Ther 68(5):835, 1988.
87. Rowley, BA: Electrical current effects on E. coli growth rates. Proc Soc Exp Biol Med 139:929, 1972.
88. Rowley, BA, et al: The influence of electrical current on an infecting microorganism in wounds. Ann NY Acad Sci 238:543, 1974.
89. Barranco, SD, et al: In vitro effect of weak direct current on Staphylococcus aureus. Clin Orthop 100:250, 1974.

90. Orida, N and Feldman, JD: Directional protrusive pseudopodial activity and motility in macrophages induced by extracellular electric fields. Cell Motil 2:243, 1982.
91. Monguio, J: Uber Die polare wirkung des galvanischen stromes auf leukozyten. Z Biol 93:553, 1933.
92. Fukushima, K, et al: Studies on galvanotaxis of human neutrophilic leukocytes and methods of its measurement. Med J Osaka Univ 4:195, 1953.
93. Dineur, E: Note sur la sensibilitie des leukocytes a l'electricite. Bulletin Seances Soc Belge Microscopic (Bruxelles) 18:113, 1891.
94. Rowley, BA, McKenna, JM, and Chase, GR: The influence of electrical current on an infecting microorganism in wounds. Ann NY Acad Sci 238:543, 1974.
95. Eberhardt, A, Szczpiorski, P, and Korytowski, G: Effect of transcutaneous electrostimulation on the cell composition of skin exudate. Acta Physiol Pol 37(1):41, 1986.
96. Kloth, LC, et al: Standards of electrotherapeutic terminology. Report of the Electrotherapy Standards Committee of the Section on Clinical Electrophysiology of the American Physical Therapy Association Washington, DC, 1989 (in press).
97. Lund, EJ: Experimental control of organic polarity by the electric current. J Exper Zool 41:155, 1925.
98. Sinyukhin, AM: Nature of the variation of the bioelectric potentials in the regeneration process of plants. Biofizika (Russ) 2:52, 1957.
99. Mathews, AP: Electrical polarity in the hydroids. Am J Physiol 8:294, 1903.
100. Lund, ET: Bioelectric Fields and Growth. University of Texas Press, Austin, 1947.
101. Burr, HS, Harvey, SC, and Taffel, M: Bioelectric correlates of wound healing. Yale J Biol Med 11:103–107, 1938.
102. Borgens, RB, Vanable, JW, and Jaffe, LF: Bioelectricity and regeneration. Initiation of regeneration frog limb by minute currents. J Exp Zool 200(3):403–416, 1977.
103. DuBois-Reymond, E: Untersuchunger Uber Tierische Elektrizitaet. 2:2. Reimer Berlin, 1860.
104. Herlitzka, A: Ein Beitrag Zur Physiologie der Regeneration. Wilhelm Roux Arch Entwick Lungsmech Org 10:126, 1910.
105. Illingworth, CM and Barker, AT: Measurement of electrical currents emerging during the regeneration of amputated finger tips in children. Clin Phys Physiol Meas 1:87, 1980.
106. Borgens, RB, Vanable, JW, and Jaffe, LF: Bioelectricity and regeneration: Large currents leave the stumps of regenerating newt limbs. Proc Natl Acad Sci (USA) 74:4528–4532, 1977.
107. Cunliffe-Barnes, T: Healing rate of human skin determined by measurement of electric potential of experimental abrasions; study of treatment with petrolatum and with petrolatum containing yeast and liver extracts. Am J Surg 69:82–88, 1945.
108. Barker, AT, Jaffe, LF, and Vanable, JW, Jr: The glabrous epidermis of cavies contains a powerful battery: Am J Physiol, 242 (Regulatory Integrative Comp Physiol) 11:R248, 1982.
109. Foulds, IS and Barker, AT: Human skin battery potentials and their possible role in wound healing. Br J Dermatol 109:515–522, 1983.
110. Becker, RO, Bachman, CH, and Friedman, H: The direct current control system a link between environment and organism. NY State J Med 62:1169, 1962.
111. Becker, RO: The bioelectric field pattern in the salamander and its stimulation by an electronic analog. IRE Trans Med Electron ME-7:202 (July), 1960.
112. Becker, RO: Search for evidence of axial current flow in peripheral nerves of salamander. Science 134:101, 1961.
113. Becker, RO: Biological Prototypes Synthetic Systems. Plenum Press, New York, 1962, p 474.
114. Becker, RO: Search for evidence of axial current flow in peripheral nerves of salamander. Science 134:101–102, 1961.
115. Becker, RO: The significance of bioelectric potentials. Paper presented at the 10th International Symposium on Bioelectrochemistry, Pont à Mousson, Oct 1–5, 1973.
116. Becker, RO: The sign of the miracle. In Becker, RO and Selden, G (eds): The Body Electric. William Morrow and Co, New York, 1985, p 72.
117. Becker, RO: Good news for mammals. In Becker, RO and Selden, G (eds): The Body Electric. William Morrow and Co, New York, 1985, p 138.
118. Nordenstrom, BE: Biologically Closed Electric Circuits: Clinical, Experimental, and Theoretical Evidence for an Additional Circulatory System. Nordic Medical Publications, Stockholm, 1983, pp 122–150.

Appendix

MANUFACTURERS OF ELECTROTHERAPEUTIC DEVICES THAT MAY PROVIDE STIMULUS VARIABLES APPROPRIATE FOR WOUND HEALING APPLICATIONS

This appendix is intended to assist the consumer of electrotherapeutic devices that may be appropriate for wound healing applications. This partial listing of manufacturers does not indicate endorsement of their products by the editors, authors, or publishers.

High Voltage, Pulsed Current Devices

Amrex Electronics, Inc.
12583 Crenshaw Boulevard
Hawthorne, CA 90250
800-221-9069

Chattanooga Corporation
P.O. Box 4287
Chattanooga, TN 37405
615-870-2281

DynaWave Corporation
2520 Kaneville Court
Geneva, IL 60134
312-232-4945

Electro-Med Health Industries, Inc.
6240 NE 4th Court
Miami, FL 33138
305-756-6013

Henley International, Inc.
104 International Boulevard
Sugar Land, TX 77478
800-237-8749

Physio Technology, Inc.
1505 SW 42nd Street
Topeka, KS 66609
800-432-2441

Rich-Mar Corporation
Box 879
Inola, OK 74036
800-762-4665

Constant Microamperage Direct Current Devices

Amrex Electronics, Inc.
12583 Crenshaw Boulevard
Hawthorne, CA 90250
800-221-9069

Electrostim USA
1851 Black Road
Joliet, IL 60435
800-231-9621

ELMED, Inc.
60 W. Fay Avenue
Addison, IL 60101
312-543-2792

Mettler Electronics Corporation
1333 South Claudina Street
Anaheim, CA 92805
800-854-9305

Low Voltage, Pulsed Milliamperage Devices (Traditional TENS)

EMPI, Inc.
1275 Grey Fox Road
St. Paul, MN 55112
800-328-2536

Medical Designs, Inc.
833 3rd Street SW
St. Paul, MN 55162
800-328-0875

Medtronic, Inc.
11558 Sorrento Valley Road
San Diego, CA 92121
800-854-1915

NeuroLogix Systems Ltd.
62-33 Woodhaven Boulevard
Rego Park, NY 11374
718-899-0450

NTRON Electronics
350 Merrydale Road
San Rafael, CA 94903
415-472-4600

Solcoor-Medical Division
8150 Leesburg Pike #700
Vienna, VA 22180
800-368-8679

Stimtech Products
E. Main Street, P.O. Box 10
Southridge, MA 01550
508-765-1582

3M Electromedicine Products
3M Center, 225-55-01
St. Paul, MN 55144-1000
612-733-7532

Low Voltage, Pulsed Microamperage Devices

Electro Medical, Inc.
18433 Amistad
Fountain Valley, CA 92708
800-422-8726

Monad Corporation
908 East Holt
Pomona, CA 91767
800-346-6623

CHAPTER 13

Role of Ultrasound in Wound Healing

Mary Dyson, B.Sc., C.Biol., M.I.Biol., Ph.D.

Ultrasound, a mechanical vibration transmitted at a frequency above the upper limit of human hearing, has been used as an adjunctive physical therapeutic modality for more than 40 years for the treatment of a variety of disorders, usually involving soft-tissue injury. Ultrasound is widely used to stimulate wound healing. Although the extent of its use in physical therapy in the United States and Canada is not known, a survey carried out in the United Kingdom in 1985 revealed that approximately 54 percent of all physical therapy treatments in the private sector and 20 percent of those in the public sector involved the use of ultrasound.[1] In the interests of efficiency and safety, the clinically significant physical properties and biologic effects of such a widely used modality should be understood by those applying it. The objectives of this chapter are (1) to describe the relevant physical properties and biologic effects of therapeutic ultrasound and (2) to describe how these effects can be employed to accelerate wound healing and other forms of tissue repair.

PHYSICS OF ULTRASOUND

Nature of Ultrasound

Ultrasound is a mechanical disturbance in which the molecules of media that can transmit it, such as biologic tissues, are made to oscillate or vibrate at a frequency above the upper limit of human hearing.

Ultrasound is transmitted in the form of compressional waves, like ripples on a pool of water.[2] These waves consist of regions where the molecules are alternately pushed together (compressed) and pulled apart (rarefied). When traveling through liquids and soft tissues, the waves are *longitudinal*; that is, molecular displacement is parallel to the direction in which the waves travel. In solids, *transverse* or shear waves, in which molecular displacement is perpendicular to the direction of wave propagation, are also transmitted. With the exception of compact bone, virtually all of the tissues of the body

TABLE 13–1. Relationship between Frequency and Wavelength in Water, Biological Fluids, and Soft Tissues*

Frequency (MHz)	Wavelength (mm)
0.50	3.0
0.75	2.0
1.00	1.5
3.00	0.5

*Velocity estimated at 1500 m/s

irradiated by therapists behave acoustically as liquids and transmit only longitudinal waves readily. It is clinically important to be aware of these two methods of transmission because shear waves generated by mode conversion at the reflecting interface between soft tissue such as the periosteum and hard tissue such as bone are absorbed readily in the soft tissue, causing localized heating and sometimes the sensation of pain.[3]

Many of the clinically relevant effects of ultrasound on tissues are related to its *frequency* (see pp. 267–268). This frequency is the number of times per second that a molecule displaced by the ultrasound completes a cycle of movement and returns to its original position. Frequencies (f) are expressed in hertz, where 1 hertz = 1 cycle per second. The time taken to complete one cycle is termed a *period* (T). The ultrasonic frequencies used in physical therapy to accelerate wound healing and other forms of tissue repair are generally in the range of 0.5 to 3.0 megahertz (MHz).

The *wavelength* (λ) is the shortest distance, measured parallel to the direction of wave propagation, between molecules that are at equivalent points of vibration in the repeated cycle of movement, which constitutes the wave. Such propagation can be visualized as the distance between two adjacent peaks of the wave. The wavelength is related to the frequency and the *velocity* (c) of the wave by the equation $\lambda = c/f$. The velocity of ultrasound in water, blood, interstitial fluid, and soft tissue is approximately 1500 meters per second. Therefore, at a frequency of 1 MHz, the wavelength is $1500/10^6$ m; that is, 1.5 mm. Examples of the relationships between the frequencies and wavelengths most commonly used in physical therapy are listed in Table 13–1.

The *amplitude* of an ultrasonic wave is the maximal disturbance caused by the wave, which increases as the intensity is increased and can be expressed either as the displacement amplitude (that is, the maximal distance that a molecule is displaced from its point of equilibrium during the passage of the wave) or as the pressure amplitude, either positive or negative, measured from zero. Because many of the clinically relevant effects of ultrasound are related to amplitude, this variable should be under the control of the therapist.

Generation of Ultrasound

The equipment used to produce therapeutic levels of ultrasound typically consists of a microcomputer-controlled high-frequency generator linked by a coaxial cable to an applicator or treatment head containing a disc of piezoelectric material (Fig. 13–1).

The term *piezoelectric* is applied to materials such as quartz and some synthetic polarized ceramics such as lead zirconate titanate (PZT), which develop surface charges when pressure is applied to them. The effect is reversible. If an alternating voltage is applied across them, they expand and contract (vibrate or oscillate) at the same frequency as the electrical oscillation, transducing electrical into mechanical energy. If

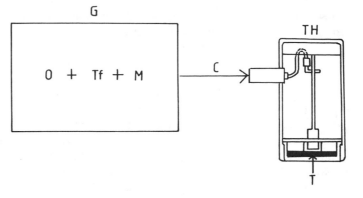

FIGURE 13-1. Block diagram illustrating the components used in the generation of therapeutic levels of ultrasound.   Key: C = coaxial cable,   G = microcomputer controlled generator, M = microcomputer, O = oscillator circuit, T =transducer, Tf = transformer, TH = treatment head or applicator.

transmitted into an elastic medium, such as the tissues and fluids of the body, at a sufficiently high frequency (greater than 20 kHz), these pressure changes produce ultrasound.

Synthetic piezoelectric ceramics are generally used as transducers instead of naturally occurring crystals such as quartz because of their better electrical and mechanical properties. Typically, they are sliced into discs about 2 or 3 mm thick and about 1 to 3 cm in diameter. One surface of the disc is mounted in contact with the deep surface of the metallic face of an applicator while the other surface is exposed to air inside the applicator. Most of the ultrasound produced by the disc is transmitted forward out of the front of the applicator. However, because the disc also vibrates laterally, some can be transmitted into the side walls of the applicator and, unless suitable precautions are taken, into the therapist. Although the energy levels involved in this *side wall irradiation*[4] are small, its effects may be cumulative. The therapist should therefore be aware of it and either avoid holding the applicator close to the transducer or wear air-trapping gloves that will reflect the ultrasound away from the therapist's hands.

Continuous and Pulsed Ultrasound

Most therapeutic ultrasound equipment can produce either continuous or pulsed ultrasound.

CONTINUOUS

When set to operate continuously, ultrasound is generally produced without interruption, although some equipment is designed to switch off temporarily if contact between the applicator and the coupling medium (p. 276) is inadequate. When this event occurs, ultrasound transmission is resumed only when adequate contact is again achieved, thus ensuring that the patient receives treatment for the desired time while protecting the transducer from damage. If ultrasound is being used primarily to heat the tissues, then continuous application is appropriate (p. 282).

PULSED

Ultrasound may be delivered in pulses (marks), typically from 0.5 to 2 milliseconds (ms) in duration, separated by pauses also lasting a few milliseconds. The term *duty cycle* is used to describe the ratio of pulse or mark duration (m) to pulse plus pause duration (m+p), and is usually quoted as a percentage:

$$m/m+p \times 100\%$$

Duty cycles of from 5 to 50 percent are available, the range varying with the equipment. The pulse-plus-pause duration is termed the *pulse repetition period*. The pulse repetition *rate* for a typical pulse repetition period of 10 ms is 100 Hz. Pulsing the ultrasound reduces the total amount of energy transmitted and thus gives protection against excessive heating, while permitting the use of sufficiently high energy levels during each pulse to produce the predominantly nonthermally induced effects (pp. 274–276), which stimulate the wound healing process.[5]

The Ultrasonic Field

Ultrasound transmitted from the applicator causes pressure variation mainly in front of it. The form of the *ultrasonic pressure field* produced depends on the size and shape of the transducer and on how it is mounted into the applicator. The pressure varies across the surface of the applicator and also according to the distance from it. The pressure changes experienced by the tissues being treated therefore depend upon their position relative to the applicator. Ultrasound is emitted from a disc-shaped transducer as a beam that is at first approximately cylindrical; this region is called the *near field* or *Fresnel zone*, and in it the energy distribution is highly variable.[6] Farther away from the transducer, the beam starts to diverge, and the energy distribution within it becomes more regular; this region is called the *far field* or *Fraunhofer zone*. The distance (d) from the transducer to the point where the far field begins can be calculated from the radius (a) of the transducer and the wavelength (λ) of the ultrasound, since $d = a^2/\lambda$.

Most ultrasonic therapy treatments are given with the target located in the near field, where nonuniformity is highest. The *beam nonuniformity ratio* (BNR) is a measure of this lack of uniformity, and is the ratio of the spatial peak intensity (I[SP]) in the near field to the spatial average intensity (I[SA]). The safest applicators to use when treating wounds are those with the lowest BNRs, since high spatial peak intensities are potentially damaging.[7]

Clinically Significant Physical Variables

To describe adequately a treatment with ultrasound, a number of physical variables should be known, recorded, and quoted. This knowledge is essential if any exposure to ultrasound is to be repeated accurately. These variables include *power, intensity, exposure duration, frequency,* and the *position of the treated tissues* relative to the applicator.

POWER

Power is the total energy in the beam, measured in watts. Since most of this energy will be absorbed and converted into heat, then provided that all other factors remain constant, the greater the power, the greater the resulting temperature increase.

INTENSITY

Intensity is the amount of energy per unit area per unit time. Although the Système International (SI) units for intensity are watts/m², applicators typically have an *effective radiating area* (ERA) of a few cm². The ERA can be determined by scanning the ultrasonic field with a pressure-sensitive detector at, for example, 5 mm in front of the face of the applicator, and calculating the area at which the power of the output is more than 5 percent of the spatial maximum at any point in the ultrasonic field at this distance.

The intensity can be *averaged* in *space* over the face of the applicator (termed spatial average or SA) or the average in *time* (temporal average or TA), a particularly important variable if the ultrasound is pulsed. The maximal or *peak* intensity can also be determined, both in *space* (SP) and in *time* (TP). When pulsed ultrasound is used, pulse average intensity, or PA (that is, the temporal average during the period of the pulse), should be stated, as well as the temporal average during the full pulse repetition cycle.

The type of intensity should be specified as follows:
If continuous: I(SATA)
If pulsed: Both I(SATA) and I(SAPA).

EXPOSURE DURATION

This duration is the total time of irradiation, usually expressed in minutes. If the ultrasound is pulsed, then either the duty cycle and pulse length (in ms) *or* the pulse length and pause length should also be noted.

FREQUENCY

The frequency of ultrasound used should be recorded (in kHz or MHz).

POSITION OF TREATED TISSUES

Because the amount of energy reaching the tissues being treated is modified by distance from the applicator and by intervening materials, both the distance of the target tissues (in mm) and their anatomic position should be noted, as should the type of coupling medium (or media) used (p. 264).

Ideally, the *ultrasonic variables measured should be those responsible for producing its clinical effects. Intensity* is the main variable involved in heating and should be recorded when thermal mechanisms are responsible for the effects observed. However, nonthermal mechanisms are also involved in producing clinically significant effects,[8] and in such circumstances other variables may be of greater relevance. The incidence of cavitation (p. 274), for example, is related to the magnitude of the pressure changes produced by the ultrasonic wave, so where effects are primarily due to cavitation, ideally the *acoustic pressure amplitude* should be measured[6] (in atmospheres, bars, or megapascals [MPa], where 1 atmosphere = 1 bar = 0.1 MPa).

APPLICATION OF ULTRASOUND

Therapeutic Ultrasound Equipment

Modern equipment typically consists of a mains electricity or battery-powered generator comprising an oscillator circuit, transformer, and controlling microcomputer, which can be linked to one of perhaps several applicators, having different ERAs and/or frequencies, by a coaxial cable that minimizes frequency distortion and interference[7] (Fig. 13–1). The equipment is designed to produce ultrasound at one or more frequencies, at variable intensities, and often in either continuous or pulsed mode.

Transmission of Ultrasound from Applicator to Patient

When ultrasound in the frequency range used therapeutically encounters a boundary or interface between two media with different acoustic properties—for example, the surface of the applicator and air, soft tissue and bone, or soft tissue and air—reflection occurs. The greater the difference in *acoustic impedance* (z), the greater the amount of energy reflected. The acoustic impedance of the medium is the product of its density (p) and the velocity of ultrasound through it (c). There is little difference between the acoustic impedance of soft tissue and water, but much more between soft tissue and bone, and even more between soft tissue and air. Consequently, there is only about 0.2 percent reflection at the interface between water and soft tissue, more than 50 percent between soft tissue and bone, and virtually complete reflection (99.9 percent) between soft tissue and air. Thus, if ultrasound is to enter the body, as it must if surface injuries are to be treated successfully, air must be excluded from its path. This is achieved by placing a *coupling* or *contact medium*, with acoustic properties similar to those of soft tissue, between the applicator and the skin or wound surface.

Selection of Coupling Medium

The ideal coupling medium would have the same acoustic impedance as skin; have excellent ultrasonic propagation properties; double as a wound dressing; and be sterile, thixotropic, nonstaining, nonirritant, chemically inert, not too rapidly absorbed, slow to evaporate, free from gas bubbles and other inclusions, transparent, and inexpensive. Because the ideal medium does not exist, choices have to be made from those available. A number of these choices are considered here, together with the ways in which they should be used.

DEGASSED WATER

If free from gas bubbles, which provide reflecting surfaces, and from impurities that might absorb the ultrasound, the acoustic properties make water an excellent contact medium,[8,9] transmitting ultrasound for considerable distances with little loss in power. A 3-mm path of water presumably attentuates 50 percent of the ultrasonic energy transmitted into it,[10] but there is neither theoretic nor practical support for this claim. A problem with the use of water as contact medium is that because of its low viscosity, water has to be held in a container within or through which it can be linked to the skin. If the region to be treated is irregular, making the maintenance of contact with the applicator and the skin difficult, and can conveniently be placed in water, then this is an appropriate method of treatment. Injuries to the ankle, foot, wrist, and hand fall into this category.

Warm degassed water is placed in a container lined with ultrasound-absorbing material, to reduce the problem of unwanted reflection. The applicator and the part of the body to be treated are submerged, care being taken to keep the water as free from gas bubbles and other impurities as possible. If there is an open wound then the water and the container should be sterile. The applicator need not touch the skin, an advantage if the site is particularly painful. If the container is sufficiently large, the applicator can be placed far enough from the target tissues for them to be in the far field (p. 262), where the spatial intensity is more uniform. If the region being treated is irregular and cannot be submerged in water, then a small balloon or a condom can be either filled with degassed water and attached by its opening to the applicator or coated with a more viscous contact medium and interposed between the applicator and the skin. This technique is difficult and has been rendered virtually obsolete now that applicators with very small ERAs (about 1 cm^2) can be applied directly to most irregular surfaces.

OILS, EMULSIONS, AND AQUEOUS GELS

These gels are more convenient to use than water because their higher viscosity means that they can be applied to the skin without being held in a container. Many media have adequate, fundamentally similar, acoustic properties.[8] Unless sterile and inert, they should not be placed over broken skin, but only over adjacent intact skin or re-epithelialized scar tissue.

AQUEOUS GEL–BASED WOUND DRESSINGS

Open wounds can most conveniently be treated via sterile wound dressings but only if these have similar acoustic properties to soft tissues and can be coupled to, and exclude air from, the wound area. An example of such a dressing is Geliperm (Geistlich Pharmaceuticals), which is a transparent polyacrylamide agar gel, impermeable to bacteria, containing 96 percent water. Geliperm has been used as a dressing for skin graft donor sites, burns, hand injuries, compound fractures, varicose ulcers, pressure sores, and following surgery for Dupuytren's contracture.[11] The hydrated sheets of Geliperm used as wound dressings are 3.3 mm thick and have been shown to transmit 95 percent of incident 1 MHz ultrasound under experimental test conditions, when measured with a tethered float radiometer.[12] Geliperm has been used satisfactorily as a combined contact medium and wound dressing in the ultrasonic treatment of chronic varicose ulcers, ligament injuries associated with abrasions, unhealed amputation stumps, and hematomas associated with surgical wounds, and is reported to be comfortable and soothing.[13] Sterile saline is applied to the injured site via a syringe, the dressing moistened on both upper and lower surfaces with more sterile saline, and then placed over the injured site, ensuring that no air is trapped between the dressing and the underlying tissue.[14] Ultrasound is transmitted into the tissue by placing the applicator on the dressing and moving it gently over the treatment area (Fig. 13-2). The application of a thin film of an aqueous gel contact medium such as Sonogel (Enraf-Nonius) or Aquason 100 (Parker Laboratories, Inc.) to the applicator eases its movement over the dressing without compromising ultrasonic transmission. (See Appendix at the end of this chapter for a list of manufacturers.)

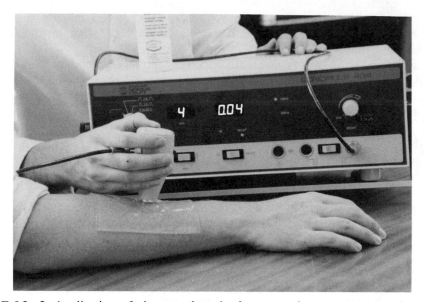

FIGURE 13–2. Application of ultrasound to the forearm, using a transparent sheet of Geli-perm as a combined sterile wound dressing and contact medium. Movement of the applicator over the surface of the Geliperm is facilitated by placing a thin layer of Sonogel between the two, as illustrated here.

Phonophoresis

Some coupling media may also be used as carriers for pharmacologically active agents whose entry into the tissues is considered to be aided by exposure to ultrasound, the process being termed *phonophoresis* or *ultrasonophoresis*. In 1967, continuous 1-MHz ultrasound at intensities of up to 1.5 W/cm^2 was shown to drive hydrocortisone ointment into the tissues of patients diagnosed as arthritic or as having some other muscle or joint pathology.[15] Of the group receiving hydrocortisone therapy in this manner, 68 percent had a marked decrease in pain and an increase in range of movement compared with 28 percent in a control group receiving ultrasound alone. More recently, patients with humeral epicondylitis and subdeltoid bursitis have also benefited from hydrocortisone applied phonophoretically.[16] Other substances that have been applied in this manner include creams such as Hirudoid (Luitpold-Werk-Munchen), lidocaine, and vasodilators such as histamine and methyl nicotinate.[4] The technique appears to be of potential clinical value, but its scientific basis requires investigation, and there is a need for further adequately controlled clinical trials of its effectiveness.

Manipulation of the Applicator

If the tissues being treated are in the near field, which is characterized by its nonuniformity (p. 262), they will be subjected to relatively large variations in spatial peak intensity (I[SP]). These peaks may be high enough to cause local injury, if the tissues are exposed to them for long enough durations. Furthermore, ultrasound passing across the various acoustic interfaces (p. 264) experiences varying amounts of reflection.

Interaction between the incident and reflected waves may produce a *standing wave field* (pp. 275–276), in which positions of maximal pressure variation (antinodes) and zero pressure variation (nodes) are static, and in which the pressure amplitudes are higher than in the absence of standing waves—that is, in a traveling wave field. Exposure to standing wave fields can cause localized tissue damage and the arrest of blood cell flow (pp. 275–276). Even if the underwater method of treatment is used and the applicator is placed in the more uniform far field, the problem of standing wave formation still remains, particularly if the water container is inadequately lined with absorbing material, and reflection can occur from its walls, as well as from the interfaces between, for example, soft tissue and bone.

The potentially damaging effects of exposure to high I(SP) and to standing waves can be minimized if the position of the applicator is continuously altered during insonation. The use of a *moving applicator technique* at all times is therefore recommended. In the interests of safety, at no time during treatment should movement of the applicator cease.

The applicator should be moved in either of the following ways, the operator selecting whichever seems more convenient:[4] (1) in short, linear movements, of a few centimeters' length, ensuring that the strokes overlap so the entire region to be treated is covered; (2) in small circular movements, again overlapping, so that the motion is essentially spiral. With both techniques, the movements should be slow and deliberate, and, if the direct-contact method is being used, care must be taken to ensure that the applicator remains in contact with the coupling medium, and through it with the underlying tissues, throughout treatment, and that no air is introduced between the applicator and the tissues.

Selection of Treatment Regimen

Selection of the most appropriate treatment regimen for a particular condition should be based whenever possible on application of the appropriate physical, biologic, and clinical concepts. In the following section, these are discussed with regard to the selection of (1) frequency, (2) onset and spacing of treatments, (3) duration of treatment, (4) pulsed or continuous treatment, and (5) intensity.

FREQUENCY

In deciding what frequency to use, assuming that the equipment available allows frequency to be varied, the therapist should consider the following: (1) the depth of the tissue to be treated; (2) differences in acoustic impedance of the tissues in the path of the beam (p. 264); and (3) the mechanisms (pp. 274–276) involved in producing the effect required. The reasons for these considerations are described subsequently.

On entering the tissues, the ultrasonic energy is gradually reduced (*attenuated*) by a combination of processes including absorption and scattering. *Absorption* is the ultimate conversion of energy in the ultrasonic beam to heat, whereas *scattering*, which is due to the inhomogeneity of the tissues, redirects the energy out of the beam.[6] The amount of attenuation depends on the type of tissues through which the ultrasound passes and the frequency of the ultrasound. Tissues with a high protein content, such as muscles and highly collagenous connective tissues, attentuate ultrasound more readily than do tissues with a high fat or water content, and the higher the frequency, the more efficient the attenuation. Thus, 3-MHz ultrasound loses half its initial intensity after passing through about 16 mm of fat or about 3 mm of muscle, while 1-MHz ultrasound travels through about 48 mm of fat, or about 9 mm of muscle, before losing half its energy[4]

TABLE 13–2. The Half Value Depth for 1 MHz and 3 MHz Ultrasound in a Range of Different Media*

Medium	1 MHz (mm)	3 MHz (mm)
1. Water	11,500.0	3833.0
2. Adipose tissue	50.0	16.5
3. Skeletal muscle (fibers parallel to sound beam)	24.6	8.0
4. Skin	11.1	4.0
5. Skeletal muscles (fibers at right angles to sound beam)	9.0	3.0
6. Tendon	6.2	2.0
7. Cartilage	6.0	2.0
8. Air	2.5	0.8
9. Compact bone	2.1	—

*From Hoogland,[4] p. 24, with permission.

(Table 13–2). Ultrasound using 3 MHz is thus more suitable for treating superficial injuries of the epidermis and collagenous dermis—that is, skin wounds—whereas 1 MHz is more suitable if the injury extends more deeply.

The mechanism producing the clinical effect(s) required should also be considered when selecting the ultrasonic frequency. Because absorption produces heating and occurs more readily at higher frequencies, 3 MHz is recommended if the effects required are in superficial tissues and are produced by a thermal mechanism. Some mechanical effects (p. 275) such as acoustic streaming also occur more readily at higher frequencies, whereas others such as stable cavitation occur more efficiently (that is, at lower energy levels) and at lower frequencies, and when these are required lower frequencies should therefore be selected.

ONSET AND SPACING OF TREATMENTS

The ultrasonic treatment of acute injuries should be commenced as soon as possible, ideally within hours of injury.[17,18] In the past, this decision was based on clinical observation and experience, but the reason for the decision is now known; early treatment can reduce the duration of the inflammatory phase of repair and in doing so accelerates the healing process (pp. 277–278).[5,14] Acute conditions are generally treated once or twice daily until symptoms such as pain and swelling are relieved, and then on alternate days until the condition is resolved.[9] In contrast, chronic conditions such as varicose ulceration (Figs. 13–3 through 13–5) are generally treated less frequently—for example, three times a week,[19]—although even one treatment a week can be effective.[20] Here treatment is prolonged throughout the proliferative phase of repair, when it has been shown that low-intensity treatment can stimulate angiogenesis[14] and fibroblast activity,[5] thus assisting in healing.

DURATION OF EACH TREATMENT

Duration is usually based empirically on the surface area to be treated. The area should be divided into zones each 1.5 times the area of the active surface (ERA; see p. 263) of the applicator, and that 1 or 2 minutes be allowed for treating each zone.[18] Thus, if the ERA of the applicator is 5 cm² and the area to be treated is estimated at 30 cm², then there would be four zones, giving a total recommended treatment time of between 4 and 8 minutes. Subsequent treatment times should be increased by 30-

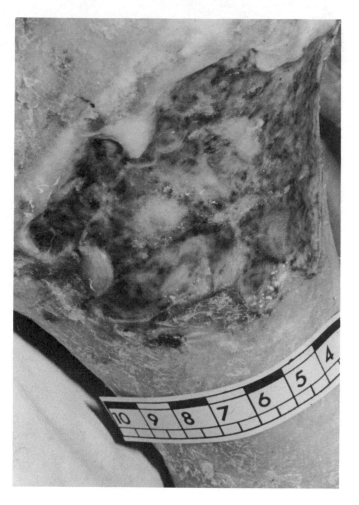

FIGURE 13–3. Varicose ulcer before treatment with ultrasound.

second intervals to a maximum of 3 minutes per zone, if progress is satisfactory.[18] Others[4] recommend a total maximal treatment time of 15 minutes, and that at least 1 minute be spent in treating an area of 1 cm².

PULSED OR CONTINUOUS TREATMENT

If heating is required, then continuous ultrasound is indicated. If, however, the local circulation is compromised and might be unable to dissipate excessive heat rapidly enough to avoid thermal injury, then pulsing can be used to reduce the I(TA), and hence the amount of heating, while keeping the I(PA) high enough to produce the nonthermal effects required.

INTENSITY

For continuous ultrasound, the following guidelines for I(SATA) can be used:

<0.3	W/cm² is considered to be **low** intensity
0.3–1.2	W/cm² is considered to be **medium** intensity
>1.2–3.0	W/cm² is considered to be **high** intensity[4]

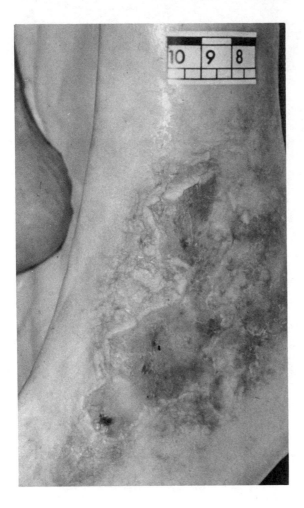

FIGURE 13–4. Appearance of varicose ulcer after 17 treatments (three per week) with ultrasound. The epidermis has extended over much of the well-vascularized granulation tissue that covers the wound bed.

In the interests of safety, the lowest I(SATA) that produces clinically beneficial effects should be used. This intensity is usually near the upper end of the "low" range for acute conditions and near the middle of the "medium" range for chronic conditions and scar tissue. For a clinically significant increase in temperature, an I(SATA) of at least 0.5 W/cm² will be needed. Primarily nonthermal effects can be achieved with lower I(SATA) intensities, obtained by pulsing the ultrasound.

The experience of trained practitioners is a valuable guide in determining appropriate treatment regimens, which are summarized in Table 13–3.[9,21–41] As more becomes understood of the mechanisms by which ultrasound produces its effects, treatment procedures are becoming less empirical and are developing a better theoretic basis. Therapists may be able to improve their treatment procedures as new information becomes available and is confirmed.

BIOPHYSICAL EFFECTS OF THERAPEUTIC ULTRASOUND

The interactions of ultrasound with tissues are the basis of its clinically significant physiologic changes, some therapeutic, stimulating healing, others potentially damaging. The physical effects that lead to these changes must be appreciated if ultrasound is

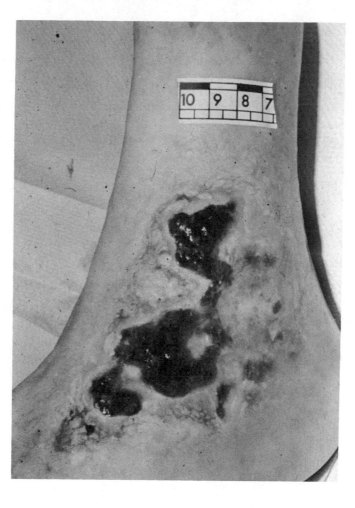

FIGURE 13–5. Appearance of ulcer 8 days later, after four additional treatments with ultrasound. Apart from a small area positioned distally, coverage of the wound surface by epidermis is complete.

to be used safely and efficiently. The object of this section is to describe these effects and their physiologic consequences.

The physical effects of ultrasound, at the levels used therapeutically, can be classified as either primarily thermal or nonthermal.

Thermal

Local tissue heating is the result of *absorption*, the amount and site of which depends on the type of tissue in the path of the beam, the efficiency of the local circulation in dissipating heat, and the frequency of the ultrasound (pp. 267–268). One of the main advantages of using ultrasound as a heating modality is that the therapist has some control over the depth at which heating occurs, since the more penetrative lower frequencies can heat deeper structures. One of the physiologic effects of ultrasonically induced heating that might be expected to stimulate wound healing is a reported increase in blood flow.[42] Raising the local temperature to between 40°C and 45°C is generally acceptable in well-vascularized tissues, but temperatures in excess of this cause thermal necrosis and must be avoided. Some anatomic structures are heated preferentially by ultrasound, including the periosteum, cortical bone joint menisci,

TABLE 13–3. A Selection of Ultrasound Regimens Used in the Treatment of Soft-Tissue Injuries*

Application	Author(s)	Type of Study	Frequency (MHz)	SATP Intensity (W/cm²)	Mode	Regimen	Outcome
Soft-tissue lesions							
Acute injuries							
Sports injuries							
Minor fractures	Patrick (1978)[17]	C	*	*	P	*	
Recent occupational soft-tissue injuries	Middlemast and Chatterjee (1978)[21]	A	1.5	0.5–2.0	P	5 times a week	Significant improvement
Subacute							
Periarthritis shoulder	Lehmann et al (1954)[22]	B	0.8/1.0	0.5–2.0	CW	5–10 min daily × 8	Significant improvement
Acute subacromial bursitis	Bearzy (1953)[23]	C	1.0	2.0–4.0	*	Up to 5 min daily × 3; then alternate days	Success with acute only
Bursitis shoulder	Newman et al (1957)[24]	B	1.0	0.8–3.0	*	5–10 min × 12	Improvement
Painful shoulder	Downing and Weinstein (1986)[25]	A	1.0	1.2–1.3	CW	6 min 3 times a week × 4	No significant difference
Subacromial bursitis	Munting (1978)[26]	A	1.5	0.5	CW	3–5 min × 10	Improvement
Chronic							
OA hip	De Preux (1952)[27]	C	0.8	1.5–2.0	*	10 min 2 times a week	Improvement
Locomotor system	Soren (1969)[28]	C	0.8	1.5–3.5	*	Alternate days	Improvement
Hemiplegic shoulder	Inaba and Piorkowski (1972)[29]	A	*	0.5–2.0	*	5 min daily × 15 min	No significant difference
Chronic arthritis	Griffin et al (1970)[30]	B	0.89/1.0	2.0	*	3 times a week × 3	0.89 MHz more successful
Plantar fascitis and Rheumatoid nodules	Clarke and Stenner (1976)[31]	C	0.75/1.5	1.0–2.5	CW	5 min ×8–10	Decreased pain
		B	3.0	1.05–2.5	CW	5 min ×8–10	Size unchanged; pain decreased

Phonophoresis							
Arthritis	Griffin et al (1967)[15]	C	1.0	1.5 max	CW	1 time a week × 9 max	Successful
Epicondylitis/bursitis	Kleinkort and Wood (1975)[16]	B	1.0	2.0 max	CW	6–9 min	Improvement
Wounds							
Episiotomies	Fieldhouse (1979)[32]	C	*	0.5–0.8	*	5 min 3 times a week × 6	Improvement
Episiotomies and surgical wounds	Ferguson (1981)[33]	C	1.0	0.5	P1:5	3 min daily × 2–4	Improvement
Episiotomies	McLaren (1984)[34]	A	*	0.5	*	5 min	Improvement
Ulcers							
Venous ulcers	Dyson et al (1976)[19]	A	3.0	1.0	P2:8	Size dependent, 3 times a week × 4	Significant improvement
Venous ulcers	Roche and West (1984)[35]	A	3.0	1.0	P2:8	Size dependent, 3 times a week × 4	Significant improvement
Pressure sores	McDiarmid et al (1985)[36]	A	3.0	0.8	P2:8	Size dependent, 3 times a week × 4	Significant improvement, dirty sores only
Scars							
Contracture after hip fixation	Lehmann et al (1961)[37]	B	*	1.0–2.5	*	5 min daily up to 3 weeks	Significant improvement
Hand scars	Bierman (1954)[38]	C	1.0	1.0–2.0	*	6–8 min, alternate days	Improvement
Dupuytren's contracture	Markham and Wood (1980)[39]	C	1.0/3.0	0.25–0.75	CW	4–10 min 1 time a week	Improvement
Dentistry							
Postinjection trismus	Brooke (1979)[40]	C	*	*	*	10 min 3 times a week × 3	Improvement
Oral surgery	El Hag et al (1985)[41]	A	3.0	0.5	P2:8	8 min × 2	Significant improvement

KEY: A = controlled trial; B = comparative study; C = descriptive report; *not specified; P = pulsed; CW = continuous wave
*Adapted from McDiarmid and Burns,[9] p 55, with permission.

fibrotic muscle tendon sheaths, and major nerve roots[42] and intermuscular interfaces.[43] Caution is indicated if any of these are in the path of the ultrasound when a tissue injury is being treated.

Because heat is normally dissipated by circulating blood, if the local circulation is poor or has been interrupted, levels of ultrasound that would be suitable for normally vascularized tissues could produce thermal damage. The presence of a reflecting interface deep to the injured tissues, such as that between soft tissue and bone, air, or a metal prosthesis, could increase the energy reaching the injured tissue and so increase heating. To reduce risk, the intensity of the incident ultrasound used should be the minimum needed to stimulate repair, and the applicator should be moved throughout treatment.

Nonthermal

Some of the physiologic changes induced by therapeutic ultrasound that can affect the healing process are primarily nonthermal in origin. The physical effects producing them include *cavitation, acoustic streaming,* and *standing wave formation.* Because thresholds are below those required for the induction of physiologically significant levels of heating, they must always be considered whenever ultrasound is used therapeutically.

CAVITATION

Under appropriate conditions, ultrasound can cause micron-sized bubbles to form at nucleation sites (discontinuities) in biologic fluids such as blood, lymph, and tissue fluid, and possibly elsewhere in the body. The ultrasonic field to which these bubbles are subsequently exposed can cause them either to vibrate in response to the cyclic pressure changes of the ultrasound (*stable cavitation*), or, if the I(SP) is high enough, to implode violently (*transient, unstable,* or *collapse cavitation*).

Transient cavitation produces localized damage and causes free radical formation. Although free radicals are produced during normal cell metabolism (for example, in aerobic respiration and phagocytosis) in quantities that can be removed by naturally occurring free radical scavengers, excessive exposure to them is dangerous and has been implicated in molecular damage and aging.[44,45] The high levels of "therapeutic" ultrasound used in the past could have induced transient cavitation and with it the petechial hemorrhaging sometimes observed.[46] Although cavitation has been detected in blood plasma exposed in a standing wave field to ultrasound at the upper extreme of the therapy range in vitro,[47] there is no evidence that it occurs in vivo at the lower intensity levels now generally used in physical therapy, provided that the consequences of standing wave formation are avoided.

In contrast, *stable* cavitation *can* be induced in soft tissues in vivo with lower I(SATP) levels[48] and may be partly responsible for the stimulation of tissue repair which exposure to ultrasound can produce. Fluid movements (microstreaming) induced around the pulsating bubbles may modify cell membrane permeability and the diffusion of metabolites and, in doing so, may be of considerable therapeutic value.[49] Unlike heating, cavitation occurs more readily at lower than at higher frequencies. If stable cavitation is required, then a low frequency (for example, 1 MHz) should be selected.

ACOUSTIC STREAMING

This streaming is the circulatory flow of fluid induced by radiation forces. When induced by ultrasound next to a small vibrating object such as a cell or bubble, the movements involved are of microscopic proportions and the process has therefore been termed *microstreaming*,[50] which results in high velocity gradients next to boundaries such as cell membranes or bubble surfaces. These gradients have high viscous forces associated with them, which can alter cell membrane structure and in consequence affect cell activity. Provided that acoustic streaming does not damage the membranes, this streaming could be of therapeutic value in facilitating the transport of ions and possibly some molecules across them.[49] Exposure of fibroblasts, cells of central importance in the repair of the dermis, to therapeutic levels of ultrasound can temporarily increase their uptake of calcium ions.[51,52] With 1-MHz ultrasound I(SP, PA) levels as low as 0.5 W/cm^2, pulsed 2 ms on, 8 ms off, have been found to be effective,[52] and it has been suggested that shear forces produced by acoustic streaming, possibly associated with stable cavitation, may be responsible for it. This effect is of considerable significance, for permeability changes, particularly to the important second messenger calcium,[53] could act as an intracellular signal for some of the events that lead to the ultrasonically induced stimulation of tissue repair—for example, the stimulation of protein synthesis by fibroblasts[54] and the increased release of wound factors from mast cells[55] and macrophages.[14] Ultrasonically induced changes in membrane permeability to sodium ions could help to explain the alterations observed in electrical activity in nerve[56] and muscle.[57] Permeability changes could also be involved in ultrasonically aided pain relief, although endorphin secretion and placebo effects (p. 280) may also play a significant role. Another clinically significant change in membrane function resulting from acoustic streaming is serotonin release from platelets.[58,59] In addition to serotonin, platelets contain chemotactic factors that promote the migration of cells essential for successful repair to the injury site.[60] If streaming can stimulate serotonin release, it may also stimulate the release of these factors, thus stimulating wound healing.

Acoustic streaming is frequently associated with cavitation[61] but can also occur in its absence as a result of radiation torque, a force by which ultrasound induces a circulatory flow of fluids and angular displacement of objects exposed to it.[50] Provided that the shear forces induced by this type of acoustic streaming are sufficient to affect membrane permeability reversibly, stable cavitation need not necessarily be involved in the ultrasonic stimulation of repair processes.

STANDING WAVE FORMATION

When ultrasound reaches an interface between two acoustically different media (for example, soft tissue and bone), some of the incident wave is reflected and the rest either absorbed or transmitted. Interaction between the incident and reflected waves can form a *standing wave* in which their superimposed pressure peaks (antinodes) are stationary in position and separated by half a wavelength. Equidistant between adjacent antinodes are loci of zero pressure, termed *nodes*. Gas bubbles collect into bands at the antinodes and cells, if free to move, at the nodes.[6] Microstreaming occurs in the fluid surrounding the bubbles, and the shear stresses imposed by this can damage the membranes of immobile cells, such as endothelial cells, located at the antinodes. If transient cavitation occurs, the cells next to the imploding bubbles will be destroyed. Standing waves produced by therapeutic intensities of ultrasound can also impede or even arrest the movement of blood cells in vivo. The cells become packed into bands centered on pressure nodes (Fig. 13–6), while the plasma continues to flow.[62] Blood cell

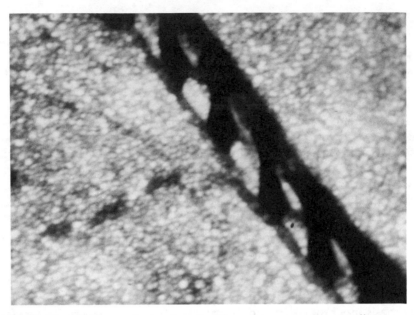

FIGURE 13–6. Photomicrograph showing the effect of exposure to a standing wave field of 3 MHz ultrasound on blood cell distribution in a small vein and adjacent artery. Note that the blood cells are packed into bands half a wavelength apart (in this case 0.25 mm) in the vein.

stasis is reversible and of little clinical significance but may temporarily reduce the efficiency of gaseous exchange. Much more serious is the damage that can be done to the endothelial cells lining the vessels: the shear stresses to which they are exposed can damage them irreversibly, to such an extent that the endothelium loses its integrity and blood clotting occurs.

Tissue damage can be avoided by ensuring that the applicator is moved continuously throughout treatment. This movement provides continuous variation in the angle of incidence of the ultrasound on any reflecting interfaces in its path, so that the positions of the nodes and antinodes constantly vary. As the positions at which mobile cells and bubbles (if present) collect changes, the circulation of blood cells can continue uninterrupted, and the possibility of endothelial damage is minimized.

EFFECTS OF THERAPEUTIC ULTRASOUND ON WOUND HEALING

The biophysical effects of ultrasound just described suggest that, if applied correctly, ultrasonic therapy should be able to produce physiologic changes that could accelerate wound healing and other forms of tissue repair. If incorrectly used, however, it would at best be ineffective and at worst deleterious, impeding repair or even causing further damage. In this section, the demonstrated effects of ultrasound on wound healing are described.

Although little is known about the direct effect of ultrasound on repair of the epidermis, considerable progress has been made in describing and understanding its effects on repair of the soft connective tissue that constitutes the dermis. To facilitate description, the repair of the dermis can be divided into three overlapping phases—

acute inflammation (early and late), proliferation, and remodeling—all of which can be affected by treatment of the injured and adjacent tissues with ultrasound.

Inflammatory Phase

As soon as soft connective tissue is injured, platelets and mast cells are activated, releasing pharmacologically active agents that initiate acute inflammation and, in part, lead to its resolution. Inflammation, the characteristics of which include pain, erythema, and swelling, is unpleasant and is often considered to be an adverse condition, for which anti-inflammatory agents are prescribed to reduce swelling and relieve pain, an appropriate course of action for chronic inflammatory conditions. Acute inflammation, however, unlike chronic inflammation, is not a disease but the normal response of tissues to injury; it is part of the healing process and as such should be accelerated rather than suppressed. Ultrasonic therapy, applied shortly after injury, can accelerate the inflammatory phase of repair,[5] and in doing so accelerate wound healing.

A single treatment of therapeutic ultrasound applied during the early inflammatory phase can stimulate the release of histamine from mast cells by degranulation.[55,63] These cells contain a wide range of chemical mediators in addition to histamine, including chemotactic agents that attract neutrophils and monocytes to the wound site.[64] Many of these agents are preformed and stored in granules; if their release is also stimulated by ultrasound, then this would help to explain why many physical therapists find ultrasonic therapy particularly valuable if applied after bleeding has stopped but during the first 24 hours after injury, that is, while still in the early part of the acute inflammatory phase of repair. Mast cell degranulation is generally triggered by membrane changes involving the increased transport of calcium ions into the cell.[64] Possibly membrane perturbation induced by ultrasonic therapy can increase calcium ion transport into mast cells, as it does in fibroblasts.[51,52]

On arriving at the site of injury, monocytes leave the blood vessels and develop into macrophages. Together with the neutrophils, they remove debris and pathogenic organisms from the wound site. Provided that the wound is not contaminated, the number of neutrophils in the wound begins to decrease after a few days, marking the end of the early part of the inflammatory phase of repair. The late part of the inflammatory phase is characterized by a continued increase in the number of macrophages, while the number of neutrophils decreases. The granules of both neutrophils and macrophages, but particularly the latter, contain chemotactic agents and growth factors that are necessary for the development of the new connective tissue at the site of the injury.[65] On their release, these agents and factors stimulate pericytes (undifferentiated mesenchymal cells), fibroblasts, and endothelial cells to produce granulation tissue at the wound site. Treatment of U937 cells (an unstimulated form of macrophage that can be maintained in vitro), with therapeutic levels of ultrasound, can result in the release of wound factors that stimulate fibroblast proliferation.[66] Treatment in the late part of the inflammatory phase, when macrophages containing these factors are gathering at the wound site, is therefore recommended, for early release of these factors could accelerate the onset of the proliferative phase of repair.

Although therapeutic ultrasound can accelerate the early inflammatory phase of repair, it is not an anti-inflammatory agent. Clinical research on the resolution of postoperative edema[63] revealed that an apparently anti-inflammatory response following low-intensity ultrasonic therapy was mainly a placebo effect. Furthermore, the same study showed that spatial average pulse average intensities (I[SAPA]) of 0.5 W/cm² and above were proinflammatory, in that they stimulated mast cell activity; this was, however, masked by its anti-inflammatory placebo-induced effects.

Proliferative Phase

This phase overlaps with, and is initiated by, the late part of the inflammatory phase of repair, generally beginning about 3 days after injury. During the proliferative phase, a highly vascularized, collagen-rich granulation tissue develops at the site of injury and, in the case of excised lesions of the skin, becomes covered superficially by epidermal cells. Granulation tissue is a temporary reparative tissue and is gradually replaced by scar tissue during the subsequent remodeling phase. This tissue is very cellular, containing macrophages (which secrete chemotactic and growth factors and in doing so control its development), pericytes, fibroblasts, and endothelial cells, together with an extracellular matrix. The matrix, secreted by cells of the granulation tissue, is rich in fibronectin (the substrate over which cells contributing to the granulation tissue migrate), Type III collagen, and hyaluronic acid.[65] Initially, the factors secreted by the macrophages are essential, for they attract the other cells of the granulation tissue to the wound area and stimulate their proliferation. Later in the proliferative phase, however, the need for them appears to be reduced, for the number of macrophages falls, while that of the fibroblasts and endothelial cells increases. The fibroblasts are of great importance in repair, for not only are they the main producers of the matrix materials, but they are also the chief contractile cells of the wound, and, as myofibroblasts, help to reduce the size of the tissue defect (that is, they are responsible for wound contraction).[67] The endothelial cells are literally vital in that they are essential for angiogenesis, forming the new blood capillaries that transport metabolites to and from the reparative tissue. There is evidence that both fibroblast activity and angiogenesis can be affected by therapeutic ultrasound in a manner conducive to the acceleration of tissue repair.

The exposure of fibroblasts in vitro to therapeutic ultrasound can stimulate them to secrete more collagen, the fibrous protein that increases the tensile strength of connective tissues.[68] This increase may be triggered by a temporary ultrasonically induced increase in their calcium ion content following reversible alterations in membrane permeability.[51,52] Shear stresses associated with acoustic streaming[52] and possibly also with stable cavitation[51] have been implicated in the production of these effects in vitro. Nonthermal levels of ultrasound can stimulate fibroblast activity in vivo,[69] but whether or not cavitation is involved remains to be determined.

Treatment with ultrasound during the inflammatory and early proliferative phases of repair can accelerate wound contraction,[70] presumably directly by its effects on the fibroblasts and indirectly by factors released from macrophages. Wound contraction, the reduction of a skin defect by the centripetal movement of the surrounding intact skin, reduces the need for scar-tissue production. During wound contraction, fibroblasts develop temporarily into myofibroblasts, specialized contractile and secretory cells,[67] and become linked together and aligned in such a way that when they contract the edges of the wound are pulled together. They resemble smooth muscle cells, and since the latter can be induced to contract by therapeutic levels of ultrasound,[71] possibly myofibroblast contraction may be affected in a similar manner. Although wound contraction can be accelerated by ultrasound, there is no evidence that the total amount of contraction is affected. No reports have been found of excessive contraction (that is, contracture) following treatment with therapeutic ultrasound; although it occurs more rapidly, the normal control mechanisms continue to operate efficiently.

In addition to numerous clinical reports (see Table 13–3), there are now quantitative data to support the hypothesis that treatment of injured skin with therapeutic ultrasound during the inflammatory and early proliferative phases of repair can accelerate healing of the dermis.[14,66] The method used is based on the observation that during repair different types of cells arrive at, and then leave, the wound site in a characteristic sequence. The first to arrive, during the inflammatory phase, are neutrophils (polymorphonuclear leukocytes) and macrophages. Provided that the wound is not contaminated, the neutrophils leave within a few days, marking the end of the early part of the inflammatory process, but the macrophages continue to increase in number. During the proliferative phase, the number of fibroblasts and endothelial cells increases, while the number of macrophages gradually falls. This sequence is shown diagrammatically in Figure 13–7. Because each group of cells reaches a maximum and then decreases, the rate of progress of repair can be quantified by assessing the relative numbers of each cell type at different times after injury.[72] By 5 days after injury, there are fewer macrophages but significantly more fibroblasts in wounds treated with ultrasound at either 1 or 3 MHz (0.5 W/cm² [SAPA], pulsed 2 ms on:8 ms off for 5 minutes daily) compared with sham-irradiated controls,[14,16] suggesting that wounds treated with ultrasound in this manner leave the inflammatory phase and enter the proliferative phase of repair more rapidly than the controls. Treatment with ultrasound can thus be shown to accelerate dermal repair.

Treatment with therapeutic ultrasound can also stimulate endothelial cell activity, in addition to affecting mast cells, macrophages, and fibroblasts. In chronically ischemic muscle, treatment with ultrasound can cause new capillaries to develop and the circulation to be restored at an accelerated rate.[73] Treatment with ultrasound during the first 4 days after injury has recently been shown to result in a statistically significant increase in the rate at which blood capillaries and other vessels develop within the granulation tissue.[74] Because angiogenic factors are present in the granules of mast cells and macrophages[75] the stimulation observed may be due, at least in part, to an accelerated

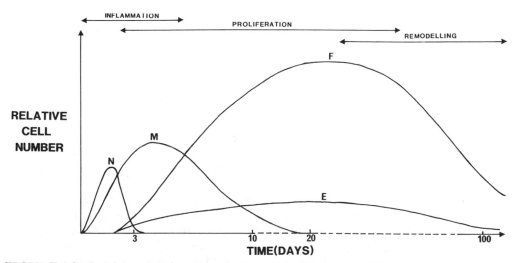

FIGURE 13–7. Diagrammatic representation of the changes in cellularity that occur in the wound bed during repair of the dermis. E = endothelial cells; F = fibroblasts (including myofibroblasts and fibrocytes); M = macrophages; N = neutrophils (polymorphonuclear leukocytes).

liberation of their release. The possibility of a direct effect on endothelial cells has not yet been investigated.

Remodeling Phase

During this phase, which overlaps with the preceding proliferative phase, the initial, apparently haphazard deposition of collagen fibers is changed. Collagen fibers are removed from some locations and newly synthesized fibers deposited in others, resulting in a more regular pattern believed to be related to the mechanical forces to which the tissue is subjected during normal activity. Furthermore, some of the Type III collagen is replaced by Type I. Ideally, remodeling should continue until the scar tissue, which replaces granulation tissue at the site of injury, becomes both structurally and functionally identical to preinjury tissue. In the case of injured dermis, this ideal state is never reached, the scar tissue remaining weaker and less elastic than uninjured dermis indefinitely.

Exposure to therapeutic levels of ultrasound during remodeling has been used in attempts to improve the mechanical properties of mature scar tissue, with limited success.[38,39] An alternative approach is to commence treatment immediately after injury, a technique that has been shown to have more dramatic effects on the mechanical properties of the scar tissue. Full-thickness skin wounds treated with therapeutic levels of ultrasound (0.5 W/cm² [SAPA], 3 MHz, pulsed 2 ms on:8 ms off for 5 minutes, three times weekly for 2 weeks) developed significantly stronger and yet more elastic scar tissue than control, sham-irradiated wounds, but remained mechanically less satisfactory than uninjured skin.[69,76] The increased strength of the treated scar tissue is believed to be due to its increased collagen content, while the increased elasticity could be related to a change in collagen fiber pattern. Scanning electron microscopy has shown that the pattern in ultrasonically treated scar tissue is that of a three-dimensional lattice resembling that of the uninjured dermis, whereas in sham-treated controls the fiber arrangement is less regular. Change in fiber angle in the lattice arrangement in response to the application of a tensile force to the tissue would permit a limited amount of elongation, followed by recoil when the force was reduced and the fibers returned to their original position; it could also increase the amount of energy that the scar tissue can absorb before rupturing.[77]

PLACEBO EFFECTS ASSOCIATED WITH THERAPEUTIC ULTRASOUND

Many patients find exposure to therapeutic ultrasound pleasant, soothing, and relaxing. There is an increasing body of evidence that, in addition to the direct, physical effects of ultrasound, there are also psychologic effects associated with the treatment, which can act as a placebo.[41,78] The exposure of surgical patients to placebo treatments can lead to lowered perception of pain, and this change is associated with changes in plasma β-endorphins.[79] Placebo effects can be beneficial, provided that pain relief does not lead the patient to inappropriate and damaging activity. The benefits derived from placebo effects should be considered as a bonus to the benefits provided directly by the therapeutic modality with which they are associated. The role of placebo effects in physical therapy is worthy of further investigation.

THE SAFE USE OF THERAPEUTIC ULTRASOUND

Although ultrasound, correctly used, has an impressive record of safety and efficiency, this modality is potentially dangerous if used inappropriately. The literature contains long lists of contraindications and precautions,[80] including irradiation of the uterus during pregnancy; the gonads; malignancies and precancerous lesions; tissues previously treated by deep x-ray or other radiation; vascular abnormalities including deep vein thrombosis, emboli, severe atherosclerosis; acute infections; the cardiac area in advanced heart disease; the eye; the stellate ganglion; hemophiliacs not covered by factor replacement; over subcutaneous bony prominences; epiphyseal plates; the spinal cord after laminectomy; subcutaneous major nerves; the cranium; and anesthetic areas; and the use of a stationary applicator technique. Certainly, the excellent safety record of ultrasonic therapy owes much to the conservative approach that such a lengthy list engenders. Although they are an excellent aid to the safe use of ultrasound, not all of the contraindications listed have been subjected to experimental verification; many appear to have been included if there is even only a remote possibility that damage might ensue.

Any invasive, interactive treatment has an element of risk; the therapist should always be aware of this and apply such treatment only if the benefit outweighs the risk. Proper assessment of benefit versus risk is only possible if the mechanisms of the treatment are understood (pp. 270–276). As more becomes known of these mechanisms, and as methods of applying ultrasound are improved, these lists should be reviewed and, when appropriate, amended.

In addition, it is recommended,[81] in the interests of safety and efficiency, that the following basic precautions be taken:

1. Use ultrasound only if adequately trained to do so.
2. Use ultrasound only to treat patients with conditions known to respond favorably to this treatment, unless it is being used experimentally.
3. Use the lowest intensity that produces the required effect, since higher intensities may be damaging.
4. Move the applicator constantly throughout treatment, to avoid the damaging effects of standing waves.
5. If the patient feels any additional pain during treatment, either reduce the intensity to a pain-free level or abandon the treatment.
6. Use properly calibrated and maintained equipment.
7. If there is any doubt, do not irradiate.

CLINICAL DECISION MAKING

The preceding sections of this chapter contain the basic information a therapist requires to decide, when treating an injured patient, (1) if ultrasound will be an effective and safe form of treatment, and (2) how it should be applied; that is, what treatment regimen should be used.

The following section summarizes the procedures to be followed and the major questions to be answered before these decisions can be reached.

Stages in Decision Making

1. **Determine the nature of the condition.** Consider if, in view of the medical history of the patient and the location of the injury, the use of ultrasound is contraindicated. See p. 281.

2. **Is the condition acute or chronic?** If acute, make use of the nonthermal (mechanical) effects of ultrasound. Set to pulsed mode so that these effects can be achieved without excessive heating. If chronic (or scar tissue), then provided that the blood supply to the regions is not compromised, ultrasound can be used as a heating modality and applied in continuous mode. However, if the blood supply is poor or interrupted, the pulsed mode should be used. See p. 269.

3. **How deep does the injury extend?** If it is superficial (less than 1 cm), select a high frequency (3 MHz). If the injury extends more deeply, select a lower frequency (e.g., 1 MHz). See pp. 267–268.

4. **Assess the size of the area to be treated.** Select the size of applicator to be used accordingly. Assuming a minimal treatment time of 1 minute/cm^2 and a maximal treatment time of 15 minutes,[4] an applicator with an ERA of 1 cm^2 is suitable. For larger areas, use a larger applicator. See pp. 268–269.

5. **Select coupling medium.** If the skin is broken, then a sterile aqueous gel-based wound dressing is indicated. If epithelialized, other materials can be used. If the area is irregular and a small applicator is not available, the region can be treated while submerged in clean, degassed water. If the area is regular, then an appropriate oil, emulsion, or gel can be used. See pp. 264–265.

6. **Select intensity.** Use the upper end of low range for acute conditions and the middle of the medium range for chronic conditions, unless the blood supply is defective, when the lowest part of the medium range is recommended. See p. 269–270.

7. **Select the duration of treatment.** A minimum of 1 minute/cm^2 for a total treatment time of 15 minutes is suggested. See p. 268–269.

8. **Assess and record response to treatment.** Modify or replace it if necessary.

SUMMARY

Ultrasonic therapy is of considerable value in accelerating wound healing, provided that ultrasound is used correctly. Ultrasound is particularly effective if treatment is commenced shortly after injury, during the inflammatory phase of repair. There is now considerable evidence that this modality can accelerate the resolution of inflammation and that, in consequence, the onset of the proliferative phase of repair is advanced. Ultrasound can produce a wide range of effects on cells and tissues. Some of these effects are potentially beneficial, while others can be harmful. Ultrasound users must be informed of them and of the mechanisms by which they are produced, if the modality is to be used with optimal efficiency and safety.

ACKNOWLEDGMENTS

I thank all the members, past and present, of the Tissue Repair Research Unit at United Medical and Dental Schools (Guy's Hospital), who have contributed to this work, the physical therapists and physicists who have provided such valuable information and advice, the manufacturers who have supplied equipment (Duffield, Electro Medical Supplies, Enraf-Nonius Delft, Magnetopulse, Mettler, S.C.I. Instruments, and T.G.S. Electronics), and the following who have provided financial support for the work on ultrasound bioeffects carried out by the research unit: Geistlich Pharmaceuticals, Johnson and Johnson, Inc., Luitpold-Werk, Magnetopulse, the Medical Research Council (Grant No. G8518373CA), and the National Fund for Research into Crippling Diseases (Grant Nos. A/8/1017 and A/8/1153).

REFERENCES

1. ter Haar, GR, Dyson, M, and Oakley, E: The use of therapeutic ultrasound by physiotherapists in Britain: 1985. Ultrasound Med Biol 13:659, 1987.
2. ter Haar, GR: Basic physics of therapeutic ultrasound. Physiotherapy 73:110, 1987.
3. Wlliams, R: Production and transmission of ultrasound. Physiotherapy 73:113, 1987.
4. Hoogland, R: Ultrasound Therapy. Enraf-Nonius, Delft, Holland, 1986.
5. Dyson, M: Mechanisms involved in therapeutic ultrasound. Physiotherapy 73:116, 1987.
6. NCRP Scientific Committee 66: Biological effects of ultrasound: Mechanisms and clinical implications. NCRP Report No. 74. National Council on Radiation Protection and Measurements, Bethesda, MD, 1983.
7. Ziskin, MC and Michlovitz, SL: Therapeutic ultrasound. In Michlovitz, SL (ed): Thermal Agents in Rehabilitation. FA Davis, Philadelphia, 1986, p 141.
8. Docker, M, Foulkes, DJ, and Patrick, MK: Ultrasound couplants for physiotherapy. Physiotherapy 68:124, 1982.
9. McDiarmid, T and Burns, PN: Clinical applications of therapeutic ultrasound. Physiotherapy 73:155, 1987.
10. Reid, DC and Cummins, GE: Efficiency of ultrasound coupling agents. Physiotherapy 63:255, 1977.
11. Woods, HE and Cottier, D (eds): Geliperm: A clear advance in healing. Conference Proceedings, John Radcliffe Hospital, Oxford, September 30–October 1, 1983. Sheffield University Printing Unit, Sheffield, 1985.
12. Shotton, C: A tethered float radiometer for measuring power from ultrasound therapy equipment. Ultrasound Med Biol 6:131, 1980.
13. Brueton, RH and Campbell, B: The use of Geliperm as a sterile coupling agent for therapeutic ultrasound. Physiotherapy 73:653, 1987.
14. Young, S: The effect of therapeutic ultrasound on the biological mechanisms involved in dermal repair. PhD Thesis, University of London, 1988.
15. Griffin, JE, et al: Patients treated with ultrasonic driven cortisone and with ultrasound alone. Phys Ther 47:594, 1967.
16. Kleinkort, JA and Wood, F: Phonophoresis with one per cent versus ten per cent hydrocortisone. Phys Ther 55:1320, 1975.
17. Patrick, MK: Applications of therapeutic pulsed ultrasound. Physiotherapy 64:169, 1978.
18. Oakley, EM: Application of continuous beam ultrasound at therapeutic levels. Physiotherapy 64:103, 1978.
19. Dyson, M, Franks, C, and Suckling, J: Stimulation of healing of varicose ulcers by ultrasound. Ultrasonics 14:232, 1976.
20. Callam, MJ, et al: A controlled trial of weekly ultrasound therapy in chronic leg ulceration. Lancet 2:204, 1987.
21. Middlemast, SJ and Chatterjee, DS: Comparison of ultrasound and thermography for soft tissue injuries. Physiotherapy 64:331, 1978.
22. Lehmann, FF, et al: Comparison of ultrasonic and microwave diathermy in the physical treatment of periarthritis of the shoulder. Arch Phys Med Rehabil 35:627, 1954.
23. Bearzy, HJ: Clinical applications of ultrasonic energy in treatment of acute and chronic subacromial bursitis. Arch Phys Med Rehabil 43:228, 1953.
24. Newman, MK, Kill, M, and Frampton, G: Effects of ultrasound alone and combined with hydrocortisone injections by needle or hypospray. Am J Phys Med 37:206, 1957.
25. Downing, DS and Weinstein, A: Ultrasound therapy of subacromial bursitis: A double blind trial. Phys Ther 66:194, 1986.

26. Munting, E: Ultrasonic therapy for painful shoulders. Physiotherapy 64:180, 1978.
27. De Preux, T: Ultrasonic wave therapy in osteoarthritis of the hip joint. Br J Phys Med 15:14, 1952.
28. Soren, A: Ultrasound treatment in diseases of the locomotor system. Med Times 97:219, 1969.
29. Inaba, MK and Piorkowski, M: Ultrasound in treatment of painful shoulders in patients with hemiplegia. Phys Ther 52:737, 1972.
30. Griffin, JE, Echternach, JL, and Bowmaker, KL: Results of frequency differences in ultrasonic therapy. Phys Ther 50:481, 1970.
31. Clarke, GR and Stenner, L: Use of therapeutic ultrasound. Physiotherapy 62:185, 1976.
32. Fieldhouse, C: Ultrasound for relief of painful episiotomy scars. Physiotherapy 65:217, 1979.
33. Ferguson, HN: Ultrasound in the treatment of surgical wounds. Physiotherapy 67:12, 1981.
34. McLaren, J: Randomised controlled trial of ultrasound therapy for the damaged perineum. Clin Phys Physiol Meas 5:40, 1984.
35. Roche, C and West, J: A controlled trial investigating the effect of ultrasound on venous ulcers referred from general practitioners. Physiotherapy 70:475, 1984.
36. McDiarmid, T, et al: Ultrasound and the treatment of pressure sores. Physiotherapy 71:66, 1985.
37. Lehmann, JF, et al: Clinical evaluation of a new approach in the treatment of contracture associated with hip fracture after internal fixation. Arch Phys Med Rehabil 42:95, 1961.
38. Bierman, W: Ultrasound in the treatment of scars. Arch Phys Med Rehabil 35:209, 1954.
39. Markham, DE and Wood, MR: Ultrasound for Dupuytren's contracture. Physiotherapy 66:55, 1980.
40. Brooke, RI: Post-injection trismus due to formation of fibrous band. Oral Surg Oral Med Oral Pathol 47:424, 1979.
41. El Hag, M, et al: The anti-inflammatory effects of dexamethasone and therapeutic ultrasound in oral surgery. Br J Oral Maxillofac Surg 23:17, 1985.
42. Lehmann, JF and Guy, AW: Ultrasound Therapy. In Reid, J and Sikov, M (eds): Interaction of Ultrasound and Biological Tissues. DHEW Publication (FDA) 73-8008. Government Printing Office, Washington, DC, 1972, p 141.
43. ter Haar, GR, and Hopewell, JW: Ultrasonic heating of mammalian tissue in vivo. Br J Cancer 45 (Suppl V):65, 1982.
44. Zoler, ML: Free radicals: The real culprits in aging? Geriatrics 40:126, 1985.
45. Balin, AK: Testing the free radical theory of aging. In Alderman, RC, and Roth GS (eds): Testing the Theories of Aging. CRC Press, Boca Raton, FL, 1982, p 137.
46. Lehmann, JF and Herrick, JF: Biologic reactions to cavitation, a consideration for ultrasonic therapy. Arch Phys Med 3:86, 1953.
47. Crum, LA, et al: Acoustic cavitation and medical ultrasound. Proc Inst Acoust 8:137, 1986.
48. ter Haar, GR and Daniels, S: Evidence of ultrasonically induced cavitation in vivo. Phys Med Biol 26:1145, 1981.
49. Dyson, M: Therapeutic applications of ultrasound. In Nyborg, WL and Ziskin, MC (eds): Biological Effects of Ultrasound (Clinics in Diagnostic Ultrasound). Churchill-Livingstone, Edinburgh, 1985, p 121.
50. Nyborg, WL: Acoustic streaming. In Mason, WP (ed): Physical Acoustics. Vol 2, Part B. Academic Press, New York, 1985, p 265.
51. Mummery, CL: The effect of ultrasound on fibroblasts in vitro. PhD Thesis, University of London, 1978.
52. Mortimer, AJ and Dyson, M: The effect of therapeutic ultrasound on calcium uptake in fibroblasts. Ultrasound Med Biol 14(6):499–506, 1988.
53. Rasmussen, H and Weismann, D: The messenger function of calcium in endocrine systems. In Litwock, C (ed): Biochemical Actions of Hormones. Vol 8. Academic Press, New York, p 1.
54. Webster, D, et al: The role of ultrasound-induced cavitation in the in vitro stimulation of protein synthesis on human fibroblasts by ultrasound. Ultrasound Med Biol 4:343, 1988.
55. Fyfe, MC and Chahl, LA: Mast cell degranulation: A possible mechanism of action of therapeutic ultrasound. Ultrasound Med Biol 8 (Suppl 1):62, 1982.
56. Madsen, PW and Gersten, JW: The effects of ultrasound on conduction velocity in peripheral nerve. Arch Phys Med Rehabil 42:645, 1961.
57. Mortimer, AJ, et al: A relationship between ultrasonic intensity and change in myocardial mechanics. Can J Physiol Pharmacol 58:67, 1980.
58. Williams, AR: Release of serotonin from platelets by acoustic streaming. J Acoust Soc Am 56:1640, 1974.
59. Williams, AR, Sykes, SM, and O'Brien, WD: Ultrasonic exposure modifies platelet morphology and function in vitro. Ultrasound Med Biol 2:311, 1976.
60. Ginsberg, M: Role of platelets in inflammation and rheumatic disease. Adv Inflamm Res 2:53, 1981.
61. Doulah, MS: Mechanisms of disintegration of biological cells in ultrasonic cavitation. Biotechnol Bioeng 19:649, 1977.
62. Dyson, M, et al: The production of blood cell stasis and endothelial cell damage in the blood vessels of chick embryos treated with ultrasound in a stationary wave field. Ultrasound Med Biol 1:133, 1974.
63. Hashish, II: The effects of ultrasound therapy on post-operative inflammation. PhD Thesis, University of London, 1986.
64. Yurt, RW: Role of the mast cell in trauma. In Dineen, P and Hildick-Smith, G (eds): The Surgical Wound. Lea and Febiger, Philadelphia, 1981, p 37.
65. Clark, RAF: Cutaneous tissue repair: Basic biologic considerations. J Am Inst Dermatol 13:701, 1985.

66. Dyson, M and Young, SR: Acceleration of tissue repair by low intensity ultrasound applied during the inflammatory phase. American Physical Therapy Association/Canadian Physical Therapy Association Joint Congress, Abstract Number RP-PL 97, 1988.
67. Gabbiani, G, Ryan, GB, and Majno, G: Presence of modified fibroblasts in granulation tissue and their possible role in wound contraction. Experientia (Basel), 27:549, 1971.
68. Harvey, W, et al: The in vitro stimulation of protein synthesis in human fibroblasts by therapeutic levels of ultrasound. Proceedings of Second Congress of Ultrasonics in Medicine. Excerpta Medica, Amsterdam, 1975, p 10.
69. Webster, DF: The effect of ultrasound on wound healing. PhD Thesis, University of London, 1980.
70. Dyson, M and Smalley, D: Effects of ultrasound on wound contraction. In Millner, R and Corbet, U (eds): Ultrasound Interactions in Biology and Medicine. Plenum, New York, 1983, p 151.
71. ter Haar, GR, Dyson, M, and Talbert, D: Ultrasonically induced contraction of mouse uterine smooth muscle in vivo. Ultrasonics 16:175, 1978.
72. Dyson, M, et al: Comparison of the effects of moist and dry conditions on dermal repair. J Invest Dermatol 91:434, 1988.
73. Hogan, RD, Burke, KM, and Franklin, TD: The effect of ultrasound on microvascular hemodynamics in skeletal muscle: Effects during ischemia. Microvasc Res 23:370, 1982.
74. Hosseinpour, AR: The effects of ultrasound on angiogenesis and wound healing. BSc Thesis, University of London, 1988.
75. Martin, BM, et al: Stimulation of nonlymphoid mesenchymal cell proliferation by a macrophage-derived growth factor. J Immunol 126:1510, 1981.
76. Dyson, M: The effect of ultrasound on the rate of wound healing and the quality of scar tissue. In Mortimer, A and Lee, N (eds): Proceedings of the International Symposium on Therapeutic Ultrasound. Manitoba. Canadian Physiotherapy Association, Winnipeg, 1981, p 110.
77. Forrester, JC: Mechanical, biochemical and architectural features of surgical repair. Adv Biol Med Phys 14:1, 1973.
78. Hashish, II: The effects of ultrasound therapy on post-operative inflammation. PhD Thesis, University of London, 1986.
79. Hargreaves, KM, Dionne, RA, and Mueller, GP: Plasma β-endorphin-like immunoreactivity, pain, and anxiety following administration of placebo in oral surgery patients. J Dent Res 62:1170, 1983.
80. Reid, DC: Possible contraindications and precautions associated with ultrasound therapy. In Mortimer, A and Lee, N (eds): Proceedings of the International Symposium on Therapeutic Ultrasound. Canadian Physiotherapy Association, Winnipeg, 1981, p 274.
81. Dyson, M: The use of ultrasound in sports physiotherapy. In Bromley, I and Watts, N (series eds): International Pespectives in Physical Therapy. Grisogono, V (volume ed): Sports Injuries. Churchill-Livingstone, Edinburgh. Accepted for publication, 1988.

Appendix

MANUFACTURERS OF PHARMACEUTICALS

Geistlich Pharmaceuticals
Newton Bank
Long Lane (A41)
Chester, CH2 3QZ
England

Parker Laboratories, Inc.
307 Washington Street
Orange, NJ 07050

B.V. Enraf-Nonius, Delft
P.O. Box 483-2600
A1 Delft, The Netherlands

Luitpold-Werk-Munchen
P.O. Box 701209
Zeilstattstrasse 9211
8000 Munchen 70
West Germany

CHAPTER 14

Role of Light in Wound Healing

Jack Cummings, Ph.D., P.T.

This chapter discusses the use of low-energy laser, ultraviolet, and infrared radiation in facilitating the healing of open wounds.

LOW-ENERGY LASER IRRADIATION

A physical agent reputed to be medically and cost effective in facilitating the healing of dermal wounds is the helium-neon (He-Ne) laser, a type of low-energy or cold laser.[1] Several scientific studies reported in the European literature provide beginning evidence that the low-powered He-Ne laser may be effective in promoting wound healing.[2,3] Although the He-Ne laser has been well received by the American medical community, introduction of these devices into the United States has been surrounded by controversy.[4,5] One factor contributing to the controversy is the paucity of American and Western research reports supporting the use of low-energy laser biostimulation studies since most of the studies are of Soviet or Eastern European origin. The results of many of the reported studies have been questioned because the methods used in the studies have not been well described, rendering the studies nonreproducible. Therefore, the United States Food and Drug Administration (FDA) has limited the use of low-energy, cold lasers to approved experimental use.[6] At present, the status of low-energy, cold lasers remains experimental.

Biophysical Properties of Laser

The biomedical laser, *l*ight *a*mplified by *s*timulated *e*mission of *r*adiation, may be classified as either high or low powered, or hot and cold, respectively. When a high-powered light beam or hot laser is directed at tissue, the basic reaction is one of destruction of tissues, which is known as *photocoagulation necrosis*. This reaction is similar to the tissue changes induced by electrical burns.[7] High-powered lasers have been used in surgery for the past 20 years. Surgical lasers are used for precision cutting and to destroy diseased tissue with very little if any damage to surrounding normal structures. Since the surgical laser cauterizes as it cuts tissue, blood loss from incisions is minimal. Today, surgical lasers are used in virtually all of the surgical disciplines. Of particular significance is the common use of lasers in ophthalmology for the repair of retinal detachments.[8,9]

In contrast to high-powered lasers, which produce an intense thermal effect, low-powered lasers have a minimal heating effect. The benefits of low-powered lasers are thought to be the photochemical and biostimulatory effects and not the thermal effects of the optically pure light. An example of a photochemical effect is the formation of free radicals (highly active intermediates in various reactions in living tissue).[7] The low-powered laser irradiation may be applied to human tissues without tissue damage resulting from intense heat. While the power of high-energy lasers may be in the 10 to 100 W/cm² range, the power emitted by low-energy lasers is measured in milliwatts (less than 1 mW) per square centimeter.[8-11]

The biostimulatory effects of low-powered lasers may result from the unique physical properties of laser light. The light we normally receive from the sun is a mixture of light waves of varying frequencies and wavelengths. However, the light generated by a laser is pure light composed of waves of the same wavelength (monochromatic) that travel in step with one another (coherence) and are nearly parallel (low divergence).[8,9]

The Helium-Neon Laser

All lasers have three components: (1) a power source, (2) an active medium, and (3) a feedback mechanism. The power source, usually electricity, can be a chemical reaction, an intense ordinary light source, or possibly another laser. The active medium is the substance in which the beam of light is generated. The active medium can be a solid such as the crystal ruby; a liquid dye; or a gas, such as argon, carbon dioxide, nitrogen, or helium-neon. The third component of the laser, the feedback mechanism, is composed of two mirrors that are placed at each end of a tube containing the active medium. The mirrors amplify the light produced by the active medium once the power source activates the medium.[7,8,11]

The active medium determines the wavelength of the laser beam, which is described in nanometers (nm). For example, the solid ruby crystal produces a beam of light having a wavelength of 694.3 nm, carbon dioxide produces coherent light with a wavelength of 10,600 nm, and the He-Ne laser light emits a wavelength of 632.8 nm (Fig. 14–1).

Power is the rate at which energy is produced and is measured in watts (J/sec). If a laser produces one pulse per second (pps), its average power, the amount of energy transferred in 1 second, will be 0.001 J/1 sec = 0.001 W or 1 mW. When the average power of a laser is 1 mW or less, the laser is classified as a low-power, low-energy, or cold laser.[10] In the case of high-powered lasers, the power may be intense enough to burn through solid objects such as metals.[7]

Power density describes the concentration of power in a specific area. It is determined by power divided by area. Therefore, a 1 mW laser beam distributed over a 1 cm² area has a power density of 1 milliwatt per square centimeter (1 mW/cm²).[10]

The beam of light is produced by the active medium through a process called *excitation*. Excitation occurs after the atoms composing the medium absorb more energy from the power source than they can normally hold. Because the atoms of the medium

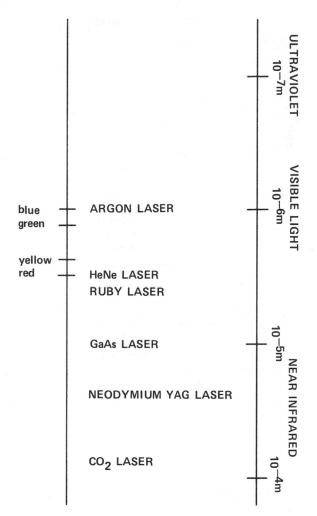

FIGURE 14–1. The visible light and infrared portions of the electromagnetic spectrum, with several types of lasers placed in their approximate location on the spectrum (From Michlovitz,[61] p. 220, with permission).

cannot hold any additional energy, they expel the energy in the form of photons. As one atom gives off energy in the form of light (photons), a chain reaction is initiated in which other atoms in the medium also release energy in the form of light. Initially, the light beams travel in random directions; however, they eventually pass back and forth between the mirrors of the feedback mechanism (Fig. 14–2). This process is called *amplification*. Ultimately, the laser beam will be emitted from one end of the laser tube, through a small opening in one of the mirrors.[11] A fiber optic cable then transmits the beam to a stylus aperture that allows the user to direct and apply the laser energy.

The He-Ne laser uses the inert gases helium and neon as the active medium. The gases are enclosed in a glass tube having a mirror at each end. Following excitation of the helium atoms by the electrical power source, the helium atoms collide with and excite the neon atoms. Once in the excited state, the neon atoms are capable of amplification.[10,11] The He-Ne laser is considered a low-energy, cold laser because it does not generate an appreciable amount of heat.

All forms of radiant (light) energy incident upon a substance will be reflected, absorbed, or transmitted at varying amounts depending upon the composition of the substance and upon the intensity, wavelength, and exposure time of the irradiation.

BASIC COMPONENTS OF A LASER

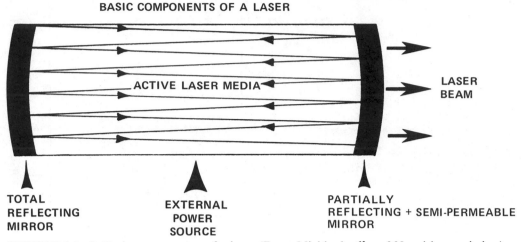

FIGURE 14–2. Basic components of a laser (From Michlovitz,[61] p. 221, with permission).

Radiant energy with long wavelengths will penetrate a substance such as skin deeper than radiant energy with shorter wavelengths.[12] The maximal penetration into the skin of radiant energy with a wavelength of 12,000 angstroms is about 3 mm, while very long waves (100,000 to 400,000 angstroms [Å]) may penetrate several centimeters of tissue.[13] Since the He-Ne laser has a relatively short wavelength of 632.8 nm, its radiant energy penetrates human skin very superficially. Research findings have shown that 99 percent of low-power irradiation is absorbed in the superficial 3.6 mm of human skin.[8]

Biostimulation Effect of Low-Energy Laser Irradiation

The nonthermal effects of low-powered lasers have been studied since the mid-1960s. To date, there have been many claims but limited research documentation regarding the effectiveness of this form of energy in decreasing inflammation,[14] controlling pain,[15–17] and healing wounds.[18,19]

A biologic principle that is used in an attempt to explain the apparent biologic response to low-energy He-Ne laser irradiation is the Arndt-Shultz biologic principle. This principle theorizes that tissues react to the amount of energy absorbed per unit time. Weak stimuli excite physiologic activity, moderately strong stimuli favor it, strong stimuli retard physiologic activity, and very strong stimuli arrest physiologic activity.[20]

Kleinkort and Foley[21] cite a third possible theory for the mechanism of action of low-powered laser biostimulation, as proposed by Moreno. Moreno postulated that low-intensity laser can stimulate energy stores via ATP formation and activation of enzyme activity leading to restoration of normal physiologic processes at the cell-organ-organism levels.

Proposed Physiologic Effects of Low-Energy Laser Irradiation

Low-energy laser irradiation with its proposed biostimulation capabilities coupled with a purported lack of any harmful side effects has been used to treat numerous medical conditions.

One of the conditions for which low-energy lasers were initially used was treatment of pain. In the 1970s, Plog[22] initiated work in the area of low-energy laser irradiation of acupuncture points for modulation of pain. In effect, Plog[22] replaced the metal acupuncture needle with the light beam. In a double-blind clinical study, Walker[23] reported pain relief accompanied by increased blood serotonin following He-Ne laser irradiation of acupuncture points in chronic pain patients. A second potential explanation for the laser irradiation modulation of pain, in addition to activating the release of serotonin, has been proposed by Muckerheide.[24] He proposes that the laser-generated spark phenomenon is capable of producing fields around nerve fibers that may either inhibit or accelerate neural transmission.

Two recent studies in the physical therapy literature on the effect of low-energy laser irradiation on sensory latencies report conflicting findings. Greathouse and associates[25] report that irradiation using a low-energy infrared laser had no significant effect on either the distal sensory latencies or on the amplitude of evoked responses of radial nerves. However, in 1988 Snyder-Mackler and Bork[16] reported a significant increase in distal radial nerve sensory latencies following He-Ne irradiation. In the Snyder-Mackler and Bork study, 40 healthy subjects with no history of right upper extremity pathology were assigned to either a treatment group or to a placebo group. Six 1-cm^2 blocks along a 12-cm segment of the right superficial radial nerve received 20-second applications of either the He-Ne laser or the placebo. The differences between pretest and post-test latencies were assessed using t-tests for correlated and independent samples. The irradiated subjects showed a statistically significant increase in latency, that corresponded to a decrease in sensory nerve conduction velocity. Snyder-Mackler and Bork[16] concluded that this finding of decreased sensory nerve conductor velocity provides information about the mechanism of the reported pain-relieving effect of He-Ne laser irradiation. Indeed, this increase in sensory latency following irradiation may help confirm the reported pain modulation provided by He-Ne irradiation.

In addition to possibly modulating pain, a second proposed physiologic effect of low-energy laser irradiation is stimulation of the immune system. One of the initial studies on the potential biostimulatory effect of low-energy laser on the immune system was reported by Kupin and associates.[26] They irradiated in vitro T and B lymphocytes obtained from 30 breast cancer or melanoma patients and 20 normal individuals. The cells were irradiated with either an apron or a He-Ne laser for periods of either 3, 5, and 10 minutes at a power density of 30 mW/cm^2. The study showed an increase in the percentage of active T cells following in vitro irradiation. Such an increase in the number of T cells may contribute to a more effective immune response.

Considering that the mechanism of wound healing involves the interaction between cells of the immune system and bacteria, Passarella and coworkers[27] investigated the potential effect of low-energy laser stimulation on such an interaction. They irradiated human lymphocytes, cultured with Salmonella bacteria, with continuous wave He-Ne laser at a power of about 12 mW to give an energy dose of 5 J/cm^2. The irradiated lymphocyte suspensions and a nonirradiated suspension were assayed immediately following irradiation of the experimental suspensions. Passarella and associates[27] concluded from this study that laser irradiation increased (1) the frequency of binding lymphocytes; (2) the affinity of the Salmonella bacteria for the lymphocytes; and (3) the actual number of lymphocyte receptor sites.

Another proposed effect of low-energy laser irradiation is the relief of protective myospasms.[28] The proposed physiologic mechanisms responsible for relieving these spasms are (1) the normalization of the sarcolemma membrane potentials of the contracting muscle and (2) reduction of arteriolar smooth muscle spasms, resulting in vasodilation. Interestingly, this vasodilation response may also explain the purported clinical effectiveness of low-energy laser irradiation in the reduction of inflammation. In fact, Kleinkort[1] states, "Laser has proved to be the modality of choice for patients with tendinitis, bursitis, and localized arthritis for treating pain and inflammation." However, in spite of this claim, additional research is needed to identify the specific physiologic mechanisms, such as autonomic interaction, responsible for the purported vasodilation and inflammation reduction associated with low-energy laser irradiation.

Proposed Effect of Low-Energy Laser Irradiation on Wound Healing

During the past 20 years, there have been numerous reports indicating that low-energy laser irradiation will facilitate the healing of open wounds. These reports include studies done in vitro on cell and tissue cultures as well as in vivo animal models and human studies.

One of the first studies that investigated the effects of low-power laser on wound healing was reported by Mester and associates[29] in 1968. They found that low-energy laser irradiation would stimulate leukocytic phagocytes and ultimately increase the healing rate of induced open wounds in rats. In a second study on rats, Mester and coworkers[2] reported an increase in healing third-degree burns induced by electrocoagulation. They reported that the optimal dose of irradiation was 1.0 J/cm^2 at 4-day intervals.

Although these studies demonstrated an increase in healing rate of irradiated wounds, the mechanisms responsible for the increase in healing were not presented. Therefore, in a controlled study designed to demonstrate the response of collagen synthesis to laser irradiation, Mester and Jasysagi-Nagy[30] irradiated incisions made in rats with the ruby laser at total dosages of up to 4.0 J/cm^2. They demonstrated an increase in the healing rate, which was associated with increased collagen synthesis. They also showed the greatest increase in collagen synthesis when the incisions were irradiated immediately following injury. In a similar study comparing He-Ne and argon laser irradiation at different dosages, Kana and colleagues[3] reported that the He-Ne laser irradiation applied at an energy density of 4 J/cm^2 was most effective in increasing the rate of healing, while the argon laser had no significant effect on the healing rate. Interestingly, they reported that He-Ne irradiation at an energy density of 10 J/cm^2 had no significant effect on the healing rate, while irradiation at 20 J/cm^2 had an inhibiting effect on wound healing.

Additional studies of potential mechanisms responsible for the increase in wound healing rate following low-energy laser irradiation have been done in vitro. In 1967, Hardy and associates[31] irradiated cultures of mouse fibroblast with four exposures of pulsed ruby laser light at a dose of 10 J/cm^2, which resulted in a fivefold increase in number of cells when contrasted with nonirradiated controls. More recently, Abergel and others[32,33] have shown an increase in procollagen synthesis in human fibroblast cultures following either helium-neon or gallium-arsenide laser irradiation. As early as 1984, Abergel and coworkers[34] postulated that the mechanisms for the acceleration of wound healing with laser biostimulation involved acceleration of the messenger RNA transcription rate of the collagen gene or other enzymatic changes following laser stimulation.

As a result of their work on stimulating collagen production by cultured human skin fibroblasts, Abergel's research group[35] extended their studies to in vivo healing of induced wounds using the hairless-mouse model. This study demonstrated increased collagen synthesis which was accompanied by increased tensile strength of irradiated wounds.

Recognizing that several studies[35,36] had indicated that collagen synthesis is regulated on the transcription level of gene expression, Sapareia's research group,[35] using a pig model, designed a study to examine the effect of He-Ne irradiation on procollagen messenger RNA levels. The results from this study are of particular significance since unlike some of the earlier animal model and human studies, the variables in the study were very well controlled. Additionally, the methods used in the study were documented in such a manner as to render the study readily reproducible. Therefore, the specifics of the study warrant detailed description. Full-thickness wounds of 1 cm² were surgically induced on the backs of pigs. Wounds were irradiated with a He-Ne laser, subjected to nonlaser irradiation (a tungsten light), or left untreated as control wounds. All wounds were cleaned with 3 percent hydrogen peroxide, treated with a topical antibiotic ointment, and covered with an occlusive dressing. Wounds receiving He-Ne irradiation were treated with a continuous wave laser (wavelength of 632.8 nm) at an average power output of 1.56 mW. Irradiation was performed at a 2.0-cm distance from the wound, which provided an area of light with a 0.5-cm radius. Irradiated wounds were treated three times a week for up to 28 days. Each treatment lasted 5 minutes. The results of this study demonstrated that procollagen messenger RNA levels were significantly increased when measured at days 17 and 28 in wounds treated with the He-Ne laser. No significant increases in messenger RNA levels were noted in either the tungsten irradiated wounds or the nonirradiated control wounds. The investigators concluded that the findings from this study support clinical observations that verify enhanced wound healing in humans subjected to low-power laser treatment.

Clinical Use of Low-Intensity Laser Irradiation in Wound Healing

There have been a number of case studies claiming that wound healing in humans can be accelerated by He-Ne laser irradiation. Unfortunately, the majority of these reports either have not reported the treatment parameters in a manner that would allow for replication of the studies or have not controlled for all variables involved in the treatment protocol.

However, Kahn,[37] reporting two case studies in which the He-Ne laser was successfully used in the management of open wounds, does quite specifically describe the irradiation variables. One case involved a 72-year-old diabetic woman with a gaping wound on the plantar surface of the left foot, measuring 2 cm deep and 3 cm long. Using 90 seconds of irradiation per square centimeter of open wound surface, Kahn[37] irradiated with an interrupted beam of light at 80 pps. The patient was treated twice weekly, with full wound closure after 10 treatments. Kahn suggests that in chronic wounds a lower pulse rate of approximately 40 pps may be more beneficial than a higher pulse rate of 80 pps.

Kahn[37] has also described a procedure for irradiating large lesions (4 to 6 cm in diameter). His technique for large lesions involves a slow traversing of the perimeter of the lesion, allowing approximately 90 seconds per linear centimeter of the perimeter. Irradiating the perimeter of the larger wounds was done in addition to blanketing the entire wound with the beam of light. Kahn reported no unwanted reactions or side effects in his case studies.

Mester and associates[38] reported on their experience using low-energy laser irradiation on wound healing in 1120 clinical cases involving ulcers as well as nonhealing wounds that did not positively respond to the usual therapeutic procedures including plastic surgery. Using either the He-Ne or argon laser they reported that 875 of the irradiated wounds healed in an average of 12 to 16 weeks. One hundred sixty wounds showed improvement, while 85 wounds did not heal. All wounds were irradiated twice a week at a dosage of 4 J/cm². From this study they concluded that healing can usually be expected in clinical cases when no general circulatory disturbances are present or when a general circulatory disturbance can be corrected. Mester and associates[38] also stated that in accordance with their experience, laser irradiation can also be applied as preparative, eventually complementary, treatment for dermatoplastic surgical interventions.

To date, most studies have been very supportive of the effectiveness of He-Ne laser irradiation for augmenting wound healing. However, Surinchak and associates[19] compared He-Ne laser irradiated versus nonirradiated surgically induced, full-thickness wounds in two animal models and found no significant differences in the healing rates. Using an argon laser, Jongsma and associates[39] found no significant differences in healing time of irradiated versus nonirradiated open wounds in rats at energy densities of either 1 J/cm² or 4 J/cm². In a study using the pig, Hunter and associates[40] irradiated surgically induced wounds with the He-Ne laser at 1 J/cm²/day (15 sec/cm²). No statistically significant increases in healing rate existed in these wounds versus nonirradiated wounds. More recently, a study by McCaughan and coworkers[41] using the argon laser on mechanically induced wounds in guinea pigs found no effect on the overall rate of wound healing at an exposure of 2.05 J/cm² with a power density of 20 mW/cm².

Clearly, all investigators do not agree regarding the efficacy of low-powered laser irradiation in the treatment of wounds. However, encouraging reports are presented in the clinical literature. Another review of laser biostimulation for the healing of open wounds has been recently completed by Enwemeka.[42] The reader is encouraged to consult this review for additional information.

A Look to the Future Use of Laser Biostimulation in Wound Healing

Although some animal model and human case studies report a positive conclusion between laser irradiation and accelerated wound healing, much confusion persists regarding the efficacy of low-energy irradiation of wounds. One reason for the confusion is the lack of definitive, clinical studies on humans in which such critical parameters as dosage are controlled. Until such studies are reported and accepted by the scientific and clinical communities, doubts concerning the efficacy of low-power laser will persist, as they should. To establish treatment parameters empirically is neither scientific nor clinically responsible.

ULTRAVIOLET IRRADIATION

Actinotherapy, the use of ultraviolet light, has been used as a healing agent for centuries; Hippocrates (460–370 B.C.) and Galen (131–201 A.D.) routinely prescribed sun baths for their patients.[21] Recently, ultraviolet irradiation has been used in the treatment of acne vulgaris, eczema, atopic dermatitis, psoriasis, and decubitus and other indolent ulcers.[43] The history of ultraviolet therapy is reviewed in detail by Licht.[44]

Physiologic Effects

Irradiation of the skin with ultraviolet light has several noticeable physiologic effects. The most obvious physiologic response is the erythema that follows exposure. According to Stillwell,[43] the primary phenomenon in the delayed production of erythema is the release of a vasodilator substance by cells of the prickle cell layer that have been damaged by the quanta of the ultraviolet light. The vasodilator substance is thought to diffuse to the subdermal layer where it causes vasodilation. The latency of the response may be several hours following exposure.

A second physiologic effect of ultraviolet irradiation is the thickening of the stratum corneum in an effort to provide some protection from subsequent ultraviolet exposures. The thickening of the stratum corneum may occur secondary to increased proliferation of epidermal cells and/or increased migration of melanocytes toward the surface. The erythemal response may lead to exfoliation of the superficial layer of skin following either an intense exposure or repeated exposures to the ultraviolet rays. Additionally, the bleached melanin within the melanocytes will be oxidized by the ultraviolet radiation, which results in a darkening of the pigment. The presence of pigmented melanin in the epidermis helps protect the deeper layers of the skin from damage by ultraviolet radiation.

A third physiologic effect of ultraviolet irradiation is the stimulation of the production of vitamin D in the skin, which is essential for normal calcium metabolism. Vitamin D increases calcium and phosphorus absorption from the gastrointestinal tract and helps to control calcium deposition in bone. A deficiency of vitamin D in children is manifested as rickets, while a deficiency in adults contributes to osteomalacia.[45] In human skin, ultraviolet irradiation of 7-dehydrocholesterol, found in sebum secreted by sebaceous glands, will result in the conversion of the steroid to vitamin D. The absorption spectrum of 7-dehydrocholesterol extends from about 2400 to 3000 Å. This maximum corresponds to a minimum in the action spectrum for erythema. Guyton[45] believes that most of the ultraviolet energy produced at these wavelengths is absorbed in superficial layers of the skin where vitamin D is produced and does not penetrate deeply enough to participate in the production of erythema.

A fourth physiologic effect of particular significance in the irradiation of wounds is the bactericidal effect of ultraviolet light. As early as 1877, Downes and Blunt[46] demonstrated that bacteria were killed by exposure to sunlight. The bactericidal effect is primarily caused by ultraviolet rays having wavelengths of 2537 Å that have been shown to destroy bacteria either by producing toxic substances or through destruction of cellular components.[47] Ultraviolet irradiation has also been used for air sterilization in surgical suites and ventilation systems for several decades.[48]

The Use of Ultraviolet Irradiation in Wound Healing

The rationale behind the use of ultraviolet irradiation in treating chronic wounds is most often based upon the bactericidal effects of ultraviolet light, and on the erythemal response, which some authors believe stimulates the healing process by initiating an inflammatory response, which is then followed by exfoliation and repair.[43,48] Although ultraviolet irradiation has been used quite extensively to facilitate wound healing, its value has been questioned.[49,50]

The bactericidal effects of ultraviolet light are well documented and accepted by the clinical community. As previously mentioned, Downes and Blunt[46] reported more than

100 years ago that bacteria could be killed by sunlight. Gates[51] studied the ultraviolet bactericidal action spectrum and determined that the maximal efficacy of inactivation of Escherichia coli occurs at 2600 Å. Because pyrimidine residues of nucleic acids absorb ultraviolet rays maximally at the same wavelength, Gates[51] concluded that the absorption of ultraviolet light by the nucleic acids is lethal to the bacteria. Based on Gate's[51] observations, Kelner[52] developed a model relating a series of events that occurred following the ultraviolet irradiation of bacteria. He proposed that following irradiation the nuclear functioning of the bacteria is inhibited with a cessation in DNA synthesis, which affects all nuclear-governed responses and leads to bacterial death.

Numerous studies have implicated interruption of DNA synthesis as responsible for the bactericidal effect of ultraviolet irradiation. However, the effects of ultraviolet light on RNA may also contribute to bacterial death following irradiation.[53]

Regardless of the specific mechanism, ultraviolet irradiation does exhibit a bactericidal effect. In open wounds, the effect is lethal to bacteria, and results in a relatively bacterial-free wound, which heals more rapidly than an infected wound.

The erythemal response to ultraviolet is also thought to stimulate wound healing by initiating an inflammatory response, which includes vasodilation and increased capillary permeability. The inflammatory response begins 2 to 6 hours after irradiation and reaches a peak between 10 and 12 hours after exposure. After the peak erythemal response has been reached, the redness and dilation of cutaneous capillaries gradually disappears with subsequent exfoliation of decaying epidermal cells that circumscribe the wound periphery.[54] The erythemal response and associated vasodilation may also facilitate the transport of cellular components, like fibroblasts, necessary for healing into the vicinity of the wound, and therefore increase the rate of healing.[54] Vasodilation would also enhance the delivery of oxygen to the wound, which in turn may increase the local metabolism and in this manner facilitate wound healing.

The possibility that ultraviolet irradiation may generate a diffusible mediator that promotes re-epithelialization in irradiated wounds as well as in wounds distant from the irradiated area was suggested by Geronemus and associates.[55] This group studied the rate of re-epithelialization of split-thickness wounds in pigs following exposure to ultraviolet light. Wounds were irradiated daily for six consecutive days with either UVB (wavelength range from 2800 Å to 3150 Å at a dosage of 400 mJ/cm^2) or UVC (wavelength range from 1800 Å to 2800 Å at a dosage of 135 mJ/cm^2). On the third through sixth days, the tissue specimens were removed from the wounds, evaluated for re-epithelialization, and compared with nonirradiated wounds on the same animals. These specimens were also compared with untreated wounds on nonirradiated pigs. Geronemus and associates[55] demonstrated that UVC and UVB promote re-epithelialization in both irradiated and nonirradiated wounds on the same animal. These findings suggest the presence of an ultraviolet-generated mediator capable of influencing wound healing distant to the site of irradiation.

Gilchrest and coworkers[56] have studied UVA-induced (wavelength range from 3200 Å to 4200 Å) histologic and biochemical changes in normal human skin. They have quantified an increase in the amount of arachidonic acid, prostaglandins, and histamine present in human skin following UVA irradiation of intact skin. They report that (1) arachidonic acid levels are at 150 percent of control values at 3 to 4 hours following irradiation; (2) a threefold to sixfold elevation in prostaglandins occurs at 3 to 6 hours after irradiation; and (3) histamine levels are 20 times greater than control values between 6 and 15 hours following exposure. These findings suggest that UVA effects are mediated in part by both epidermal and dermal cells with the subsequent release of arachidonic acid, prostaglandins, and histamine. Although this study was done on intact skin, the documented release of these substances following irradiation may help explain the findings of Geronemus and colleagues.[55] However, additional research is needed to identify and substantiate that these substances are released either from irradiated wounds or from irradiated intact skin on the periphery of wounds, and that they act as diffusible mediators to influence wound healing at sites distant to the irradiated wound.

Another somewhat distant effect that ultraviolet irradiation has on wound healing is mediated through the production of vitamin D in the skin. Vitamin D, as previously noted, is instrumental in the uptake of calcium and phosphorus from the gastrointestinal tract. Calcium and phosphorus, in turn, are important in the wound-healing process. Without vitamin D and the proper absorption of calcium and phosphorus from the gastrointestinal tract, the wound-healing process would be inhibited.

Technique of Application, Indications, and Contraindications

One technique for the application of ultraviolet light for wound healing is described by Scott,[54] who advocates the use of ultraviolet in the treatment of indolent ulcers, particularly when there is little or no sign of healing. Scott[54] emphasizes that the reaction of the skin to the irradiation should be tested on normal skin adjacent to the ulcer. After determining the ultraviolet exposure time needed to produce a first-degree erythemal reaction, Scott[54] recommends a dosage from 20 to 100 times the first-degree erythemal reaction. According to Scott,[54] "within reasonable limits, the greater the reaction, the quicker the ulcer heals." He notes that ulcers may be treated with general treatment lamps or with local ultraviolet lamps, although a local lamp is preferred.

Freytes and associates,[47] using the technique of Scott,[57] reported satisfactory results of ultraviolet irradiation in the treatment of indolent ulcers in three cases. The wounds were treated with a Kromeyer lamp until the ulcers were almost completely healed. Also using Scott's technique, Wills and associates[58] irradiated pressure sores twice weekly at doses of 2.5 times the minimal erythemal dose (second-degree erythema). In subsequent treatments, they increased the dosage by 50 percent over the previous doses in order to maintain production of a second-degree erythema. Therefore, those patients receiving a full 8 weeks of treatment had a final exposure of approximately 7 minutes and 30 seconds. In this study, Wills and associates[58] report a significant ($p < 0.02$) increase in mean healing time of irradiated wounds when compared with nonirradiated control wounds.

The possibility that the ultraviolet irradiation of infected wounds could be simultaneously and effectively used with transparent dressings has recently been suggested by MacKinnon and Cleek.[59] Although the investigators stated that ultraviolet rays apparently did not penetrate the two types of transparent dressings tested in their study, they emphasized that the results of the study were inconclusive regarding the bactericidal effects of ultraviolet light on a wound covered by a transparent dressing, since a bactericidal effect may occur even when a minimal erythemal response is not produced.

Contraindications to ultraviolet therapy pervade the literature and are reviewed by Scott.[54] The application of ultraviolet rays may exacerbate some conditions and should be avoided during the acute onset of psoriasis, lupus erythematosus, herpes simplex, acute eczema, and other conditions. Some of the general conditions in which irradiation should be used with caution include cardiac or renal failure, hyperthyroidism, pulmonary tuberculosis, and diabetes.[54] As when using any physical agent, certain precautions must be taken to protect the patient from possible injury from overdose. With ultraviolet irradiation, the patient and operator must be screened from the ultraviolet source except during the actual time of the therapeutic exposure. Also the eyes must be shielded by wearing dark glasses that protect against misdirected or reflected rays.[43]

Future Use of Ultraviolet Light in Wound Healing

The use of ultraviolet irradiation in the treatment of wounds has experienced periods of popularity and decline. With the availability of topical antibiotics and other agents, such as the low-energy laser, for the treatment of wounds, the use of ultraviolet irradiation is not currently in vogue. However, the capabilities and the historic successes of ultraviolet therapy should be understood and appreciated by today's clinicians. Ultraviolet therapy may be proved to be an important adjunct to other forms of wound management in the future.

INFRARED IRRADIATION

Infrared irradiation is a form of radiant energy that provides superficial dry heat. The energy for clinical use falls within both the near-infrared and far-infrared regions of the electromagnetic spectrum. Since near infrared lamps emit light within the 7600 to 15,000 Å wavelength range and have some visible light, they are often referred to as luminous lamps. Far-infrared lamps emit light within the 15,000 to 125,000 Å range of the electromagnetic spectrum. Because negligible light is emitted from these lamps, they are also called nonluminous lamps. The depth of skin penetration by light from nonluminous lamps is approximately 2 mm compared with 5 to 10 mm for light emitted from luminous infrared lamps. The output of infrared lamps is determined by the wattage. The intensity of the irradiation is usually controlled by varying the distance of the lamp from the skin. This distance is usually between 45 and 60 cm.[60] The duration of each treatment is typically 20 to 30 minutes since the maximal dilatation effect on cutaneous arterial circulation is not attained in less than 20 minutes.[61]

The physiologic effects of infrared irradiation are associated with a local increase in skin temperature that accompanies the irradiation. According to Stillwell,[62] this local healing effect leads to an increase in the local metabolic rate with an increase in quantity of metabolites and increased heat generated by the tissues. The metabolites in turn lead to an increase in capillary blood flow and an increase in capillary hydrostatic pressure.

Infrared irradiation has also been used to facilitate the healing of open wounds. The rationale for using infrared to treat open wounds is the local heating effect that is accompanied by vasodilation. As discussed in the section on ultraviolet irradiation, it is thought that vasodilation may facilitate wound healing through mobilization of fibroblasts, and so on. Unfortunately, heat from infrared irradiation usually has a dehydrating effect on wound tissues, which may inhibit the healing process and actually contribute to additional tissue destruction.

The future use of infrared irradiation in the healing of open wounds is bleak. There are no well-controlled studies that indicate that infrared is an effective adjunct in facilitating the healing process of chronic wounds. Also, the development of the low-powered laser, with its convenience of application and the recent potential that the laser has demonstrated in facilitating wound healing, renders treatment of chronic wounds with infrared radiation obsolete.

CASE STUDIES

A 27-year-old man presented with a diagnosis of diabetes mellitus established when he was 17. Ever since the diagnosis was made 10 years ago, he has been plagued with a diabetic dermal ulcer on the medial aspect of his right ankle. During the past 10 years, the wound has been treated using various modalities including topical medicaments, whirlpool baths, dressings, and hyperbaric oxygen. Unfortunately, none of the treatments resulted in total wound closure, which, at times, almost occurred. The patient now presents with a wound that has surface area dimensions of 3.7 cm long × 2.4 cm wide × 3 mm deep. This State II ulcer is beefy-red, which indicates well-developed granulation tissue. Treatment of the wound consisted of daily He-Ne continuous laser with the aperture held 1 cm from the wound. Each square centimeter of wound surface was exposed for 30 seconds, three times a week for a total of 32 treatments. Weekly tracings of the wound area dimensions showed a weekly reduction in size. This reduction was evidenced by epithelial cell migration across the wound, which became evident after the first 10 days of treatment. Epithelialization and closure were complete after 32 treatments.

A 53-year-old woman with a primary diagnosis of multiple sclerosis had been wheelchair bound for 3 months, during which time she developed a pressure sore over the right ischial tuberosity. The Stage III wound, which measured 2 cm wide × 2.5 cm long × 1 cm deep, had a purulent drainage and a foul odor. A culture of the wound fluid indicated that infection was present chiefly by Pseudomonas aeruginosa. Ultraviolet treatments were administered three times weekly for 2 weeks, with a portable cold quartz lamp centered over the wound and held 2 cm from the skin surface. An exposure time equal to 2.5 times the pre-established minimal erythemal dose was used for the first exposure with subsequent exposure times increased by 50 percent. After six treatments, another culture revealed that the colony count of the infecting organism was within normal limits.

SUMMARY

Various forms of light have been used through the ages to facilitate wound healing. While ultraviolet and infrared irradiation have been traditionally used for wound healing, neither agent has provided consistent, positive results. However, the results of numerous basic science and clinical studies indicate that a relatively new type of light, low-energy laser irradiation, may be effective in facilitating the healing of open wounds. Although more definitive studies need to be done in this area, low-energy laser irradiation may be the wave of the future in the healing of open wounds.

REFERENCES

1. Kleinkort, JA and Foley, RA: Laser: A preliminary report on its use in physical therapy. Clin Man Phys Ther 2(4):30, 1982.
2. Mester, E, et al: Effect of laser rays on wound healing. Am J Surg 122:532, 1971.
3. Kana, JS, et al: The effect of low power density laser radiation on the healing of open skin wounds in rats. Arch Surg 116:293, 1981.
4. FDA Tightens Laser Law Enforcement. Progress Report of the American Physical Therapy Association 12(5):1, 1983.
5. Laser Sales Suspended, Resume. Progress Report of the American Physical Therapy Association 12(7):1, 1983.

6. Fact Sheet: Laser Biostimulation. Division of Consumer Affairs, Office of Training and Assistance, Center for Devices and Radiological Health, Food and Drug Administration, US Department of Health and Human Services, Rockville, MD, 1984.
7. Goldman, L: Basic Reactions in Tissue. In Goldman, T (ed): The Biomedical Laser. Springer-Verlag, New York, 1981.
8. Goldman, L and Rockwell, JR: Lasers in Medicine. Gordon and Breach Science Publishers, New York, 1971, pp 44–62.
9. Dynatron 1120 Operator's Manual. Dynatronics Corp, Salt Lake City, UT.
10. Seitz, LM and Kleinkort, JA: Low-power laser: Its applications in physical therapy. In Michlovitz SL (ed): Thermal Agents in Rehabilitation. FA Davis, Philadelphia, 1986, pp 217–238.
11. McKie, R: Lasers. Franklin Watts, New York, 1983.
12. Brown, R: Lasers: Tools of Modern Technology. Doubleday, New York, 1968, pp 126–131.
13. Stillwell, GK: Therapeutic heat and cold. In Krusen, FH (ed): Handbook of Physical Medicine and Rehabilitation, ed 2. WB Saunders, Philadelphia, 1971, p 240.
14. Plog, FMW: Biophysical application of the laser beam. In Koebner, HK (ed): Lasers in Medicine. John Wiley and Sons, New York, 1980, pp 21–37.
15. Welgel, A, Pothman, R, and Stux, G: Acupuncture Therapy with Laser Beam. Reviews and Abstracts. Seventh World Congress of Acupuncture. Columbo, Sri Lanka, October 1981.
16. Snyder-Mackler, L and Bork, CE: Effect of helium-neon laser irradiation on peripheral sensory nerve latency. Phys Ther 68:223, 1988.
17. Snyder-Mackler, L, et al: The effect of helium-neon laser on musculoskeletal trigger points. Phys Ther 66:1087, 1986.
18. Mester, E: Clinical result of wound healing stimulation with laser and experimental studies of the action mechanism. Proc Laser '75 Opto Elektronics Conference, Munich, 1976, pp 190–213.
19. Surinchak, JS, et al: Effects of low-level energy lasers on the healing of full-thickness skin defects. Lasers Surg Med 2:267, 1983.
20. Griffin, JE and Karselis, TC: Introduction to the electromagnetic and acoustic spectra. In Griffin, JE and Karselis, TC (eds): Physical Agents for Physical Therapists, ed 2. Charles C Thomas, Springfield, IL, 1982, pp 34–35.
21. Kleinkort, JA and Foley, RA: Laser acupuncture: Its use in phsyical therapy. American Journal of Acupuncture 12:51, 1984.
22. Plog, FMW: Biophysical application of the laser beam. In Goldman, T (ed): The Biomedical Laser. Springer-Verlag, New York, 1981, pp 314–315.
23. Walker, J: Relief from chronic pain by low powered laser irradiation. Neurosci Lett 43:339, 1983.
24. Muckerheide, MC: Laser medical technology for the twenty-first century. In Goldman, L (ed): The Biomedical Laser. Springer-Verlag, New York, 1981, pp 313–324.
25. Greathouse, D, Currier, D, and Gilmore, R: Effects of clinical infrared laser on superficial radial nerve conduction. Phys Ther 65:1184, 1985.
26. Kupin, IV, et al: Potentiating effects of laser radiation on some immunological traits. Neoplasm 29:403, 1982.
27. Passarella, S, et al: Quantitative analysis of lymphocytes-salmonella interaction and effects of lymphocyte irradiation by helium-neon laser. Biochem Biophys Res Commun 130:546, 1985.
28. Kleinkort, J and Foley, R: Laser acupuncture: Its use in physical therapy. American Journal of Acupuncture 12:51, 1984.
29. Mester, E, et al: The stimulating effect of low power laser rays on biological systems. Laser Rev 1:3, 1968.
30. Mester, E and Jasysagi-Nagy, E: The effects of laser radiation on wound healing and collagen synthesis. Studia Biophysica 35:227, 1973.
31. Hardy, LB, et al: Effect of ruby laser radiation on mouse fibroblast culture. Fed Proc 26:668, 1967.
32. Abergel, RP: Low energy lasers stimulate collagen production in human skin fibroblast cultures. Presented at 1st Canadian Low Powered Medical Laser Conference, Toronto, 1985.
33. Abergel, RP, et al: Biostimulation of wound healing by lasers: Experimental approaches in animal models and fibroblast cultures. J Dermatol Surg Oncol 13:127, 1987.
34. Abergel, RP, et al: Biostimulation of procollagen production by low-energy lasers in human skin fibroblast cultures. J Invest Dermatol 82:395, 1984.
35. Sapareia, D, et al: Demonstration of elevated type I and type II procollagen in RNA levels in cutaneous wounds treated with helium-neon laser. Biochem Biophys Res Commun 138:1123, 1986.
36. Liau, G, Yamada, Y, and deCrombrugghe, B: Coordinate regulation of the levels of type III and type I collagen messenger RNA in most but not all mouse fibroblasts. J Biochem 260:531–536, 1985.
37. Kahn, J: Case reports: Open wound management with the HeNe (6328AU) cold laser. J Orthop Sports Phys Ther 6:203, 1984.
38. Mester, E, Mester, AF, and Mester A: The biomedical effects of laser application. Lasers Surg Med 5:31, 1985.
39. Jongsma, FHM, et al: Is closure of open skin wounds in rats accelerated by Argon laser exposure? Lasers Surg Med 3:75, 1983.
40. Hunter, J, et al: Effects of low energy laser on wound healing in a porcine model. Lasers Surg Med 3:285, 1984.

41. McCaughan, JS, et al: Effect of low-dose argon irradiation on rate of wound closure. Lasers Surg Med 5:607, 1985.
42. Enwemeka, CS: Laser biostimulation of healing wounds: Specific effects and mechanisms of action. Orthop Sports Phys Ther 9:333, 1988.
43. Stillwell, GK: Ultraviolet therapy. In Krusen, FH (ed): Handbook of Physical Medicine and Rehabilitation, ed 2. WB Saunders, Philadelphia, 1971, pp 350–351.
44. Licht, S: History of ultraviolet therapy. In Stillwell, GK (ed): Therapeutic Electricity and Ultraviolet Radiation, ed 3. Williams and Wilkins, Baltimore, 1983, pp 1–69.
45. Guyton, AC: Vitamin and mineral metabolism. In Guyton, AC (ed): Textbook of Medical Physiology. WB Saunders, Philadelphia, 1976, pp 983–984.
46. Downes, A and Blunt, T: Researches on the effect of light on bacteria and other organisms. Proc Royal Soc Lond 26:488, 1877.
47. Freytes, HA, Fernandez, B, and Fleming, WC: Ultraviolet light in the treatment of indolent ulcers. South Med J 58:223, 1965.
48. Scott, BO: Clinical uses of ultraviolet radiation. In Licht, E (ed): Therapeutic Electricity and Ultraviolet Radiation, ed 2. Waverly Bros, Baltimore, 1967, pp 335–378.
49. Wilkinson, DS: Trophic ulcers and pressure sores: Medical and dermatological aspects. Physiotherapy 54:278, 1968.
50. Fugill, GC: Pressure sores. Physiotherapy 6:46, 1980.
51. Gates, FL: Discussion and corespondence on nuclear derivatives and the lethal action of ultraviolet light. Science 68:479–480, 1928.
52. Kelner, A: Growth, respiration and nuclear acid synthesis in ultraviolet-irradiated and in photoactivated escherichia coli. J Bacteriol 65:252–262, 1953.
53. Painter, RB: The action of ultraviolet light on mammalian cells. In Giese, A (ed): Photophysiology. Vol 5. Academic Press, New York, 1970, pp 177–179.
54. Scott, BO: Clinical uses of ultraviolet radiation. In Stillwell, GK (ed): Therapeutic Electricity and Ultraviolet Radiation. Williams and Wilkins, Baltimore, 1983, pp 228–262.
55. Geronemus, R, et al: The effect of UVC and UVB on epidermal wound healing. Clin Res 50:586A, 1982.
56. Gilchrest, BA, et al: Longwave ultraviolet (UVA) induced histologic and biochemical changes in normal skin. Clin Res 30:586A, 1982.
57. Scott, BO: The Principles and Practice of Electrotherapy and Actinotherapy. Charles Thomas, Springfield, IL, 1959, pp 254–301.
58. Wills, EE, et al: A randomized placebo-controlled trial of ultraviolet light in the treatment of superficial pressure sores. J Am Geriatr Soc 31:131, 1983.
59. MacKinnon, JL and Cleek, PL: The penetration of ultraviolet light through transparent dressings. A case report. Phys Ther 64:204, 1984.
60. Michlovitz, SL: Biophysical principles of heating and superficial heat agents. In Michlovitz, SL (ed): Thermal Agents in Rehabilitation. FA Davis, Philadelphia, 1986, pp 99–118.
61. Stillwell, GK: Therapeutic Heat and Cold. In Krusen, FH (ed): Handbook of Physical Medicine and Rehabilitation, ed 2. WB Saunders, Philadelphia, 1971.

CHAPTER 15

Use of Hyperbaric Oxygen in Wound Healing

Susan Kravitz, M.S., P.T.

Clinicians and researchers have examined the effects of breathing varying percentages of oxygen and carbon dioxide on tissue healing.[1] Additional investigation has been done to determine the effects of varying oxygen tension on wound metabolism and collagen synthesis.[2] Bone and soft-tissue wounds have healed with the use of hyperbaric oxygen, which reportedly provided the environment for enhanced healing of hypoxic tissue.[3] The administration of hyperbaric oxygen has increased in the past 15 to 20 years although work with hyperbaric medicine has been recognized for more than 100 years.[4]

The objectives of this chapter are to (1) review wound healing literature pertinent to the use of hyperbaric oxygen; (2) present the physical principles and biophysical effects of topical hyperbaric oxygen; (3) discuss the clinical methods of applying the topical oxygen; (4) identify clinical conditions for which local hyperbaric oxygen has been shown effective; (5) discuss indications, contraindications, and guidelines for the safe and effective use of topical hyperbaric oxygen; and (6) discuss clinical decision making models for determining the appropriateness of this modality.

OVERVIEW

During the past 25 years, the utilization of hyperbaric oxygen for treatment of dermal ulcers has increased and a number of clinical studies have supported its efficacy. Slack and associates[5] used hyperbaric oxygen to treat patients with a variety of ischemic and vascular disorders. Treatment outcomes were most encouraging with patients who had traumatic ischemic lesions and varicose ulcerations. Some patients showed temporary improvement; however, those with severe ischemic disease and with severe Raynaud's disease did not respond well. Deleterious responses are also reported by Bird and Telfer,[6] who showed a reduction of limb blood flow with use of hyperbaric oxygen. Slack[7] used hyperbaric oxygen on 250 patients with osteomyelitis, clostridial infections, acute traumatic ischemia, decubitis ulcers, varicose ulcers, and carbon monoxide poisoning. Treatment was reported to be beneficial for these disorders, and patients did not develop oxygen toxicity. In the same study, other patients with carcinoma, peripheral vascular disease, and nontraumatic acute ischemia secondary to thrombosis or embolism did not respond well to treatment with hyperbaric oxygenation. Slack[7] suggested that additional research was needed to support the use of hyperbaric oxygen treatment for wound care.

Copeman and Ashfield[8] treated dermal lesions in scleroderma patients with secondary Raynaud's phenomenon in a whole body hyperbaric oxygen chamber at 2.0 atmospheres. They reported improvement in the Raynaud's symptoms as well as more rapid healing of skin ulcers, and improvement of all patients was maintained for more than 1 month following treatment. Fischer[9] provided hyperbaric treatment to patients with a variety of skin ulcers in controlled and uncontrolled trials. Wounds of patients in the uncontrolled trials included diabetic ulcers, venous stasis ulcers, pressure sores, lesions from mechanical trauma, and lesions associated with occlusive vascular disease or osteomyelitis. The control groups consisted of six patients with bilateral lower extremity skin ulcers. Ulcers on one leg of each patient were initially treated with other conservative methods, while ulcers on the opposite leg were treated with hyperbaric oxygen. Eventually, bilateral ulcers on all six patients received hyperbaric oxygen. From the results of all trials, Fischer reported that hyperbaric oxygen was more successful than other traditional treatments in aiding the healing of a variety of wounds. Only those patients with underlying osteomyelitis and those with ischemic lesions healed poorly in these trials.

In 1975, Fischer[10] performed additional studies with hyperbaric oxygen on patients with burns, pressure sores, venous stasis ulcers, postsurgical infected wounds, rheumatoid arthritis with ulcer complications, and one case of dermal ulcers secondary to hypergammaglobulinemia. Wounds of most patients in the study healed satisfactorily, but in one case of rheumatoid arthritis and in the case of hypergammaglobulinemia, healing did not occur. All patients benefited from a dramatic decrease in infection and edema. Fischer[10] employed topical hyperbaric extremity chambers that covered the entire involved limb. These portable topical chambers were reported to be convenient and eliminated the possibility of oxygen toxicity that sometimes developed when oxygen application was confined to smaller areas of the body.

Heng[11] reported the effects of local hyperbaric oxygen therapy on leg ulcers including wounds of ischemic etiology. Once again, favorable results were achieved without the risks of oxygen toxicity to patients. Hyperbaric oxygen administered percutaneously at lower tension than systemic oxygen was observed to aid in the development of profuse tissue granulation, which appeared to aid oxygen diffusion to the tissues.

Upson[12] treated two patients with topical hyperbaric oxygen. The first had developed progressive leg ulcers, while the second suffered an abscess following a thrombectomy. Both patients were afflicted with many medical problems including peripheral vascular disease; atherosclerotic heart disease; and other complications of vascular origin. Hyperbaric oxygen treatment applied to their recalcitrant ischemic wounds was successful. Upson[12] concluded that the use of the topical hyperbaric oxygen was warranted in the treatment and prevention of ulcers on ischemic legs.

Jackson and colleagues[13] presented findings from their experience with topical hyperbaric oxygen and pinch grafting. Patients were treated for stasis ulcers that had existed from 4 months to 10 years. Wound care commenced with daily topical hyperbaric oxygen treatments followed by pinch grafting after periods of 3 days to 2 weeks into the treatment period. The researchers made follow-up examinations 8 to 28 months later, noting that pinch grafts of three patients healed without complication. One patient lost the pinch grafts because of infection but did go on to heal with the assistance of hyperbaric oxygen. Ulceration did not recur in this patient for at least 16 months after healing. The use of hyperbaric oxygen for the initial treatment of these wounds seemed to increase granulation and to decrease necrotic debris in the ulcer bed. All patients were observed to require shorter hospital stays than did similar patients not treated with hyperbaric oxygen and none complained of side effects.

Kwiecinski[14] found positive results from the use of topical hyperbaric oxygen on one patient with a post-traumatic ulcer on the lower extremity complicated by Cushing's syndrome. A decrease in edema as well as tissue granulation only a few days after beginning the treatment occurred in this case. The investigator suggested that topical hyperbaric oxygen treatment is appropriate for persistent foot ulceration when good vascularization is present.

Regardless of the origin of skin lesions, they ultimately cause emotional distress and physical disablement to their victims.[15] Individuals troubled with dermal lesions are often hospitalized or confined to extended-care facilities for lengthy stays. In many cases, they have endured years of unsatisfactory and costly treatment.[16] The aforementioned studies suggest that oxygen applied topically under pressure may augment plasma pO_2 levels in vessels permeating wound tissue. If hemoglobin levels are within normal limits (12 to 18 g/100 ml of blood), an increase in oxygen tension may be achieved by raising the pO_2 in the circulating blood. Oxygen partial pressure increases when the amount of oxygen carried in the plasma increases. Unfortunately, many of the clinical studies cited above were not well designed and had no control groups. More studies with control groups or blind/double-blind design, or both, are needed to lend additional credibility to the hyperoxic method of wound care.

PHYSICAL PRINCIPLES

Physics of Gases

Proper employment of topical oxygen under variations in atmospheric pressure requires knowledge of the effects of pressure changes upon human tissue. To appreciate the impact these changes have on tissues, one must first understand the gas laws of Boyle and Henry.[17]

Measured on a gauge, normal gas pressure is expressed either as zero atmospheres or as one atmosphere absolute. Normal atmospheric pressure is 14.7 pounds per square inch or 760 millimeters of mercury (mmHg) at sea level. Hyperbaric oxygen is pressurized oxygen with characteristics similar to other gases under pressure.

According to Boyle's law, the volume of a gas varies inversely with its pressure when mass and temperature remain constant. Henry's law states that, given a constant temperature, the solubility of a gas is proportional to the pressure of the gas to which a liquid is exposed. The use of a pure oxygen atmosphere in a hyperbaric chamber creates a passive diffusion gradient.[18] This gradient is found by dividing the gas pressure difference in the oxygen chamber by the diffusion distance. The rate of net oxygen diffusion in the chamber is directly proportional to the gradient. Boyle's law, Henry's law, and the passive diffusion gradient interact and cause oxygen to diffuse into tissues and skin lesions. This diffusion causes an increase in the tissue oxygen tension.[19]

Venous Hydrostatic Pressure

The human upright posture is in continuous conflict with gravity. As we stand or sit erect, our peripheral venous system functions with the aid of a compensatory antigravity venous return mechanism. Whether young or old, humans are vulnerable to vascular breakdown. In the upright position, hydrostatic pressure is created in the large veins by gravitational force that exerts pressure on the blood confined to a liquid column. This pressure increases from the feet upward over a measurable gradient.

The squeezing action of contracting muscles in the legs creates a pumping effect responsible for driving the blood from vessels in the lower extremities toward the heart. This driving process is assisted by the venous valve system, which acts as a backflow check to maintain blood distribution and a pressure gradient throughout the venous circulatory system. An incompetent valve within the system allows retrograde blood flow, which compromises the efficiency of the muscle pump mechanism.

Poorly functioning venous valves allow retrograde blood flow, which in turn increases hydrostatic pressure at the bottom of the venous liquid column, causing an increased volume of edema fluid to move from the vascular bed to the surrounding tissues. If edema remains in the tissues, interruption of fluid and metabolic exchange occurs across the capillary wall, eventually bringing about tissue destruction.[20]

Exogenous Pressure Variations

Hyperbaric oxygen systems administer oxygen to the tissues under low or high pressure. Topical low pressure systems operate at a constant low pressure level, while higher pressure systems intermittently elevate the chamber pressure up to a maximum followed by a drop in pressure during a release phase. Using a local chamber with constant low pressure applied at 0 to 12 mmHg, depending on the patient's tolerance, Olejniczak and Zielinksi[21] suggested that treatment should not exceed 20 minutes daily because they theorized that more time in the chamber could induce lymphedema. In the care of 11 lower leg ulcers, Diamond and associates[22] applied topical oxygen via a local hyperbaric chamber at a constant pressure of 22 mmHg and a flow of 4 liters per minute to four patients. Seven additional patients were subsequently treated in a similar manner with topical hyperbaric oxygen and with standard wound care. Therapy was administered for 90 minutes, twice daily. Treatment time varied from 6 days to 2 months. Hyperbaric treatment was terminated in 9 of the 11 patients when ulcers were completely healed. Two patients achieved either superficial healing of tissues or a reduction in the diameter of the wounds. Oxygen applied in this manner allowed the partial pressure of oxygen (pO_2) to increase without obstructing capillary flow.

In a similar study performed by Lehman and associates,[23] hyperbaric oxygen was administered to human bites. This study used a topical intermittent hyperbaric, humidified oxygen unit cycling pure oxygen at a pressure of 50 mmHg, applied twice daily for 90 minutes each session. Twenty-seven patients received standard care without hyperbaric oxygen, while 16 patients received supplemental topical hyperbaric oxygen. Random selection of patients was based only on hyperbaric oxygen unit availability. The researchers believed that this method of selection eliminated bias. Patients were discharged once their lesions were free of cellulitis and pain, and demonstrated improved granulation. For patients with severe infections, hyperbaric oxygen shortened hospitalization by as much as 9 days.

Full body chambers have also been successful in treating skin wounds. Bass[24] applied oxygen at 2 atmospheres pressure for 2 hours daily, 5 days a week, to heal varicose leg ulcers. He reported rapid, visible healing in some patients and minimal effectiveness in others. To study the effects of hyperbaric oxygen on bacterial pathogens, Watt[25] studied oxygen supplied at 2.5 atmospheres for 2½ hours, twice daily to patients with a variety of disabilities including peripheral vascular disease, traumatic ischemia, gas gangrene, and pyogenic infections. Treatment was administered at 3 atmospheres to patients with severe wound infections. Accelerated healing in pyogenic infections and dramatic recovery of wounds resulting from toxemia in gas gangrene, burns, electric shock, and vascular injury were noted. Hyperbaric oxygen also appeared to eliminate sepsis and promoted healing of grafts.

BIOPHYSICAL EFFECTS

The interaction of hyperbaric oxygen applied under intermittent pressure to hypoxic tissue produces five effects: (1) improvement in the oxygen tension within the tissues of an open wound, (2) collagen synthesis, (3) revascularization, (4) retardation of bacterial growth, and (5) reduction of edema.

Capillary partial pressure of oxygen (pO_2) of intact tissue is 100 mmHg. In the presence of a wound, the pO_2 over the capillary in ambient air (21 percent oxygen) is 80 mmHg, and the pO_2 measurement in the dead space of the wound nears zero.[26] The reductions in partial pressures at a wound site indicate tissue hypoxia. The goal of hyperbaric oxygen therapy is to augment plasma pO_2 in the vessels of hypoxic wound tissue so an oxygen gradient between the tissues and the capillary system is re-established, permitting increased diffusion of oxygen into the hypoxic tissues.

Fischer[10] found that capillary pO_2 at the site of a wound increased from 76 to 79 mmHg to 115 to 120 mmHg following exposure to hyperbaric oxygen. Under these conditions, tissue hypoxia is reversed and the arterial oxygen tension is raised, making more oxygen available to the wound tissues in which blood flow and oxygen diffusion are usually below normal.[27] Gruber and colleagues[28] found that oxygen penetrated the skin to the superficial dermis when it was applied at 1 atmosphere, and as a result, the growth of viable tissue increased to maintain skin grafts. Gruber and associates[28] measured the oxygen concentration at the dermal layer in abdominal skin specimens that were removed in surgical patients. Electrodes placed in the tissue specimens were used to measure the tissue oxygen tension values. A rise in the pO_2 value indicated that oxygen had permeated the tissues. Tissue oxygen tension in five skin specimens ranged from 10 to 25 mmHg. When oxygen was applied at 3 atmospheres, pO_2 reached 100 mmHg in four of five specimens. The pO_2 of the deep dermis did not change in response to hyperbaric oxygen applied at 3 atmospheres.

Collagen Synthesis

The synthesis of collagen is possible only in the presence of oxygen. Oxygen stimulates formation of new granulation tissue by enhancing fibroblastic production of collagen.[29] Oxygen invites additional fibroblastic migration to the wound. Epithelialization has also been observed to be accelerated under hyperbaric oxygen treatment.[30]

Revascularization

Poor wound vascularity retards healing, but healing improves with the application of hyperbaric oxygen.[31] Intermittent hyperbaric oxygenation has been shown to enhance capillary revascularization in burn wounds. In addition, capillary blood flow is enhanced as indicated by an increase in measured oxygen tension following hyperbaric oxygen treatment.[32]

Silver[33] has discussed macrophage function and angiogenesis, and Knighton and colleagues[34] have reported that blood vessel formation is dependent on tissue oxygen gradients as well as macrophage function. Thus, the macrophage may be a key cell in the initiation of angiogenesis because angioblasts have been shown to follow a gradient of angiogenic factor produced by hypoxic macrophages. In this regard, macrophages function best in a hypoxic state rather than in a fully oxygenated or totally anoxic state. If the normal tissue oxygen gradient is eliminated artificially, or if a macrophage-free tissue space is created, angiogenesis may be halted temporarily or permanently.[35] Thus, periods of hyperbaric oxygenation may maintain the relative hypoxic environment needed to stimulate new blood vessel growth. The findings of Heng and colleagues[36] seem to support this assumption, as does the observation that new vessels grow toward the center of a wound where maximal hypoxia exists[33] and where fibroblasts are laying collagen down to develop granulation tissue, which fills the wound from the base toward the epidermal surface.[36] Additional investigation is needed to determine if the use of hyperbaric oxygen stimulates tissue reparative processes at some optimal time in the healing process.

Bactericidal Effects

Topical hyperbaric oxygen is beneficial in suppressing growth of bacteria such as Staphylococcus aureus.[21] Anaerobic bacteria are found on normal human skin. These microbes are killed by high oxygen tension. Fischer[10] showed that oxygen-saturated tissues produce elevated redox potentials, the main active barrier against bacterial growth. Inhibition of anaerobic organisms, such as Pseudomonas, often present in lesions, may be enhanced by the application of acetic acid soaks during hyperbaric oxygen treatments.[37] Bornside[38] exposed 20 species of aerobic and facultative anaerobic bacteria and Sacina lutea to 100 percent oxygen at 3 atmospheres. A bactericidal effect occurred in 102 strains of the 20 species involved. The percentage of different organisms destroyed was directly related to the duration of oxygen application. Sacina lutea began dying after only 6 hours of exposure while organisms such as Pseudomonas aeruginosa took from 1 to 2 full days to show any significant decline under this exposure. Beltran-ena[39] has indicated a bacteriostatic effect on a wide variety of anaerobic bacteria and on some aerobic microorganisms as a result of increasing pO_2. Diamond and associates[22] found suppression of bacterial growth in wounds of all patients receiving hyperbaric oxygen treatment in conjunction with conservative wound care consisting of ointments and/or antibiotics.

Edema Reduction

Edema may accumulate in tissues deprived of an adequate blood supply. The potential for tissue regenerative changes decreases if anoxia remains long enough for necrosis to develop. Hyperbaric oxygen has been reported to aid in decreasing edema when used in the recovery stages following replantation of severed limbs.[40] In severe cases of edema, serum albumin may be intentionally elevated parenterally to reduce interstitial edema by increasing the plasma colloid osmotic pressure. In addition, Beltranena[39] has documented that increased partial pressure of oxygen acts adrenergically to relieve edema by decreasing external pressure around blood vessel walls.

Intermittent positive-pressure applied during hyperbaric oxygen treatment also contributes to edema reduction by elevating the tissue pressure in the affected area. The rise in tissue pressure increases venous blood and lymphatic flow facilitating the movement of tissue fluids out of the affected tissues.

INSTRUMENTATION AND APPLICATION OF METHODS

Hyperbaric chambers have been manufactured in a variety of sizes. Two types of units, monoplace and multiplace, are full body chambers.[39] Multiplace chambers can accommodate several patients, who breathe pure oxygen from masks at ambient air pressures. The monoplace chamber is a hermetically sealed total body, single patient unit; it produces pure oxygen under pressure.

A number of portable hyperbaric oxygen devices are available commercially and use local applicators rather than total body exposure for the treatment of localized wounds. They are lightweight and their components are easy to move and adjust. One type of applicator is used for extremity treatment, while another is used to treat wounds located on the torso, hips, and sacrum.

Figure 15–1 illustrates the components of a topical hyperbaric oxygen chamber used for extremity application.* This chamber is bivalved and hermetically sealed. An oxygen source delivers oxygen to the chamber through rubber tubing at flow rates ranging from 1 to 4 liters per minute. This chamber is constructed of two nondisposable rigid Plexiglas components (Fig. 15–1). Accessory controls allow oxygen to be delivered

---

*Topox Pulsed Hyperbaric Oxygen Extremity Chamber. Topox Therapeutic Rentals, Inc., 634 Summit Avenue, Jersey City, NJ 07306.

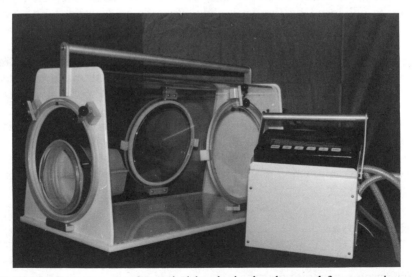

FIGURE 15–1. Components of a topical hyerbaric chamber used for extremity applications (Courtesy of Topox Corporation, Jersey City, NJ).

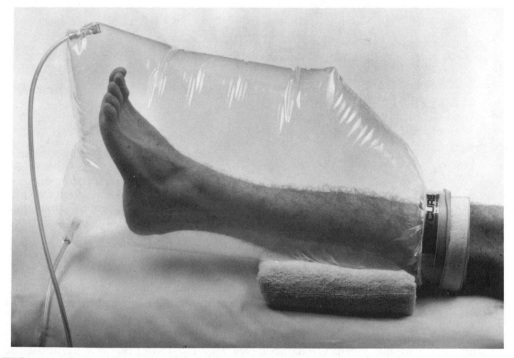

FIGURE 15–2. A disposable soft plastic chamber used for extremity applications (Courtesy of Concord Laboratories, Keene, NH).

with a fine mist at pulsed (intermittent) pressure of up to 50 mmHg during a compression phase lasting 15 seconds and a decompression phase to zero lasting 2 seconds. Latex sleeves attach to the chamber and surround the involved extremity, creating a seal around the limb.

Disposable one-piece chambers* made of soft plastic are placed over the involved extremity (Fig. 15–2). Oxygen is delivered to the wound at a constant flow regulated within a range of 22 to 28 mmHg. These chambers may be disposed of when the practitioner determines that the extent of wound healing is satisfactory.

The sacral chambers illustrated in Figures 15–3 and 15–4 vary in design and require slightly different methods of application. Both chambers deliver a constant flow of oxygen at approximately 4 liters per minute. The sacral chamber in Figure 15–3 allows a pressure of 38 mmHg, and the chamber in Figure 15–4 allows a pressure of 24 mmHg. If the chambers exceed their maximal pressure, a valve will release the excess pressure.

Application Methods

The procedure used in applying local extremity chambers varies slightly, depending on the device. The soft plastic bag (boot) is placed over the arm or leg to be treated. The boot collar is positioned approximately 1½ inches from the top of the latex sleeve, which

---

*Concord Oxycare Topical Oxygen Treatment System. Concord Laboratories, Inc., Keene, NH 03431.

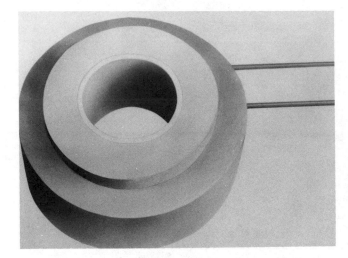

FIGURE 15–3. A sacral chamber consisting of a rubber cushion. The aperature diameter in the cushion is selected according to the wound dimensions (Courtesy of Topox Corporation, Jersey City, NJ).

is cut to match the extremity circumference and secured by Velcro straps. A rubber tube attaches the bag to the pressure gauge. During treatment, the bag must be stabilized to prevent fluctuations in pressure. When treatment is terminated, the strap is loosened, the bag and latex sleeve removed, and the bag discarded.

Application of the Plexiglas chamber (see Fig. 15–1) is preceded by antiseptic cleansing of the unit. The size of the latex sleeve used to seal the chamber aperture through which the patient's extremity is placed, is determined by measuring the circumference of the involved extremity at approximately 5 inches proximal to the lesion. The perimeter of the sleeve is attached to a Plexiglas ring that is temporarily removed from the chamber opening for this purpose. The snugly fitting sleeve with the Plexiglas ring attached to it is then slid over the patient's involved extremity, and the ring is aligned into the aperture grooves of the unit. Foam pieces of appropriate sizes may be placed along the extremity to hold it in place inside the chamber. When the Plexiglas compo-

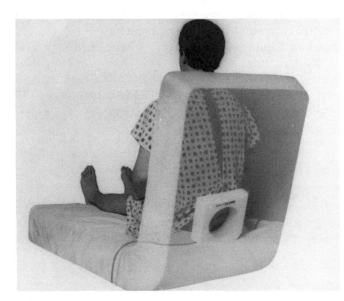

FIGURE 15–4. A sacral chamber consisted of a rubber cushion with a transparent window for wound visualization (Courtesy of Concord Laboratories, Keene, NH).

nents are clamped together, two side ports may be opened to gain accessibility for checking or changing the position of the extremity in the chamber. To maintain a moist environment in the chamber, a container attached to the outside of the chamber is filled three-quarters full with distilled water. Controls attached to the outside of the chamber allow release of humidified oxygen into the chamber. Additional adjustments on the control box allow setting of treatment pressure.

Application of the sacral chamber shown in Figure 15–3 is performed by placing the aperture of the rubber cushion over the wound. The size of the chamber opening surrounding the wound may be selected from three different ring sizes—small, medium, and large. The smallest ring that fits around the wound perimeter without contacting the wound edge is the appropriate choice. A tight seal of the applicator against the skin is achieved by securing it to the patient with body straps. The patient may be positioned prone, sidelying, supine, or sitting, depending on the area requiring treatment.

The sacral chamber shown in Figure 15–4 is a rubber cushion with an aperture slightly larger than the wound. The seal is obtained by the patient resting his or her body weight against the cushion, which is positioned on a bed or chair. A binder may be used to improve the cushion-to-skin seal if a tight seal is difficult to obtain. The outer surface of the cushion, which does not make patient contact, is transparent so that the wound and surrounding tissues may be observed during treatment. Both sacral chambers are connected to the flowmeter and pressure gauge with separate hoses.

CLINICAL USES OF HYPERBARIC OXYGEN

Decubitis Ulcers

Decubitis ulcers are a debilitating consequence of prolonged, excessive pressure applied to the skin of individuals. These wounds occur secondary to contracture, paralysis, fracture, general debilitation, and various other conditions that may require an extended period of immobility. The ulcers occur over areas of the body where bony prominences protrude, especially at the hip, sacrum, ischial tuberosities, malleoli, and heels. They commonly arise in areas where body weight, in combination with shearing forces or stretching of the skin, increases the vulnerability to skin breakdown, especially if the skin is subjected to repeated exposure to fecal matter and/or skin maceration from moisture and urea contained in urine.

A few studies have reported successful outcomes following the use of topical hyperbaric oxygen for treating decubitis ulcers.[9,10,41,42] Torelli[41] employed hyperbaric oxygen for treating decubitis ulcers in patients confined to nursing homes. Topical oxygen was successful in healing wounds in combination with standard medical care of the lesions.

Rosenthal and Schurman[42] used hyperbaric oxygen on 18 patients with 38 pressure sores. They reported that total wound closure occurred in 58 percent of cases, and closure of 50 percent or more of the original wound size occurred in 13 percent of the cases. Fischer[9] treated 26 cases of pressure sores located on the hip and sacral areas with hyperbaric oxygen and observed that sores of up to 2.5 cm diameter required an average of 16 days of treatment to heal. Larger sores measuring from 3 to 6 cm in diameter took 8 weeks to heal, and ulcers larger than 6 cm in diameter, which were repaired surgically, healed after hyperbaric oxygen reportedly helped to suppress bacterial growth. In another study by Fischer,[10] pressure sores on the ankle, heel, and medial aspect of the knee treated with hyperbaric oxygen all developed well-vascularized tissue between 2 weeks and 2 months.

Venous Insufficiency Ulcers

The etiology of venous ulcers helps to explain why these wounds may be difficult to heal. These wounds develop when chronic tissue hypoxia secondary to venous insufficiency causes cell death and tissue necrosis in the presence of edema. The ulcers occur predominantly on the distal, gravity-dependent areas of the lower extremities. Fischer[9] observed that hyperbaric oxygen enhanced healing of venous insufficiency ulcers in an average of 15 days in 16 patients who had had their lesions between 5 months and 24 years. All ulcers had been unsuccessfully treated by other therapies before being treated with hyperbaric oxygen. One sore, which had been in existence for 24 years, took 30 days to heal. In a study involving three cases of venous ulcers that had existed from 6 months to 35 years, Fischer[10] observed that healing in each case, which took 2 to 7 weeks for wound closure, was accompanied by a gradual reduction in edema and inflammation and a progressive development of tissue granulation.

DIABETIC ULCERS

Singer and colleagues[43] used portable hyperbaric oxygen to treat 65 patients with lower-extremity diabetic ulcers. Fifteen patients were treated with hyperbaric oxygen and 50 patients were selected as a control group. The control group was treated with conservative methods that were not described. No amputations were performed in the control group. The patients receiving hyperbaric oxygen required a significantly shorter time in bed than did the control group (62 days opposed to 138 days). Ulcers located on the toes, heels, and forefoot appeared to heal at different rates. Even after minor toe amputations, confinement to bed was still considered short in comparison to time already spent in bed by the patient. When patients lacked complications such as gangrene or abscesses, treatment time was still shorter, and patients quickly gained the ability to lead independent lives.

Sourifman and associates[44] reported a beneficial outcome in a single case following treatment of a diabetic heel ulcer with hyperbaric oxygen. The patient, relying on daily doses of insulin for her 20-year diabetic condition, had received a left below-the-knee amputation from diabetic complications. The ulcer on the right heel existed in the presence of considerable soft-tissue swelling as well as bone degeneration and cultures of Proteus and Pseudomonas. The patient received hyperbaric oxygen treatment at 2 atmospheres for 1½ hours, twice daily. After 2 months of hyperoxic therapy, surgical debridement was followed by a pedicle flap procedure. After receiving 10 postoperative hyperbaric oxygen treatments, the ulcer healed and the patient was discharged from the hospital. No conclusion was made in this case as to whether healing was enhanced by debridement, surgical flap procedure, hyperoxic therapy, or from all three interventions.

Ignacio and colleagues[45] noticed higher than expected success in healing diabetic ulcers when they used topical hyperbaric oxygen. They treated 17 severe diabetics for 6 days a week, twice a day at 16 to 20 mmHg pressure for 45 minutes per session. Although they also treated several other types of lesions, they found that the diabetic patients healed very well, considering the severity of their disease. Although the study design did not permit objective reporting of results, the authors did stress the importance of determining whether wound pathogens are present. They also speculated that hyperbaric oxygen in conjunction with other conventional wound-care methods may help to reduce the need for amputation.

Burns

Burn wounds have distinguishing characteristics that are different from mechanical lesions. Hunt and coworkers[46] have noted that burns became edematous during the period of vascular impairment, with little inflammatory change during the first few days. In one case, they reported that the pO_2 level in the edematous tissue below the burn eschar was about one-half the normal value. With oxygenation, capillary budding occurs, leading to formation of new tissue granulation. Some evidence exists that shows that repair of burn wound tissue is partly dependent on maintaining tissue oxygen tension at or near the normal range of 0 to 20 mmHg.[47]

Studies on rats have demonstrated that topical application of humidified oxygen to third-degree burns enhances collagen growth.[48] In other studies, Kaufman and associates[49] increased tissue oxygen tension and humidity, which appeared to accelerate the healing of burns. This study also demonstrated that collagen fibers in wounds treated with hyperoxic therapy developed diameters greater than collagen fibers in wounds that were not treated with hyperbaric oxygen. Maintaining wound moisture during hyperbaric oxygen treatments by humidifying the interior of the hermetically sealed chamber may assist healing of burn wounds.

Frostbite

Although local hyperbaric oxygen has reportedly been used for treatment of frostbite injuries, no reference was found in peer-reviewed literature that specifically addressed this application.[50] That hyperbaric oxygen treatment may contribute to the prevention of amputation in frostbite cases is only speculative. Further research is needed to justify the use of hyperbaric oxygen for such cases.

Infected Wounds

Recent clinical research has supported the theory that hyperbaric oxygen can eliminate wound infections. Lehman and coworkers[23] have reported positive treatment outcomes using hyperbaric oxygen as an adjunct treatment of human bite infections of the hand. Following acute-care procedures and debridement, patients were referred for hyperoxic therapy. Twenty-seven patients received standard care, while 16 received hyperbaric oxygen as a supplementary treatment. Three other patients with osteomyelitis were reviewed separately. The equipment used in the study was a portable, humidified, pulsed hyperbaric oxygen chamber that allowed the arm to be hermetically sealed during treatment. Applied at a pulsed pressure of 50 mmHg, 100 percent oxygen was cycled into the chamber every 30 seconds for 90 minutes, twice daily. Hyperbaric oxygen produced bactericidal effects as evidenced by lower culture counts and decreased hospital stays in patients with severe infections (mean = 4.7 days) compared with hospital stays of patients who did not receive hyperbaric oxygen therapy (mean = 11.2 days). Culture counts revealed that hyperoxic therapy produced bactericidal effects on anaerobic organisms found in the wounds, which were predominantly those of mouth flora. In addition, the authors observed that there was no significant response to hyperbaric oxygen treatment in patients with superficial wounds that were moderately infected.

Hyperbaric oxygen has also been used by Gorecki[51] to treat infected bedsores of 9 months' duration. The ulcers, measuring 1.0 by 1.5 inches and 1.0 by 2.0 inches, were located at the sacrum and right hip, respectively. A makeshift chamber consisted of oxygen delivered through tubing to an inverted funnel connected to the patient's body with sponge material fitting the body contour and sealing the funnel aperture. Oxygen flowing at 12 to 15 liters per minute was applied at a pressure of 15 mmHg for 15 minutes three or four times daily. All wounds healed after approximately 4 weeks of treatment. Gradual healing was accompanied by a clearing of infection and progressive epithelialization.

PRECAUTIONS AND CONTRAINDICATIONS

When hyperbaric oxygen is applied systematically under excessively high tensions, oxygen toxicity may pose a serious problem.[52] McFarlane and Wermuth[53] investigated the efficacy of hyperbaric oxygen in preventing tissue necrosis following skin flaps and grafts in animal model experiments. Subsequent to flap or graft surgical procedures, groups of rats were totally exposed to oxygen at 1 atmosphere for 6 hours a day for 5 days, 2 atmospheres for 4 hours a day for 3 days, or 3 atmospheres for 4 hours a day for 2 to 5 days. Oxygen applied at three atmospheres was fatal to rats on the second and fifth days. The investigators reported that applying oxygen under high pressures created oxygen toxicity, which was fatal within short periods of time. Oxygen toxicity is a potential problem when oxygen is applied under high pressure in a full body chamber but not when applied locally.

In contrast, Kaufman and Hurwitz[54] did not find significant improvement on healing skin flaps in rats with whole body exposure to hyperbaric oxygen. They noted the dangers of oxygen toxicity resulting from systemic treatment applications. Perrins[55] observed that full body hyperbaric oxygen given to patients at 2 or 3 atmospheres pressure for 2 hours, four times a day, for 2 to 3 days, halted or reversed the deterioration of skin flaps. Two flaps failed, one from ischemia and one from infection.

Isolating extremity wounds by treating them with a portable topical hyperbaric chamber has eliminated the danger of oxygen toxicity.[23] Avoidance of this complication is possible because the chambers used can restrict the pressurized pure oxygen to a local wound site on an extremity; oxygen will not travel throughout the body.[10] Systemic delivery of oxygen to chronic wound tissues is rarely necessary but, when it is, only a professional health-care provider with special training should provide treatment.

Certain conditions, including lung cysts and chronic obstructive lung disease, are contraindicated for systemic hyperbaric oxygen treatment.[56] Some pregnant women treated for emboli in a full body chamber have aborted during the procedure.[57] In addition, individuals undergoing narcotic withdrawal are poor candidates for the full chamber treatment because of their vulnerability to toxic reactions.[58]

Topical hyperbaric oxygen applied under positive pulsed pressures should not be used in the presence of acute thrombophlebitis because the pressure variations may dislodge the thrombus. Treatment of severe ischemic wounds with topical hyperbaric oxygen may be ineffective, because the ability of the tissues to take up oxygen may be compromised. Treatment success may depend on the degree of wound tissue ischemia and ability of the tissues to take up oxygen.

Certain precautions should be considered before using topical hyperbaric oxygen chambers. Antiseptic cleansing of the involved limb[59,60] and of the Plexiglas nondisposable chamber before and after every treatment is required to prevent cross-infection from microbes that may linger in the unit.[59] If Pseudomonas bacteria are present in the wound, the practitioner may opt to apply acetic acid dressings before using hyperbaric oxygen.[59] The acid is reported to increase pH and to suppress the growth of bacteria in an oxygen-saturated environment.[39] When a humidifier is available to use with the hyperbaric chamber, it must be properly filled with distilled water and adjusted to prevent wound tissues from drying or from causing static sparks from friction created in the chamber or from electrical malfunction outside the chamber.[61] Because oxygen is a highly flammable gas, the therapist must avoid administering hyperbaric oxygen near any device that could emit mechanical or electrical sparks or direct flames. For the same reason, cigarette smoking is never permitted near oxygen tanks or chambers.

Finally, the therapist needs to consider the patient's emotional status. The individual who is unable to remain relatively immobile during treatment may pull the arm or leg from the portable extremity chamber or displace the seal of the sacral chamber. Care must always be taken to ensure the patient's well-being, and a clear explanation of the advantages and procedures of treatment often assists in achieving success.

CLINICAL DECISION MAKING

In making a decision for hyperbaric oxygen treatment, the following factors must be considered: (1) the anatomic location and size of the wound, (2) the patient's ability to assume and maintain the treatment position, (3) the circulatory status of the involved region, (4) the patient's general medical condition, and (5) the patient's emotional status.

Wounds that are larger than the area of the portable chamber warrant a full body chamber. If a full body chamber is unavailable or contraindicated, selection of another modality is necessary. When the site of tissue destruction is confined to the distal two thirds of the extremities or when it is located in areas where the sacral chamber can create an effective seal, the topical hyperbaric unit is a viable option. In cases of venous stasis ulcers and pressure sores or wounds in which edema and indurated tissue are present, an intermittent topical oxygen chamber may be the best modality. In this situation, affected tissue is not only diffused with pure oxygen under pressure, which serves to increase tissue oxygen tension, but also the tissues are flushed by the intermittent positive pressure, which serves to increase tissue pressure.

To use the portable unit, a patient must be able to assume a comfortable position that also accommodates the unit. The Plexiglas chamber requires the patient to be in a supine or long-sitting posture. Less rigid chambers may allow modified positioning, but the patient must still maintain a fixed position for the treatment duration. The patient treated by means of the sacral or torso chamber will be in a prone, semiprone, or sidelying posture, depending on the location of the lesion. The sacral chamber may be used for various body areas, including the hip, torso, and upper leg (where the extremity chamber cannot reach) as long as the aperture of the chamber is sealed around the periphery of the wound.

Before selecting hyperbaric oxygen for tissue healing, the therapist must consider the patient's circulatory system status. Blood should be perfusing through the wound tissues for hyperbaric oxygen to be of value. Oxygen applied to tissues that have impaired blood perfusion provides little or no benefit to wound healing. Hyperbaric oxygen may assist in preventing necrosis of macerated and/or eroding tissue surrounding the wound. In addition, hyperoxic therapy may be used to keep tissue damage to a minimum in a more proximal extremity wound when performing other medical or surgical procedures on distal circulatory problems. For example, a patient with distal lower extremity ulcers secondary to diabetes and poor circulation in the foot may benefit from hyperbaric oxygen to the more proximal wound before amputation of the distal part of the extremity.

Medical status plays a leading role in choosing a physical modality for wound healing, especially with the chronically ill, immobilized patient. When deciding on hyperbaric oxygen, the health-care professional must review these cases for the possibility of embolism, which is a contraindication for treatment with hyperbaric oxygen. Patients with fragile small vessels secondary to steroidal therapy may be vulnerable to blood vessel rupture when oxygen is applied to the tissues under pressure. Hyperbaric oxygen treatment is not the therapy of choice for patients suffering from peripheral arterial disease with severe vasospasm.[62]

The mental status of the patient must also be taken into consideration. Patients suffering from certain emotional problems or mental deficiencies may be unable to maintain the necessary treatment position long enough to benefit from treatment. Patients suffering from paranoia may be fearful of the device and may therefore be better candidates for other therapies. If these individuals can be supervised and/or calmed, however, portable hyperbaric oxygen may be an excellent adjunct therapy, especially for those chronic wounds having low pO_2.

Hyperbaric Oxygen with Other Modalities

Hyperbaric oxygen is used as an adjunct treatment in tissue repair. When used in conjunction with wet-to-dry dressings in the care for chronic skin ulcers, treatment with hyperbaric oxygen has achieved success. However, precautionary measures, such as soaking the bandages, should be taken to prevent loss of newly granulated tissue during removal of the dressing. Hyperbaric oxygen has also been used with enzymes and oral antibiotics and has been reported to be a successful debriding agent before surgical intervention such as skin grafting.[22] In addition, hyperbaric oxygen and whirlpool treatments have been used alternatively, particularly following debridement procedures.[12] Once a wound is clean of necrotic tissue, whirlpool sessions may be discontinued and hyperbaric oxygen continued alone until the wound is free of infection and healed.

Table 15–1 illustrates some patient examples that address the decision-making factors mentioned in this section. To further illustrate this decision-making process, a single, more indepth case study follows.

CASE STUDY

The following case study provides a decision-making example of the use of topical hyperbaric oxygen on a venous stasis ulcer.

S.P. is a 62-year-old woman diagnosed with a severe venous stasis ulcer on the left lower leg. The wound has been present for 10 years. Three years before developing the ulcer, S.P. experienced significant edema of both ankles. She also experienced constant pain in the left leg, which caused insomnia and a great deal of stress.

Past treatment of her wound consisted of a variety of methods, none of which

TABLE 15-1. Three Case Studies that Use Appropriate
Hyperbaric Oxygen Chambers for the Wound Healing Process

Case	Decision/Rationale	Outcome
27-year-old man, 1 month post L4–L5 spinal fusion with spontaneous hematoma rupture with positive Staphylococcus aureus wound 6.2 cm long × 3.4 cm wide × 3.0 cm deep	Sacral chamber at 38 mmHg. Chamber fits this area. Higher pressure to send more oxygen to the deeper tissue regions and to aid circulation. Patient unable to sit for prolonged periods	Total lesion healing 2 months after hyperbaric oxygen treatments started: 53 treatments; after 20th, on outpatient basis
57-year-old woman, 3 years post right below-the-knee amputation with onset of cellulitis of right stump; wound size 5.8 cm long × 3.2 cm wide × 6 cm deep; wound drainage with Staphylococcus aureus infection with stump edema	Intermittent pressure Plexiglas chamber at 0 to 50 mmHg pressure; intermittent to aid circulation and decrease edema. Higher pressure for bactericidal effect	After 25 treatments, wound 3.8 cm long × 2 cm wide × 2.4 cm deep. No bacteria, surgical closure, 5 more HBO sessions. Total closure by end of 17 days in hospital
19-year-old man with traumatic lesion right great toe 3 cm long × 2 cm wide; no bacteria or edema; extremity sensitive to excesses of pressure on limb	Constant pressure disposable extremity chamber at 38 mmHg. Circulation in extremity initially good. Less pressure over injured extremity	Total healing after 7 treatments. No surgical intervention necessary

HBO = hyperbaric oxygen

produced significant or lasting relief. Initial treatments began in the spring, with 6 months of sulfa sticks applied to the lesion, followed by numerous ointments. Cortisone treatments were intermittently administered for short periods of time over a year. Subsequently, she was treated with an Unna's boot applied every 2 weeks for 2 years. During this time, the ulcer's dimensions reduced in size, and the Unna's boot treatment was replaced by an elastic bandage. After a few months, the ulcer again increased in size. The patient was then seen by a vascular surgeon, who recommended skin grafting. S.P. refused this option and attempted to treat herself for the next 2 years. Unsuccessful, she sought assistance from a dermatologist and spent the next year and a half cleansing the wound, as she once again wore an elastic bandage. Finally, under the direction of the dermatologist, she was referred to a physical therapist for instruction in a home program of topical pulsed hyperbaric oxygen.

When the patient was seen for the first time by the physical therapist, a tracing of the ulcer was taken and transferred onto graph paper. The volume of the wound was determined by placing sterile water in the wound and measuring it with a graduated cylinder. The area of the ulcer measured 1700 cm² and had a depth of 9 mm. Tissue granulation was almost nonexistent, and a culture was positive for Staphylococcus and Pseudomonas.

Treatment of the left lower leg consisted of cleansing the limb with a povidone-iodine solution between hyperbaric treatments. The patient also applied acetic acid soaks to the wound during the period when Pseudomonas was present. Initially, the patient was able to tolerate hyperbaric oxygen treatment only once a day because of severe leg pain; after the first 2 months, she tolerated the therapy twice for 90 minutes.

The compression phase was adjusted to 50 mmHg for 15 seconds followed by decompression to 0 mmHg in 2 seconds. Oxygen was supplied by large tanks delivered to the patient's home; each tank provided approximately eight treatments.

When not receiving hyperbaric oxygen treatment, the patient wore dry dressings and an Ace bandage for compression. Topical oxygen therapy continued until the ulcer was superficially covered by epithelial cells and an outline of the wound measured 20 mm² in area across the newly granulated tissue.

Within the first month of treatment, S.P. suffered considerably less pain and was able to sleep through most nights. Tissue granulation improved, ulcer depth decreased, and pain diminished until she was ambulatory without discomfort and returned to her normal activities. At the end of the treatment program, the patient was fitted with a compression stocking for the left lower extremity to help maintain circulation and prevent recurrence of edema. Hyperbaric oxygen therapy was discontinued after 1½ years of treatment. A follow-up visit by the patient 16 months later showed that the ulcer had remained closed. The therapist speculated that healing took as long as it did not only because of the depth and area of the lesion but also because S.P. was so active that her leg was in a gravity-dependent position for most of her waking time.

SUMMARY

Hyperbaric oxygen may be used under appropriate conditions alone and as an adjunct to other treatments in healing dermal ulcers. Therapists may use topical portable hyperbaric oxygen chambers to treat a variety of wounds in many different areas of the body. Effects of hyperbaric oxygen include improved collagen synthesis, revascularization, and bacterial reduction or elimination. Edema reduction, probably occurring from intermittent compression, is another desirable effect. Such positive results seen in select patients provide the best rationale for using this modality. Relief of relative hypoxia in the damaged tissue and stimulation of epithelial formation provide further justification for using hyperbaric oxygen to heal chronic wounds.

Before beginning any treatment program, the therapist must obtain a full account of the patient's physical and mental condition. Correct techniques in applying topical hyperbaric oxygen are necessary to achieve positive treatment outcomes.

In reviewing literature pertaining to hyperbaric oxygen for wound care, the clinician must be attentive to treatment protocol and reported results. Many studies have not fully detailed wound types, bacterial population, controls, and other medical factors. Further research can aid in determining the future of this modality.

REFERENCES

1. Stephens, FO and Hunt, TK: Effect of changes in inspired oxygen and carbon dioxide tensions on wound tensile strengths. Ann Surg 173:515, 1971.
2. Hunt, TK and Pai, MP: The effect of varying ambient oxygen tensions on wound metabolism and collagen synthesis. Surg Gynecol Obstet 135:561, 1975.
3. Davis, J, Dunn, JM, and Heinback, R: Indications for hyperbaric oxygen therapy. Texas Med 76:44, 1980.
4. Norkool, BM: Current concepts of hyperbaric oxygenation and its application in critical care. Heart Lung 8(4):728, 1979.
5. Slack, WK, Thomas, DA, and De Jode, LR: In Brown, IW and Cox, BG (eds): Proceedings of the Third International Conference on Hyperbaric Medicine. National Academy of Sciences—National Research Council, Publication No. 1404, Washington, DC, 1966, pp 621–624.
6. Bird, AD and Telfer, ABM: Effect of hyperbaric oxygen on limb circulation. Lancet 1:355, 1965.

7. Slack, WK: A hyperbaric unit for your hospital? Hosp Pract 1(3):42–47, 1966.
8. Copeman, PWM and Ashfield, R: Raynaud's phenomenon in scleroderma treated with hyperbaric oxygen. Proc R Soc Med 60:30, 1967.
9. Fischer, BH: Topical hyperbaric oxygen treatment of pressure sores and skin ulcers. Lancet 2:405–409, 1969.
10. Fischer, BH: Treatment of ulcers on the legs with hyperbaric oxygen. J Dermatol Surg 1:57, 1975.
11. Heng, M: Local hyperbaric oxygen administration for leg ulcers. Br J Dermatol 109:232, 1983.
12. Upson, AV: Topical hyperbaric oxygenation in the treatment of recalcitrant open wounds—a clinical report. Phys Ther 66:1411, 1966.
13. Jackson, B, et al: Topical hyperbaric oxygen therapy. Presented at the Scientific Study area at 1987 A.A.D. Meeting. Veterans Administration Hospital, Memphis, Tennessee, and University of Tennessee. Unpublished material, 1987.
14. Kwiecinski, MG: Therapeutic value of hyperbaric oxygen in lower extremity ulcerations. J Foot Surg 26:394, 1987.
15. Camp, R: Leg ulcers. Nurs Times 73:25, 1977.
16. Kravitz, S: Comparison of whirlpool and hyperbaric oxygen in the healing of venous stasis ulcers. Study submitted for Master's thesis, New York University. Unpublished material, 1984.
17. Pittinger, CB: Hyperbaric Oxygenation. Charles C Thomas, Springfield, IL, 1966, p 10.
18. Hunt, TK, Zederfeldt, B, and Goldstick, TK: Oxygen and healing. J Surg 118:521, 1962.
19. Hunt, TK, Juha, N, and Zederfeldt, B: Role of oxygen in repair process. Acta Chir Scand 138:109, 1972.
20. Haeger, K: The treatment of venous ulcers of the leg. Geriatrics 19:160, 1964.
21. Olejniczak, S and Zielinski, A: Low hyperbaric therapy in the management of leg ulcers. Mich Med 74(32):707–712, 1975.
22. Diamond, E, et al: The effect of hyperbaric oxygen on lower extremity ulcers. J Podiatr Assoc 72:184, 1982.
23. Lehman, WL, Jr, et al: Human bite infections of the hand: Adjunct treatment with hyperbaric oxygen. Infect Surg 4(6):460, 1985.
24. Bass, BH: The treatment of varicose leg ulcers by hyperbaric oxygen. Postgrad Med J 46:407, 1970.
25. Watt, J: Surgical applications of hyperbaric oxygen therapy in the Royal Navy. Proc R Soc Med 64:877, 1971.
26. Knighton, DR, et al: Regulation of repair: Hypoxic control of macrophage mediated angiogenesis. In Hing, TK, et al (eds): Soft and Hard Tissue Repair—Biological and Clinical Aspects. Praeger, New York, 1984, p 41.
27. Lanpier, EH and Brown, IW: The physiological basis for hyperbaric therapy. In Fundamentals of Hyperbaric Medicine. National Academy of Sciences, National Research Council, Committee on Hyperbaric Oxygenation, Publication No 1298, National Academy of Sciences, Washington, DC, 1966, pp 33–55.
28. Gruber, RP, et al: Skin permeability to oxygen and hyperbaric oxygen. Arch Surg 101:69, 1970.
29. Underfriend, S: Formation of hydroxyproline in collagen. Science 152:1335, 1966.
30. Winter, GD and Perrins, JD: Effects of hyperbaric oxygen treatment on epidermal regeneration. Proceedings of the Fourth International Congress on Hyperbaric Medicine. Edited by J Wada and T Iwa. Igaku Shoin, Tokyo, 1970, p 363.
31. Niinikoski, PB, Rajamaki, A, and Kulonen, E: Healing of open wounds: Effects of oxygen, distributed blood supply and hyperemia by infrared radiation. Acta Chir Scand 137:399, 1971.
32. Ketchum, SA, III, Thomas, AN, and Hall, AD: Angiographic studies of the effect of hyperbaric oxygen on burn wound revascularization. Proceedings of the Fourth International Congress on Hyperbaric Medicine. Edited by J Wada and T Iwa. Igaku Shain, Tokyo, 1970, p 388.
33. Silver, IA: Oxygen and tissue repair, an environment for healing: The role of occlusion. Proc R Soc Med 88:16, 1987.
34. Knighton, DR, Silver, IA, and Hunt, TK: Regulation of wound-healing angiogenesis—Effect of oxygen gradients and inspired oxygen concentration. Surgery 90(2):262, 1981.
35. Banda, MH, Hunt, TK, and Silver, IA: CIBA Symposium on Fibrosis, 1985.
36. Heng, MCY, Pilgrim, JP, and Beck, FWS: A simplified hyperbaric oxygen technique for leg ulcers. Clin Res 30:262, 1982.
37. Hitchcock, CR: Acetic acid inhibits pseudomonas during hyperbaric oxygen treatment. Hennepin County Medical Center, Minneapolis, MN, p 41.
38. Bornside, GH: Bactericidal effect of hyperbaric oxygen determined by direct exposure. Proc Soc Exp Biol Med 130:1165, 1969.
39. Beltranena, H: Medical and surgical indications of hyperbaric oxygenation. J Am Osteopathol Assoc 81:331, 1982.
40. Shanghai Sixth People's Hospital, China: Hyperbaric oxygen therapy in replantation of severed limbs. Chin Med J 1:197, 1975.
41. Torelli, M: Topical oxygen for decubitus ulcers. Am J Nurs 73:494, 1978.
42. Rosenthal, AM and Schurman, A: Hyperbaric treatment of pressure sores. Arch Phys Med Rehabil 52:413, 1971.
43. Singer, P, et al: Concerning the initial results from the treatment of diabetic gangrene with a chamber for local high pressure oxygen treatment. Berlitz Translation Service, Berlitz School of Language of America, Central Institute for Cardiac and Circulatory Research, Berlin, 1978.

44. Sourifman, HA, Thomas, MP, and Epstein, DL: Hyperbaric oxygenation and ulcer treatment: A case report. J Am Podiatr Assoc 71:381, 1981.
45. Ignacio, DR, et al: Treatment of extensive limb ulcers with the use of topical hyperbaric oxygen therapy. Greater Southeast Community Hospital, Washington, DC, 1983.
46. Hunt, TK, Sheldon, G, and Fuchs, R: Physiologic mechanisms of repair of burns. Burns 1:212, 1974.
47. Kernahan, DA, Zingg, W, and Kay, WW: The effect of hyperbaric oxygen on the survival of experimental skin flaps. Plast Reconstr Surg 36:19, 1965.
48. Kaufman, T, et al: The microclimate chamber: The effect of continuous topical administration of 96% oxygen and 75% relative humidity on the healing rate of experimental deep burns. J Trauma 23(9):806, 1983.
49. Kaufman, T, et al: Acceleration of wound healing and contraction of experimental deep burns by topical oxygen. Surg Forum 34:112, 1983.
50. Howard, PE: Gonic man healing remarkably. Foster's Daily Democrat, Dover, NH, February 4, 1983.
51. Gorecki, Z: Oxygen under pressure applied directly to bedsores: Case report. J Am Geriatr Soc 12:1147, 1964.
52. Barnard, EEP: Oxygen toxicity. Proc R Soc Med 64:10, 1971.
53. McFarlane, RM and Wermuth, RE: The use of hyperbaric oxygen to prevent necrosis in experimental pedicle flaps and composite skin grafts. Plast Reconstr Surg 37:422, 1986.
54. Kaufman, T and Hurwitz, DJ: Systemic and local oxygen effects on rat axial pattern flap survival. Chir Plastica 7:308, 1983.
55. Perrins, DJD: Hyperbaric oxygenation of ischemic skin flaps and pedicles. In Brown, IW and Cox, BG (eds): Proceedings of the Third International Conference on Hyperbaric Medicine. National Academy of Sciences — National Research Council, Publication No. 1404, Washington, DC, 1966, pp 613–620.
56. Gunby, P: Hyperbaric oxygenation therapy now making 'careful comeback.' JAMA 246:1057–1058, 1981.
57. Gunby, P: HBO: New chambers, some growing pains. JAMA 246(11):1171–1177, 1981.
58. Gunby, O: HBO can interact with preexisting patient conditions. JAMA 246(10):1177–1178, 1981.
59. Topox Therapeutic Rentals: Procedures Manual for the Topox Hyperbaric Oxygen Systems. Jersey City, NJ.
60. B & F Medical Products: Topical High Oxygen Pressure Sleeve — Tissue Trauma Therapy Device #64390. Toledo, OH.
61. McLaren, CAB: Patient safety. Proc R Soc Med 64:876, 1971.
62. Baffes, TG, et al: Administration of hyperbaric oxygen in an individual high pressure chamber. Surgery 60:319, 1966.

Appendix

MANUFACTURERS OF HYPERBARIC EQUIPMENT

B & F Medical Products, Inc.,
1421 N. Expressway Drive
Toledo, OH 43608
(419)729-0606

Concord Laboratories, Inc.
Keene, NH 03431
(800)258-5361

Topox Therapeutic Rentals, Inc.
634 Summit Avenue
Jersey City, NJ 07306
(201)798-0636

INDEX

A page number in *italics* indicates a figure. A "*t*" following a page number indicates a table.